Treatments for Anxiety

Also Available from Bloomsbury Academic

Prescription for Inequality: Exploring the Social Determinants of Health of At-Risk Groups

Jillian M. Duquaine-Watson

Medical Firsts: Innovations and Milestones That Changed the World

Tish Davidson

Wellness around the World: An International Encyclopedia of Health Indicators, Practices, and Issues

Brenda S. Gardenour Walter, Editor

Treatments for Anxiety

Fact versus Fiction

Myrna Chandler Goldstein and Mark A. Goldstein, MD

BLOOMSBURY ACADEMIC
NEW YORK · LONDON · OXFORD · NEW DELHI · SYDNEY

BLOOMSBURY ACADEMIC
Bloomsbury Publishing Inc
1385 Broadway, New York, NY 10018, USA
50 Bedford Square, London, WC1B 3DP, UK
29 Earlsfort Terrace, Dublin 2, Ireland

BLOOMSBURY, BLOOMSBURY ACADEMIC and the Diana logo are trademarks of Bloomsbury Publishing Plc

First published in the United States of America 2024

This book discusses treatments (including types of medication and mental health therapies), diagnostic tests for various symptoms and mental health disorders, and organizations. The authors have made every effort to present accurate and up-to-date information. However, the information in this book is not intended to recommend or endorse particular treatments or organizations, or substitute for the care or medical advice of a qualified health professional, or used to alter any medical therapy without a medical doctor's advice. Specific situations may require specific therapeutic approaches not included in this book. For those reasons, we recommend that readers follow the advice of qualified health care professionals directly involved in their care. Readers who suspect they may have specific medical problems should consult a physician about any suggestions made in this book.

Library of Congress Cataloging-in-Publication Data

Names: Goldstein, Myrna Chandler, 1948- author. | Goldstein, Mark A. (Mark Allan), 1947- author.
Title: Treatments for anxiety : fact versus fiction / Myrna Chandler Goldstein and Mark A. Goldstein, MD.
Description: New York: Bloomsbury Academic, 2024. | Includes bibliographical references and index. | Audience: Ages 17- 21 | Audience: Grades 10-12
Identifiers: LCCN 2023052669 (print) | LCCN 2023052670 (ebook) | ISBN 9781440881022 (hb) | ISBN 9798765121429 (paperback) | ISBN 9781440881039 (epdf) | ISBN 9798765111802 (ebook)
Subjects: LCSH: Anxiety disorders–Popular works. | Anxiety disorders–Treatment–Popular works. | Anxiety in adolescence–Popular works.
Classification: LCC RC531 .G653 2024 (print) | LCC RC531 (ebook) | DDC 616.85/22–dc23/eng/20240117
LC record available at https://lccn.loc.gov/2023052669
LC ebook record available at https://lccn.loc.gov/2023052670

ISBN: HB: 978-1-4408-8102-2
ePDF: 978-1-4408-8103-9
eBook: 979-8-7651-1180-2

Typeset by Deanta Global Publishing Services, Chennai, India
Printed and bound in Great Britain

To find out more about our authors and books visit www.bloomsbury.com and sign up for our newsletters.

We dedicate this book to the loving memory of our two sisters:
Beryl Helaine Chandler
October 24, 1944–October 29, 1970
Frances Goldstein Landers
February 7, 1936–December 12, 1995
May Their Memory Be a Blessing

Contents

Acknowledgments   viii

Preface   ix

Introduction to Anxiety Disorders   1

Acupressure   11

Acupuncture   21

Animal Therapy   31

Benzodiazepines   41

Beta-Blockers   59

Buspirone   69

Cannabis and CBD   79

Cognitive Behavioral Therapy   89

Exercise   99

Gabapentin   109

Herbal Medicine   119

Hydroxyzine   135

Hypnosis   145

Magnesium   155

Melatonin   165

Mindfulness Meditation   177

Mirtazapine   187

Music Therapy   197

Probiotics   207

Psilocybin   217

Reflexology   229

Selective Serotonin Reuptake Inhibitors   239

Serotonin and Norepinephrine Reuptake Inhibitors   263

Tai Chi   275

Vitamin D   285

Notes   295

Index   323

About the Authors   331

Acknowledgments

We would like to thank our editor, Maxine Taylor, who has edited most of our recent books. Tirelessly dedicated, Maxine has repeatedly offered excellent suggestions and advice.

Preface

Anxiety, My Story

Myrna Chandler Goldstein

Like millions of other Americans, I suffer from anxiety. No, it is not the debilitating form of anxiety that causes some to retreat inside their homes, afraid to venture outside. For those poor souls, living outside their cloistered bubble causes anxiety levels to skyrocket to unbearable levels. I have a milder form of anxiety that periodically challenges my ability to maintain an even keel.

In retrospect, it is evident that the first hints of my anxiety appeared when my older sister, Beryl H. Chandler, was killed shortly after she turned twenty-six. At the time, I was only twenty-two years old. Though I clearly would have benefited from some therapy and/or medication, especially since anxiety and depression were common in my family, no suggestions were made. Decades later, when my father, Craig A. Chandler, fought a valiant two-year battle against leukemia, my anxiety again emerged. But, it did not become a daily threat until my mother, Sarah D. Chandler, was diagnosed with recurrent breast cancer early in the fall of 2004. To cope with my anxiety, I sought the help of a psychiatrist who prescribed therapy and medication. Though I am no longer a "nervous Nellie," I still have days when I am more nervous than usual, and there are specific events that may easily trigger anxiety, such as driving too fast in heavy traffic, shopping in overcrowded stores, and preparing for potentially upsetting medical appointments.

And, I am far from alone. According to the Anxiety and Depression Association of America, anxiety disorders are the most common mental illness in the United States. Every year, they affect about forty million adults eighteen years of age and older or 18.1 percent of the population. People with anxiety disorders are three to five times more likely to visit a physician and six times more likely to be hospitalized for a psychiatric problem. In addition, people with anxiety disorders are often dealing with depression. Almost half of the people diagnosed with depression have an anxiety disorder.

It is important to note that not all cases of anxiety are the same. There are various forms of this medical problem, which are addressed in the introduction to this book. In addition, people dealing with anxiety fall across the spectrum in terms of disability. While many are completely disabled and are generally unable to complete some of the basic tasks of daily living, significant numbers are able to lead relatively normal lives. Thus, for more than thirty years, I have worked as a reporter/correspondent/researcher and writer. During this time, I have written thousands of articles and authored or coauthored many books.

It was while researching and writing our most recent book on the management of physical pain, which I cowrote with my husband, Mark A. Goldstein, MD, that I realized that I also wanted to address psychological pain. Ironically, some of the entries of the book were written during the Covid-19 pandemic. At first, we heard continuous reports of all the physical problems associated with Covid-19. And, they were truly daunting. As the months passed, we heard more about the psychological tolls from social distancing, isolation, and virtual education. Two of our grandchildren who live in San Francisco studied virtually for months; our three grandchildren who were then living in Washington, DC were virtual for over a year. We were grateful they all had access to virtual education; many children, who lacked some form of internet access, were not as fortunate. Rates of psychological illnesses in Mark's adolescent and young adults medical practice, especially anxiety and depression, rose exponentially. Moreover, there are also anecdotal reports of increasing rates of suicide and attempted suicide.

This book addresses scores of potential traditional and integrative treatments for anxiety. Each entry presents published scientific research on a specific treatment and evaluates it's actual proven or disproven efficacy. Only treatments in which there are actual published scientific studies are included; no hearsay speculation is presented. The goal is to help people dealing with anxiety to make informed decisions about their treatment options, thus enabling them to obtain the maximum degree of relief as soon as possible.

Anxiety, My Experience

Mark A. Goldstein, MD

When I first started seeing adolescent patients in the late 1970s, few complained of mental health symptoms and even fewer reported being anxious. By the time I retired a few years ago, up to one half of the patients I cared for had a mental health complaint, and many of those adolescents were anxious. As a result, I had to treat many teens for anxiety.

Adolescents face many stressors, including those that are relatively new. One generation ago, no one would have thought about climate anxiety, especially in adolescents. This anxiety is characterized by heightened emotional, mental, or somatic distress that is in response to dangerous changes in the climate system. It is apparent now that teens do experience panic attacks, insomnia, and obsessive thinking from the global climate crisis and the threat of environmental disaster. When added to the other stressors that all adolescents deal with, this additional issue could affect their mental health, leading to an anxiety disorder. And, of course, the Covid pandemic transformed many emotionally stable adolescents into anxious ones. Now, several years later, many continue to be anxious.

Although the levels clearly vary from person to person, everyone experiences some degree of anxiety. Before an examination, even a quiz, many teens are anxious. Receiving test grades is also anxiety-provoking, especially among those who fear less than ideal outcomes. From adolescence into young adulthood, worries and fears are part of the process of normal development. Physical symptoms of anxiety may include a rapid heartbeat, increased perspiration, and stronger muscle tension. Normal everyday anxiety should be short-lived and resolve on its own.

An adolescent with an anxiety disorder may have worries that he or she is unable to stop or control. Many teens are preoccupied with academic issues and how they perform in comparison to their fellow students. As they strive for perfection, they often focus on their mistakes or shortcomings. Some have health concerns, such as obsessive worrying about contracting illness. Parents and teachers may observe these teens reporting headaches, stomachaches, avoiding certain activities, such as sleepovers, and/or poor school performance. Some may become irritable and/or have explosive behavioral issues; others may eat more or less food than in the past. And, some adolescents may report suicidal thoughts or even suicidal behaviors, such as cutting. Anxiety that is more serious is persistent, excessive, and results in the impairment of daily activities. For example, if an adolescent avoids attending school because of issues with academics, the teachers, students, or other concerns, he or she may have an anxiety disorder.

Even though everyone experiences some anxiety, researchers have yet to determine exactly why certain teens develop an anxiety disorder. It is known that in some teens there are interacting biological, psychological, and social factors that trigger anxiety disorders. Most importantly, there is probably no one factor that causes this medical problem.

There is good research demonstrating that genetic factors play an important role in determining which adolescents will have a problem with anxiety. Researchers found that generalized anxiety disorder aggregates in families. And, two large-scale twin studies determined that generalized anxiety disorder has a familial genetic risk. It is also known that children of parents who have an anxiety disorder are at increased risk of developing one themselves. In fact, there is strong evidence children who have a parent or parents with anxiety disorders have two to three times the risk.

Likewise, environmental factors are important in the etiology of anxiety disorders. In a twin study of adolescent monozygotic (one egg) and dizygotic (two eggs) twins, researchers based in Montréal, Canada, found a "social contagion" of anxiety between one teen and the other regardless of gender or zygosity. But this only occurred in same-sex twins of either gender.

A Swedish study of 2,508 twins suggests that a gene associated with anxiety is awakened during adolescence. It is generally believed that there is no single gene that directs the onset of anxiety. Rather, it may well be the cumulative effect of many genes that make an individual more vulnerable to an anxiety disorder.

There are other reasons adolescents may become anxious. In some adolescents, neurobiological factors may be linked to the onset of anxiety disorders. Imbalances between elevated amygdala activity and other brain networks, such as the ventral prefrontal cortex, seen during adolescence may activate an anxiety disorder. Even parenting style may be related to anxiety disorders. Parents who are over protective, anxious, or possibly overly critical may be factors that increase the risk of anxiety disorders in children. Children who observe and experience life learn psychological information that is integral to their development. Whether they realize it or not, parents are role models. If they display anxious behaviors, their children may well model these actions.

According to the National Institutes of Health, 31.9 percent of adolescents have an anxiety disorder. Of these, 8.3 percent are severely impaired. But, female adolescents have a higher risk than males. The risk for females is 38 percent, while it is 26.1 percent for males. All cases of anxiety are not the same. In the introduction to this book, the various types of anxiety are addressed. And, adolescents dealing with anxiety fall across the spectrum in terms of disability. While some are almost completely disabled and are unable to complete some of the basic tasks of daily life, significant numbers are able to lead relatively normal lives, although they may be subject to other issues, such as substance abuse.

This book discusses twenty-five traditional and integrative types of treatment for anxiety. Obviously, some of the entries include multiple varieties. Each entry presents published scientific research on a specific type of treatment and evaluates its actual proven or disproven efficacy. Only treatments in which there are published scientific studies are included; no hearsay speculation is presented. The goal is to help teens (and their parents) dealing with anxiety make informed decisions about the treatment options, thus enabling them to obtain the maximum degree of relief as soon as possible.

Introduction to Anxiety Disorders

There are several different types of anxiety disorders. Though they may differ from one another in a number of ways, they are all characterized by feelings of excessive and intense concern, worry, dread, and uneasiness. People with anxiety feel far more than the everyday worries many people experience and far greater than the circumstances warrant. It is much more than distress about a test at school, a particularly hard problem at work, or a relationship problem. It is persistent and overwhelming. As a result, it is not uncommon for anxiety disorders to interfere with the activities of daily life, such as schoolwork, job performance, and relationships. Without proper treatment, which may include therapy, medication, and a host of other modalities, anxieties may easily spiral out of control and result in profound disability.

And, the statistics are truly daunting. It has been estimated that in a given year, over 19 percent of the adults in the United States experience an anxiety disorder, with the prevalence higher among females. At some point in their lives, more than 31 percent of US adults have an anxiety disorder. Among these adults, about 43.5 percent have a mild impairment. An estimated 33.4 percent have a moderate impairment, and 22.8 percent have a serious impairment. The prevalence among adolescents thirteen to eighteen years is also high, with 31.9 percent having an anxiety disorder; an estimated 8.3 percent have a severe impairment. As with adults, the prevalence is higher among female adolescents than males.[1]

Common Anxiety Disorders

The most common and better researched types of anxiety are agoraphobia, generalized anxiety disorder, obsessive-compulsive disorder, panic disorder, phobias, post-traumatic stress disorder, separation anxiety disorder, and social anxiety disorder (social phobia). It is not uncommon for people to have more than one type of anxiety. All types of anxiety have a number of symptoms, including feelings of nervousness, restlessness, and impending doom, increased heart rate, rapid breathing, sweating, trembling, feeling weak or tired, trouble concentrating on other concerns, sleeping problems, poor concentration, and gastrointestinal upset. The following are specific symptoms associated with the various types of anxiety.

Agoraphobia

Agoraphobia is a type of anxiety disorder in which people fear and tend to avoid places or situations that may make them feel trapped or panicked, sometimes precipitating heart palpitations and breathing problems. People with agoraphobia normally have a fear of two or more of the following situations: using public transportation, being in open spaces, being in closed spaces, standing in line or being in a crowd, and being outside the home alone. In the most debilitating cases, people are housebound.

Generalized Anxiety Disorder

Frequently seen accompanied by another anxiety disorder and/or depression, generalized anxiety disorder (GAD) is a persistent and intense concern that is out of proportion to the actual circumstances and often impacts the individual's physical well-being. For example, people with GAD may be more likely to suffer from such problems as intense headaches or migraines or gastrointestinal upset. People with GAD tend to be on edge and irritable; they may have trouble concentrating and falling and staying asleep.

Panic Disorder

With panic disorder, people have repeated episodes of feelings of intense anxiety that escalates very quickly to a panic attack. During the episodes, people may experience heart palpitations, chest pain, shortness of breath, and feelings of impending doom. Because they are concerned about the possibility of a future attack, whenever possible, people with panic disorder try to avoid places and environments where these have occurred in the past. These attacks may take place as often as several times a day, but they also happen as infrequently as a few times a year.

Phobias

Phobias are characterized by feelings of intense nervousness when one is exposed to a specific object or situation. In the vast majority of cases, this response is completely out of proportion to the potential danger that the individual may face. As a result, active measures may be taken to avoid the phobia trigger. Examples of phobias are the fear of being inside a closed elevator, on an upper floor of a tall building, in a crowded room, or being terrified by insects, such as spiders, or crawling animals, such as snakes. And, it is not uncommon for people to fear traveling in a plane or receiving an injection from a medical provider.

Post-Traumatic Stress Disorder

When some people witness or experience an exceedingly traumatic event, such as combat in war, a devastating car accident, a life-changing sexual assault, or domestic violence, they may develop post-traumatic stress disorder (PTSD). But, this disorder may also emerge following an unexplained event such as a sudden death. With PTSD, people do not recover from the traumatic event; they remain anxious and seriously debilitated; they may have flashbacks, nightmares, and frightening thoughts. They may avoid places or events that may be reminders. They may be easily startled and feel excessively tense; they may lose interest in activities they once enjoyed. And, they may find it difficult to remember specific details about the event; they may even feel guilt that they did not attempt to prevent the trauma.

Separation Anxiety Disorder

Children with separation anxiety disorder feel far more concern about separation from parents and others who assume parental roles than might be expected by their level of development. But, adults may also have this disorder. They fear being apart from people to whom they are close. Like children dealing with separation anxiety, they often worry that something bad may happen if they are not together. So, they dread being apart and avoid separating whenever possible.

Social Anxiety Disorder

Also known as social phobia, social anxiety disorder is the intense nervousness, embarrassment, self-consciousness, and self-doubt some people feel in social situations. They may have heart palpitations, gastrointestinal upset, rigid body posture, difficulty making eye contact, and they may speak in a very soft voice. People with social anxiety disorder spend an excessive amount of their time thinking about being judged or viewed negatively by others. Because of these feelings, people with social anxiety will attempt to avoid social settings. For some people, it prevents them from working, attending school, or completing everyday activities.

Risk Factors for Anxiety

Though the risk factors vary according to the specific type of anxiety, all types of anxiety have certain risks. Adults with anxiety tend to have been shy children who were uncomfortable in new settings. Often, they were exposed to stressful, traumatic, and/or negative life situations or environmental events such as divorce or death of a parent. And, biological relatives frequently have a history of anxiety and/or other psychiatric problems. In addition, anxiety may be triggered or aggravated by physical problems, such as thyroid disease or heart arrhythmias, and substances, such as products containing caffeine and medicine designed to keep people awake.

Diagnosing an Anxiety Disorder

Trained mental health practitioners often diagnose anxiety disorders simply by discussing the symptoms with a patient. No additional testing may be necessary. But, it is not uncommon for practitioners to administer a diagnostic test. These may also be used by other health practitioners who may screen their patients for mental health problems during a routine check-up. A variety of these screening tests were used by the researchers in the studies mentioned in this book. The following are brief descriptions of many of these tests. Of the studies listed, the Hamilton Anxiety Scale, also referred to as the Hamilton Anxiety Rating Scale and the Hamilton Rating Scale for Anxiety, was the most frequently used.

Clinical Global Impression Scale

The Clinical Global Impression (CGI) Scale is a standardized assessment scale for determining the effects of mental health treatment among psychiatric patients. It has been widely used in mental health clinical trials. The scale consists of three separate global subscales. The first, Severity of Illness, compares the severity of the patient's illness to other people with the same problem. The scale is rated from 1 to 7. The higher the number, the more severe the symptoms. A score of 4 is defined as a moderate degree of illness. The second subscale, Global Improvement, allows a practitioner to determine the level of improvement. Again, the ratings are between one and seven, with one being "very much improved" and seven being a patient who is much worse. A rating of four denotes a patient who has not improved. The third subscale, the Efficacy Index, helps practitioners to understand the benefits of treatment and the severity of any side effects. This grid-shaped index uses the y-axis to measure the therapeutic effect and the x-axis measures side effects. Side effects may range from none to those that are so severe that they outweigh any benefits of the treatment. Within the mental health and scientific communities, not everyone agrees that this scale is the best way to evaluate the benefits of mental health treatment. Many object to the fact that it compares a patient to other patients, a process that is at least somewhat subjective.

Depression and Anxiety Stress Scales

There are two types of Depression and Anxiety Stress Scales—DASS-42 and DASS-21. The DASS-42 is a self-reporting scale designed to measure the negative emotional states of depression, anxiety, and stress. The scale is suitable for clinical settings, where it may be used to help diagnose depression, anxiety, and stress and to monitor any progress, as well as in nonclinical settings, where it may serve as a mental health screener. For each of the questions, the respondent selects between the answers never, sometimes, often, and almost always. People with lower scores are more likely to have normal levels of depression, anxiety, and stress; the higher the scores, the more the risk for one of these problems. The DASS-21 is a shortened form of the DASS-42. Both tests primarily evaluate the degree of symptomatology.

Faces Anxiety Scale

The Faces Anxiety Scale is a simple scale consisting of several faces that begin with a neutral no anxiety face and gradually increase to an extremely anxious face. Apparently, many patients, even those who are critically ill in intensive care units, are able to respond to the faces more easily than to some other brief and easily assessed measures of anxiety.

Generalized Anxiety Disorder Scale

A test used in many different types of medical practices and other settings, the Generalized Anxiety Disorder Scale (GAD—7) consists of seven questions and asks people to note whether, during the previous two weeks, they have felt bothered by a number of factors such as anxiety and nervousness and if they have felt on the edge or had a problem relaxing. People who may have GAD, panic disorder, social anxiety, or PTSD are asked to respond in one of four ways—not at all (zero points), several days (one point), more than half of the days (two points), and nearly every day (three points). People with GAD usually have scores of 10 or greater; people without GAD tend to have scores lower than 10. It is recommended that healthcare providers use this tool as an integral component of their usual screening processes. It will measure longitudinal changes and track the progress of treatment.

Hamilton Anxiety Rating Scale

One of the first scales developed to measure the severity of anxiety symptoms, the Hamilton Anxiety Rating Scale (HAM-A) is still widely used in both clinical and research settings. The HAM-A consists of fourteen items, each defined by a series of symptoms and measures both psychic anxiety or psychic stress and somatic anxiety or physical complaints associated with anxiety. People being tested for anxiety rate each item between zero (not present) and four (severe). Total scores range from 0 through 56. People with scores of 17 or lower are considered to have mild anxiety; people with scores between 18 and 24 are thought to have mild to moderate anxiety, people with scores between 25 and 30 have moderate to severe anxiety, and people with scores between 31 and 56 have very severe symptoms.

Hospital Anxiety and Depression Scale

Developed decades ago, the Hospital and Anxiety Depression Scale (HADS) has become a common tool to measure anxiety and depression in a general medical population of patients. It is frequently used for clinical practice and research. The HADS is a simple, easy, and quick method to assess for anxiety and depression; it focuses on symptoms. For example, one question asks if the person is restless and has a desire "to be on the move." Another question asks about "feelings of panic." Requiring only a few minutes to complete, the HADS includes seven questions on anxiety and seven on depression, which are scored separately. People respond to the questions with answers from zero to three. For both types of scores, a total of 8 to 10 means a mild degree of illness, a score between 11 and 14 means a moderate degree, and a score between 15 and 21 means a severe degree. A score of 7 or lower probably means that there is little evidence of illness.

Panic Disorder Severity Scale

The Panic Disorder Severity Scale is a self-report scale that measures the severity of panic attacks and panic disorder symptoms. It is appropriate for use with adolescents who are thirteen years old and adults. It should not be used with those under the age of thirteen years. The scale assesses the overall severity of panic disorder at baseline, and it provides a profile of the severity of the different panic disorder symptoms. It is considered an excellent tool to monitor if a patient's symptoms are improving or further deteriorating. The scale consists of ten items, each rated on a five-point scale. Zero means never; one means occasionally; two means half of the time; three means most of the time; and four means all of the time. The items ask about a variety of symptoms associated with panic disorder, such as panic frequency, distress during panic, panic-focused anticipatory anxiety, phobic avoidance of situations, phobic avoidance of physical sensations, impairment of work functioning, and impairment of social functioning. Total scores range from 0 to 40. To obtain an average score, the total score may be divided by the number of completed answers. Higher total scores indicate a greater severity of symptoms.

PTSD Checklist

The PTSD Checklist is a twenty-item self-report that assesses and measures the presence and severity of PTSD symptoms during the previous month. It serves as a screening tool for PTSD and assists in making a provisional diagnosis of PTSD. It may also be used as a tool to assess if the patient is benefiting from treatment or if the condition is becoming more serious. The PTSD checklist should, however, be combined with a clinical interview. People who suspect they might have PTSD should answer the questions, which may be completed in five to ten minutes. The checklist may also be administered by a professional or para-professional in person or over the phone. Often, patients answer the questions before meeting with a mental health provider or at the very beginning of a meeting. Each question is answered in one of the following ways—Not at all,

A Little bit, Moderately, Quite a bit, or Extremely. Total scores may range from 0 to 80. People with very low scores probably do not have PTSD, and people with low scores may have mild cases. The cutoff for diagnosing PTSD is usually 31–33. However, to help identify those people who clearly need treatment, it is best to have a trained mental health specialist make that decision. Though it may change the psychometric properties of the PTSD Checklist, the one-month time frame may be altered to meet the specific needs of the individual patient.

Spielberger's State-Trait Anxiety Inventory

A commonly used tool, Spielberger's State-Trait Anxiety Inventory (STAI), which is also known as the State-Trait Anxiety Inventory, measures both an anxiety response to a situation and anxiety that is part of a person's overall personality or situational anxiety versus personal anxiety. (The Form Y is the most popular form of the test and the one discussed here.) With a total of forty questions, twenty for state anxiety (STAI-S) and twenty for trait anxiety (STAI-T), the STAI is used in both clinical and research settings on people who have at least a sixth-grade reading level. All of the questions are rated on a four-point scale from "Almost Never" to "Almost Always." The higher the score, the greater the level of anxiety. The range of scores for each section is 20 to 80. People with scores between 20 and 37 are considered to have either low or no anxiety; people with scores between 38 and 44 are thought to have moderate levels of anxiety; and people with scores between 45 and 80 have high levels of anxiety. An example of a state anxiety item is, "I am tense; I am worried," and an example of a trait anxiety item is, "I worry too much over something that really doesn't matter."

Yale-Brown Obsessive Compulsive Scale

The Yale-Brown Obsessive Compulsive Scale (Y-BOCS) is a ten-item checklist that is designed to determine the severity of obsessive-compulsive disorder (OCD). It measures such factors as the time spent on obsessions and compulsions, the degree of interference and control, and the level of subjective distress. Individuals who think they might have OCD or clinicians who are evaluating their patients rate each of the questions between zero and four, with zero being no symptoms and four as the most extreme. After the checklist is completed, the scores are tallied. If a person has a total score between 0 and 7, he or she has a subclinical degree of OCD, and a score between 8 and 15 represents mild OCD. A person with a score between 32 and 40 has extreme OCD. A similar test, known as the Children's Yale-Brown Obsessive Compulsive Scale (Child Y-BOSC), may be used for children.

It should be noted that a number of the treatments discussed in this book were initially developed for problems other than anxiety. The use of a medication for something for which it was not intended is called the "off-label" use. Examples of this are the two entries on beta-blockers and gabapentin. Beta-blockers are a commonly prescribed medication used to slow the heart, and gabapentin is a frequently prescribed medication for seizures.

Acupressure

Introduction

A type of traditional Chinese medicine that was developed more than 5,000 years ago, acupressure focuses on applying light to firm pressure to specific parts of the body, known as acupressure points or acupoints. Most often, this pressure is applied using fingers, fingernails, knuckles, and palms, but some acupressure practitioners use elbows, toes, or specialized tools. The seemingly endless number of pressure points on the body follow specific channels, known as meridians or pathways. It is believed that there are twelve major meridians that connect specific organs, organizing a system of communication throughout the body. The meridians begin at the fingertips, connect to the brain, and then to the organs associated with specific meridians. According to the theory behind acupressure, when these meridians are blocked, qi or energy is unable to flow properly and may cause pain and/or illness. The release of this energy to flow throughout the meridians promotes relaxation, healing, and the restoration of proper function. In this way, the theory behind acupressure is very similar to that associated with acupuncture. They both direct pressure to the same points. Acupuncture uses needles, and an acupressure practitioner places pressure.

There are many acupressure points that are directly involved in treating anxiety. Placing pressure on these points naturally calms the nervous system, which reduces anxiety. So, when an acupressure practitioner wants to reduce the anxiety of a client, he or she will place pressure on one or more of these points. Located at the crown of the head, one common acupoint for anxiety is DU-20. To find DU-20, place a finger at the top of each ear and follow an imaginary line upward until the fingers meet. The meeting point is DU-20. Another frequently cited anxiety acupoint and used in a few trials later in this entry is Yintang; it is located between the eyebrows.

There are several types of acupressure. The most common three are shiatsu, Tui Na, and Jin Shin Jyutsu. Probably the best known type is shiatsu, which is Japanese for finger pressure. A shiatsu practitioner applies vigorous, firm pressure to points for three to five seconds. Tui Na is similar to traditional massage with various types of pressure applied to the body. And, in Jin Shin Jyutsu, the practitioner places gentle pressure on twenty-six specific energy points throughout the body. Acupressure is performed on clients who should wear loose, comfortable clothing; no skin needs to be exposed, and no oils are used.

Regulation, Administration, and Costs

In the United States, there is no national regulation of acupressure. Rather, it is regulated and licensed at the state level, most likely in a way similar to massage therapy. In fact, many massage therapy programs offer specific training in acupressure, as do specialized Chinese medicine or acupressure schools. And, bodywork and Chinese medicine practitioners may formally or informally study acupressure and incorporate it into their practices. The National Certification Board of Therapeutic Massage and Bodywork may well be a source of additional information.

An acupressure practitioner may work in a home or office setting; he or she may work in a holistic healing practice, fitness center, spa, or salon. Wherever the location, an acupressure session normally begins with a brief discussion about the client and his or her health concerns. The actual acupressure session, which may continue for as long as sixty or ninety minutes, is typically performed while the client lies on a massage table. During the sessions, clients are encouraged to breathe slowly and deeply and to practice guided imagery (focusing on positive images) or visualization (imagining what you want to achieve).

An acupressure session costs about the same as a massage and varies according to location and length. Obviously, a longer session in a more expensive area of the country will cost more than a shorter session in a less expensive area. On average, costs should be around $80 to $120 for sixty minutes. While it is a good idea to check with insurers, most likely acupressure sessions will not be covered.

Side Effects and Risks

Acupressure offers a wonderful, relaxing, soothing method to relieve anxiety. Though there should be no pain, because of the possibility of microscopic tears in the muscles, there may be a little delayed soreness. Because energy work is so calming, care should be taken when rising from the table and returning to a standing position. It is possible to become light-headed.

Acupressure must be used with care during pregnancy. Certain points are believed to stimulate uterine contractions. Pressure should never be directed to areas with burns or swelling, recent radiation, rashes, stitches, infections, wounds, varicose veins, contagious diseases of the skin, cancerous tumors, or active cancer that may have spread to the bones. People with certain medical problems, such as heart disease, high blood pressure, bone disease, spinal injury, a bleeding disorder, uncontrolled blood pressure, and diabetes, may wish to discuss acupressure with their healthcare providers before scheduling an appointment, as should people taking anticoagulant or antiplatelet medications.

Research Findings

Acupressure Seems to Help Ease Anxiety

In a systematic review and meta-analysis published in the *Journal of Integrative and Complementary Medicine,* researchers from Taiwan and Japan evaluated the ability of acupressure to reduce anxiety. They located twenty-seven randomized controlled studies with at least one control group that met their criteria and were published between 2003 and 2020. Eight studies were conducted in Iran, six were from China, and the others were from Taiwan, Australia, Malaysia, India, Turkey, Japan, Italy, and the United States. Nine trials included preoperative patients, nine had other types of inpatients, and nine had outpatient departments or community-dwelling adults. Nine trials used a single acupoint, six used two acupoints, and the others used multiple acupoints. In most trials, the practitioner pressed the acupoints with fingers. The duration of the interventions ranged from one treatment to three months, with most studies providing only one treatment. The treatments lasted from two to twenty minutes. Two trials mentioned adverse events, such as hypotension, dizziness, palpitations, and headaches. Six trials noted no adverse events. Eight trials had a low-bias risk, and thirteen had some bias concerns. The researchers found that acupressure effectively reduced anxiety among people in very different life situations. Acupressure with fingers was better than with equipment, and long duration acupressure did not yield better results. While the researchers acknowledged that their findings were encouraging, they noted that because of "the substantial heterogeneity across studies" the results should be interpreted with caution.[1]

In a systematic review and meta-analysis published in *Acupuncture in Medicine*, researchers from Hong Kong also assessed the efficacy of acupressure for anxiety. The researchers found seven randomized controlled trials with 451 subjects that met their criteria for review and five with 314 subjects that met their criteria for meta-analysis. Sample sizes ranged from 36 to 100. Three studies targeted the elderly, while the remaining studies recruited subjects with an average age of thirty-five years or older. Six studies had subjects with physical problems, such as hip fractures and abdominal and renal illnesses. Four trials had one acupoint, two trials had two acupoints, and one trial had three acupoints. The duration of acupressure ranged from ten to thirty minutes, and the acupressure was delivered by people with different backgrounds. Three trials had research personnel, three trials employed allied health professionals, and one trial involved an acupuncturist. All seven studies employed a sham site near the true acupoints, which blinded the participants to the actual intervention. No adverse events were reported. All of the studies were considered to be at low risk for bias. The researchers determined that acupressure provided immediate relief for pretreatment anxiety and reduced anxiety in both emergency and hospital settings. One study even found that applying acupressure to the healthy parents of children undergoing an operation diminished parental anxiety. It should be noted that only one of the trials included a follow-up assessment. As a result, all of the results are restricted to the ability of acupressure to deliver immediate relief from anxiety.[2]

Acupressure Appears Useful for Preoperative Cesarean Section Anxiety

In a randomized, single-blind clinical trial published in the *Journal of Acupuncture and Meridian Studies*, researchers from Iran investigated the ability of acupressure to calm the anxiety of women about to deliver by cesarean section. Sixty women facing surgery were divided into two groups of thirty. The women in the intervention group received continuous and simultaneous acupressure at the Yintang (between the eyebrows) and HE-7 (inside the wrist) acupoints for five minutes before surgery; the women in the control groups received five minutes of sham acupressure. Using the Spielberger's State-Trait Anxiety Inventory, the women had two assessments of their anxiety—one assessment was about an hour before surgery and the other was immediately after the intervention. Anxiety levels were ranked from 20 to 80, ranging from the absence of anxiety to the most intense level of anxiety. The researchers learned that while there was no significant difference between the women's anxiety scores before the intervention, after the intervention, there was a statistically significant difference. The mean anxiety scores of the women in the intervention group were 65.66 before the intervention and 52.93 after the intervention; the mean anxiety scores of the women in the control group were 65.33 before the intervention and 67.46 after the intervention. The researchers concluded that acupressure on the Yintang and HE-7 acupoints decreased anxiety levels, and "it may be used as a preoperative routine nursing care."[3]

Acupressure Reduced Anxiety in Patients Having Thoracoscopic Surgery

In a randomized, controlled trial published in the *International Journal of Environmental Research and Public Health*, researchers from Taiwan evaluated the ability of acupressure to reduce anxiety in patients about to undergo thoracoscopic surgery. One hundred hospitalized patients undergoing thoracoscopic (chest) surgery were assigned to an intervention group ($n = 49$) or a control group ($n = 51$). The patients were enrolled from the cardiothoracic ward of a medical center in central Taiwan; they had a mean age of 60.97 years, and the majority were women. The participants in the intervention group received acupressure treatment to two acupoints, Neiguan (inner arm near wrist) and Shenmen (triangular fossa of the ear). Acupressure was performed by a researcher trained by two experts; assessments were conducted four times, two times before the surgery. While the subjects in both groups had mild to moderate postoperative anxiety, the subjects in the control group had higher levels of anxiety. The researchers observed "an obvious decline" in anxiety in the subjects who were treated with acupressure, and "the effectiveness of acupressure in reducing anxiety appeared to increase with time." And, they concluded that "acupressure is an easy-to-practice, noninvasive complementary treatment that can reduce anxiety in patients undergoing thoracoscopic surgery."[4]

Acupressure, Hypnosis, and Audiovisual Aids Reduce Anxiety in Children Receiving Local Anesthesia

In a randomized, cross-sectional clinical trial published in the *International Journal of Clinical Pediatric Dentistry*, researchers from India tested the ability of acupressure, hypnosis, and audiovisual aids to relieve the anxiety of children receiving local anesthesia before dental treatment. Anxiety among children during dentistry is common and poses an ongoing challenge for dental professionals. The cohort consisted of 200 apparently healthy children between the ages of six and ten years old. They were divided into four groups of fifty—acupressure, hypnosis, audiovisual aids, and control. The children in the acupressure group had a sustained amount of pressure for two to three minutes to the He Gu (L14) acupoint, which is found on the back of the hand between the base of the thumb and index finger. During hypnosis, the children were told to imagine a pleasant experience or being in a soothing place, and during audiovisual aids the children saw some of their favorite programming. The children in the control group had none of these techniques. Levels of anxiety were measured before, during, and after administration of the local anesthetic. The researchers found that when compared to the control group, all three intervention groups had significant reductions in anxiety rates at different time intervals. The researchers noted that their interventions reduced pulse rates, respiratory rates, and levels of anxiety, and their interventions were "cost-effective, non-invasive, and non-pharmaceutical without any side effects."[5]

Acupressure Appears to Help the Anxiety Associated with Hemodialysis

In an open-label, randomized, controlled trial published in the *International Journal of Nursing Studies*, researchers from Malaysia wanted to determine if acupressure would help the anxiety, depression, and stress associated with hemodialysis for end-stage renal disease. The initial cohort consisted of 108 hemodialysis patients who were being treated at one of three hemodialysis centers. The trial, which was carried out from January to March 2014, had fifty-four patients in the intervention group and fifty-four in the control group. The patients ranged in age from twenty-eight to seventy-seven years, with a mean age of 58.08 years; 57.2 percent were male. The most prevalent comorbid diseases were hypertension and diabetes. More than half of the patients had varying degrees of anxiety ranging from mild to extremely severe. Both groups of patients received routine care, but those in the acupressure group also received fifteen minutes of acupressure three times per week for three weeks. Three acupoints were selected: the previously noted Yintang and Shenmen, as well as Taixi, near the protruding bone inside the ankle. The treatments and the characteristics of the patients at all three centers were similar. A few acupressure side effects were observed, such as hypotension, dizziness, palpitations, and headache. Assessments were made with the Depression Anxiety Stress Scales and the General Health Questionnaire. The researchers found that the acupressure group had significantly lower scores on the measures of anxiety, depression, stress, and general psychological distress than the control group. The researchers concluded that "further studies with large-scale, methodologically robust design are recommended in order to produce strong evidence for application of cost-effective acupressure intervention to promote patients' psychological wellbeing."[6]

Hand Shiatsu Massage Seems Helpful for the Anxiety Experienced by Burn Patients

In a randomized trial published in the *World Journal of Plastic Surgery*, researchers from Iran examined the ability of hand shiatsu massage to ease the anxiety of burn patients during dressing changes. The cohort consisted of sixty burn patients with underlying pain. Though they suffered from burn injuries on 10 to 45 percent of their bodies, their hands had healthy areas for hand shiatsu. The patients were placed in one of two groups—hand shiatsu (hand acupressure) and control. Those in the intervention group had ten minutes of shiatsu on each hand. Levels of pain anxiety were assessed before and after shiatsu with the Burn Specific Pain Anxiety Scale. The researchers learned that there was a statistically significant reduction between the before and after pain anxiety scores in the intervention group; no such difference was seen in the control group. And, they concluded that twenty minutes of hand shiatsu "in conjunction with analgesic medications could control the anxiety of burn patients."[7]

Acupressure Does Not Appear to Reduce Anxiety with Acute Injuries

In a prospective three-arm randomized, placebo-controlled trial published in the *Clinical Journal of Sport Medicine*, researchers from New Zealand wanted to learn if the optimal management of the pain and anxiety of sports injuries should include acupressure. The study, which was based at a sports injury clinic in Dunedin, New Zealand, included seventy-nine athletes who sustained a sports-related musculoskeletal injury. On the same day that they sustained their injury, the athletes were treated with three minutes of acupressure ($n = 29$), sham acupressure ($n = 27$), or no acupressure ($n = 23$). Acupressure treatment was on the active point along the long intestine meridian on the dorsum or back of the hand. The sham treatment was given on a non-active point of the palm of the hand. Pain and anxiety were measured immediately before and after the treatment. The athletes described their perceptions of pain relief, anxiety relief, and satisfaction with the treatment, and willingness to have the treatment again. While the researchers learned that the acupressure reduced the pain, it did not have any effect on anxiety. All three groups had essentially the same levels of anxiety. "Three minutes of acupressure was effective in decreasing pain intensity in athletes who sustained an acute musculoskeletal sport injury when measured with VAS [visual analog scale], but did not change anxiety levels."[8]

Students with Mild Anxiety May Benefit Most from Acupressure

In a trial published in the *International Journal of Prevention and Treatment*, researchers from Japan wanted to learn which college students with anxiety benefited most from self-administered acupressure. They initially hypothesized that the students with the highest levels of anxiety would obtain the greatest benefits. The cohort consisted of thirty-three male and sixteen female college students, with a mean age of 30.6 years, who were majoring in acupuncture and moxibustion medicine. They were divided into four groups—less anxious, slightly anxious, mildly anxious, and highly anxious. The subjects were taught how to perform five sessions of self-administered acupressure. Each session included pressing six acupressure points on the neck—three on each side— for five seconds. Before and after acupressure, all of the subjects completed the Tension and Anxiety subscale of the Japanese version of the Profile of Mood States short form. The researchers learned that a single session of self-administered acupressure significantly reduced anxiety. However, in contrast to the researchers' hypothesis, the most improvement was seen in the mildly anxious students. "These results suggest that the association between baseline anxiety level and the magnitude of decrease in anxiety during self-administered acupressure course are not linear." As a result of these findings, the researchers concluded that even those with milder forms of anxiety may benefit from self-administered acupressure.[9]

References and Further Readings

Abadi, Foziyeh, Faezeh Abadi, Zhila Fereidouni et al. "Effect of Acupressure on Preoperative Cesarean Section Anxiety." *Journal of Acupuncture and Meridian Studies* 11, no. 6 (2018): 361–6.

Au, Doreen W., Hector W. Tsang, Paul, P. Ling et al. "Effects of Acupressure on Anxiety: A Systematic Review and Meta-Analysis." *Acupuncture in Medicine* 33, no. 5 (October 2015): 353.

Chen, Su-Ru, Wen-Hsian Hou, Jung-Nien Lai et al. "Effects of Acupressure on Anxiety: A Systematic Review and Meta-Analysis." *Journal of Integrative and Complementary Medicine* 28, no. 1 (January 2022): 25–35.

Erappa, U., S. Konde, M. Agarwal et al. "Comparative Evaluation of Efficacy of Hypnosis, Acupressure and Audiovisual Aids in Reducing the Anxiety of Children During Administration of Local Anesthesia." *International Journal of Clinical Pediatric Dentistry* 14, no. Supplement 2 (2021): S186–S192.

Honda, Y., A. Tsuda, S. Horiuchi, and S. Aoki. "Baseline Anxiety Level as Efficacy Moderator for Self-Administered Acupressure for Anxiety Reduction." *International Journal of Prevention and Treatment* 2, no. 3 (2013): 41–5.

Hmwe, N. T. T., P. Subramanian, L. P. Tan, and W. K. Chong. "The Effects of Acupressure on Depression, Anxiety and Stress in Patients with Hemodialysis: A Randomized Controlled Trial." *International Journal of Nursing Studies* 52 (2015): 509–18.

Hsu, Hsing-Chi, Kai-Yu Tseng, Hsin-Yuan Fang et al. "The Effects of Acupressure on Improving Health and Reducing Cost for Patients Undergoing Thoracoscopic Surgery." *International Journal of Environmental Research and Public Health* 19 (2022): 1869.

Macznik, Aleksandra K., Anthony G. Schneiders, Josie Athens, and S. John Sullivan. "Does Acupressure Hit the Mark? A Three-Arm Randomized Placebo-Controlled Trial of Acupressure for Pain and Anxiety Relief in Athletes with Acute Musculoskeletal Sports Injuries." *Clinical Journal of Sport Medicine* 27, no. 4 (July 2017): 338–43.

Mohaddes Ardabili, F., S. Purhajari, T. Najafi Ghzeljeh, and H. Haghani. "The Effect of Shiatsu Massage on Underlying Anxiety in Burn Patients." *World Journal of Plastic Surgery* 4, no. 1 (January 2015): 36–9.

Acupuncture

Introduction

A key component of traditional Chinese medicine (TCM), acupuncture, which has been studied and practiced for over 2,500 years, is a technique in which practitioners insert fine needles into the skin to treat a host of different medical problems. While most often used for pain, acupuncture is now widely used for stress management, overall wellness, infertility, smoking cessation, diabetes, depression, nausea, and, of course, the various types of anxiety.

According to TCM, each person has a flow of energy or life force, known as *chi* or *qi* (chee), that travels throughout the body in pathways or meridians. When these pathways are blocked, problems occur. Inserting fine needles into specific points on these meridians and manipulating them manually or stimulating them with small electrical currents, a procedure known as electroacupuncture, unblock these pathways, foster the restoration of health, support the immune system, and promote circulation. The insertion of the needles is a minimally invasive method of stimulating nerve-rich areas of the skin, which, in turn, influences various functions of the body. By restoring the body's balance, acupuncture enables the body to naturally heal itself.

An article published in the journal *Acupuncture in Medicine* described the findings of the National Health Interview Survey (NHIS), administered in 2002, 2007, and 2012, on the use of complementary health approaches in the United States. According to the NHIS, in 2002, 2007, and 2012, respectively, 4.2 percent, 6.3 percent, and 6.4 percent of the US adults had used acupuncture with 1.1 percent, 1.4 percent, and 1.7 percent of the US adults doing so during the preceding twelve months. During the same time period, the number of licensed acupuncturists in the United States increased from 12,000 to 27,835. Still, the overall use of acupuncture among the US. adults remains relatively low, only 1.7 percent.[1]

Regulation, Administration, and Costs

There do not appear to be any national regulations for the practice of acupuncture. Most, but not all, states have their own regulations. They tend to require that nonphysician acupuncturists pass an examination conducted by the National Certification Commission for Acupuncture and Oriental Medicine.

Depending upon the area to be treated, during a treatment, patients sit in a chair or lay on their backs, stomachs, or sides on a padded table. Several acupuncture needles, which are very thin, are inserted at various points. After insertion, the acupuncturist may twirl the needles or apply heat or mild electrical pulses. The needles remain in place for at least fifteen or twenty minutes, often for longer. There is no discomfort when the needles are removed. Expect a typical acupuncture session to take thirty minutes to one hour. Initially, treatments might be held once or twice a week. After the primary problem improves, maintenance treatments may be less often, such as once or twice a month. Responses to acupuncture vary. Some people experience improvement after only one treatment; others may require many treatments. Of course, acupuncture is not an effective anxiety treatment for everyone.

Insurance coverage for acupuncture is inconsistent, and the insurers that do cover acupuncture tend to have fairly strict guidelines. While rates vary according to location, without insurance, a typical acupuncture session may cost $100 or more. Expect a first session, which probably includes a brief medical history, to be more expensive.

Side Effects and Risks

When visiting a trained, certified acupuncture practitioner who uses disposable, sterile needles, the risk of side effects and problems is low. Still, on occasion, people have soreness, mild aching, especially at the base of the needle, and minor bleeding at the insertion site of the needles. There are some people who should be more cautious before visiting an acupuncturist. For example, people who have a bleeding disorder or are taking a blood-thinning medication have an increased risk of bleeding during insertion of the needles. The electrical current used by some acupuncturists may interfere with the operation of a pacemaker. And, stimulating certain acupuncture points may increase the risk of triggering labor in pregnant women.

Research Findings

Acupuncture Seems to Benefit People with Anxiety

In a double-blinded, randomized, controlled clinical trial published in the journal *Complementary Therapies in Clinical Practice*, researchers from Portugal investigated the use of acupuncture and electroacupuncture for the treatment of anxiety. The cohort consisted of fifty-six adults between the ages of twenty-one and eighty-two years with a diagnosed anxiety disorder; 85.71 percent were female. The cohort was divided into three groups—acupuncture ($n = 23$), electroacupuncture ($n = 20$), and control ($n = 13$). For ten weeks, the subject in the intervention groups had weekly thirty-minute treatments. Throughout the trial, the researchers used levels of cortisol, the Beck Anxiety Inventory, the Generalized Anxiety Disorder Assessment, and the Overall Anxiety Severity and Impairment Scale to assess levels of anxiety. The researchers learned that by the fifth treatment, the subjects in both treatment groups experienced a "marked decrease" in anxiety scores. Although more modest, the decrease continued until the last treatment. Both treatment protocols were effective even among those subjects not taking anxiolytic medication. The anxiety levels of the subjects in the control group remained stable or increased. All of the results were statistically significant. The researchers concluded that "acupuncture and electroacupuncture are effective in treating anxiety on their own or as adjuncts to pharmacological therapy."[2]

Acupuncture May Help People with Parkinson Disease-Related Anxiety

In a randomized, double-blind, clinical trial published in the journal *JAMA Network Open*, researchers from China studied the usefulness of acupuncture for people dealing with Parkinson disease-related anxiety. The initial cohort consisted of seventy subjects, including thirty-four women and thirty-six men. They were placed in an acupuncture group or a sham acupuncture group. All of the subjects received treatments three times per week for eight weeks. Sixty-four subjects (91 percent) completed the intervention and an eight-week follow-up; they had a mean age of 61.84 years. The Hamilton Anxiety Scale was used to determine levels of anxiety. At the end of the trial, there was no significant difference between the levels of anxiety in the two groups. Both treatments significantly reduced levels of anxiety. However, two months after the trial ended, the subjects in the acupuncture group still had significantly more improvement and far better improvement than those in the sham group. The researchers commented that they thought the initial improvement was a placebo effect. TCM is highly regarded in China. The subjects could have simply assumed that they were receiving an effective treatment. "It can be preliminarily concluded that although there is a certain placebo effect in the short term—the placebo effect of acupuncture in the present study disappeared over time; its therapeutic effect was maintained long-term."[3]

Acupuncture Appears to Be Useful for Anxiety in Children and Adolescents

In a randomized, pilot trial published in the *Journal of Paediatrics and Child Health,* researchers from Alberta, Canada, examined the ability of acupuncture to help children and adolescents with anxiety. The cohort consisted of nineteen children and adolescents between the ages of eight and sixteen years; ten were placed in the acupuncture treatment group and nine in the control group. At baseline, when the children were assessed, there were no significant demographic differences between the groups and both had similar levels of anxiety. All of the children in the treatment group completed five weekly acupuncture treatments, which were tailored to meet the specific needs of each individual child. At the end of the five weeks, the children in both groups were evaluated. It was then that the children in the control group also received five weekly acupuncture treatments and were assessed again. The researchers learned that the children in the treatment group had significant improvements in anxiety. There were four reported side effects from four separate subjects—dizzy feeling, needle pain, headache, and fatigue. And, after the subjects in the control group had their series of treatments, they also experienced significant improvement. The researchers commented that their findings "provided promising results on the potential use of acupuncture to treat children and adolescents with general anxiety."[4]

Acupuncture Appears Useful for Preoperative Anxiety

In a prospective clinical trial published in the journal *Acupuncture in Medicine,* researchers from Germany and Canada studied the ability of auricular (ear) acupuncture to ease preoperative anxiety, a condition they term as preoperative anxiety syndrome, in patients scheduled for elective ambulatory gynecological surgery. Thirty-two patients with a mean age of thirty-seven years were in the acupuncture group and thirty patients with a mean age of thirty-six years had the usual care. At baseline, both groups had similar demographic parameters and the tendency to feel anxiety, also known as trait anxiety. During the course of the study, the patients who received auricular acupuncture had initial reductions of anxiety of about 14 percent on the evening before the surgery, but anxiety levels increased again immediately before the surgery; the patients who received no intervention had increases in levels of anxiety, and the levels were significantly higher at the final measurement than the first measurement. The researchers concluded that "AA [auricular acupuncture] was well accepted by patients as a treatment for preoperative anxiety."[5]

In a randomized controlled trial published in the journal *Anaesthesia*, researchers from the UK examined the effect of acupuncture at the EX-HN3 (Yintang) point on preoperative anxiety levels in neurosurgical patients. (The Yintang point is located between the eyebrows.) According to the researchers, preoperative anxiety is very common among people awaiting neurosurgery. In fact, it is experienced by 23 to 73 percent of patients. It may begin as soon as the surgical procedure is planned and tends to increase over time. The cohort consisted of 124 patients 16 years of age or older; 62 were placed in a treatment group and 62 served as controls. The researchers measured the anxiety levels with two tools—a shortened form of the Spielberger State-Trait Anxiety Inventory score and the Amsterdam Pre-Operative Anxiety and Information Scale. Before their surgeries, thirty-three in the acupuncture group and twenty-nine in the control group had significant levels of anxiety. The patients in the intervention group received thirty minutes of acupuncture at the EX-HN3 acupoint. The Spielberger measure found a 14 percent reduction in anxiety in the acupuncture group and the Amsterdam measure observed an even more notable 30 percent reduction. No changes in anxiety were noted in the control group. The researchers concluded that "acupuncture is a cheap, well-tolerated procedure that is simple to administer and has no prolonged effect on conscious levels, it should be considered a useful therapy for the anxious patient in the immediate preoperative period."[6]

It Is Not Clear If Acupuncture Is Useful for Post-Traumatic Stress Disorder

In a systematic review published in the journal *Evidence-Based Complementary and Alternative Medicine*, researchers from Korea and Alexandria, Virginia, evaluated the use of acupuncture for post-traumatic stress disorder. Unfortunately, the researchers were only able to locate four randomized controlled trials and two uncontrolled clinical trials that met their criteria. One randomized controlled trial was from the United States; the other studies were from China. All of the randomized controlled trials had parallel group designs. The four randomized controlled trials included 543 patients with PTSD; the two uncontrolled trials had 103 patients with earthquake-related PTSD. All six studies reported adverse events, such as pain and bleeding, but no event was serious. According to the researchers, while a "high quality" randomized controlled trial and a meta-analysis determined that acupuncture was effective for PTSD, the results of the other studies were not as definitive. So, they were unable to note with a degree of certainty if acupuncture would help PTSD. "Further qualified trials are needed to confirm whether acupuncture is effective for PTSD."[7]

Acupuncture Failed to Significantly Relieve the Anxiety Experienced by People with Irritable Bowel Syndrome

In a single-blind, randomized, sham-controlled trial published in the *Journal of Gastroenterology and Hepatology*, researchers from Hong Kong evaluated the use of acupuncture for anxiety in people with irritable bowel syndrome; according to these researchers, people with irritable bowel syndrome have five times the rates of anxiety than those without this syndrome. The initial cohort consisted of eighty patients with comorbid generalized anxiety disorder and irritable bowel syndrome; the mean age of the subjects was 51.61 years, and about half were female. The two groups had similar demographic and clinical characteristics. For ten weeks, they received either weekly electroacupuncture ($n = 40$) or sham acupuncture ($n = 40$). The patients were assessed at baseline, immediately after the end of the intervention, and at a six-week follow-up. Two patients in the sham group failed to complete the study. The researchers learned that about one-third of the electroacupuncture patients and one-fourth of the sham patients showed improvement, but the difference did not reach statistical significance. The researchers concluded that their "findings failed to support the effectiveness of electroacupuncture for comorbid generalized anxiety disorder and irritable bowel syndrome."[8]

While Acupuncture Seems Useful for Pre-Examination Anxiety in Students, Students Receiving Sham Acupuncture and No Intervention also Improve

In a trial published in the *World Journal of Acupuncture*, researchers from China investigated the ability of acupuncture to ease sleep disturbances caused by pre-examination (pre-exam) anxiety in undergraduates. The cohort consisted of sixty undergraduates who had sleep problems associated with final exam anxiety; they were divided into three groups of twenty. The students in one group had traditional acupuncture treatments; a second group had scalp acupuncture treatments; and third group served as the control. For both acupuncture groups, treatments began four weeks before exams and were conducted five days per week. There were two-day breaks between each series of five treatments. After one week of treatment, the anxiety scores of all the groups were slightly lower. After two weeks, the scores in the treatment groups continued to drop while the control group scores remained about the same. After four weeks, the scores in the treatment groups dropped dramatically, and the scores of those in the control group were only a little lower. One week post-treatment, the scores in the treatment groups remained low, and the scores in the control group were considerably lower, though not as low as the treatment groups. Regarding their anxiety symptoms, the researchers determined that 100 percent of the students in the treatment groups were cured, markedly improved, or improved; 83.3 percent of those in the control group experienced some level of improvement. Though the scalp treatment group had better scores than the traditional acupuncture group, the differences between them were not significant.[9]

In a randomized study published in the online journal *PLoS ONE*, researchers from Germany and Canada wanted to learn if auricular acupuncture would reduce exam anxiety among medical students. The cohort consisted of forty-four medical students in Germany; they were all Caucasian and thirty-five were females. In a crossover manner, the students received auricular acupuncture treatments, a placebo, or no treatment before three comparable oral anatomy exams. Thus, all of the students participated once in each protocol. A licensed acupuncturist with more than five years of experience applied the acupuncture points. Though the placebo treatments appeared to be actual acupuncture, they were designed to have no effect. The students in the no intervention group participated in group discussions. Pre-exam anxiety was measured the evening prior to the exam, before the intervention, after the intervention, and immediately before the exam; these measurements were conducted using a visual analogue scale (VAS) and the German version of the Spielberger's State-Trait Anxiety Inventory. When compared to placebo and no intervention, the exam anxiety of those who had actual acupuncture decreased by up to 20 percent. The largest effect was seen with the VAS the evening after the intervention on the day before the exam. When compared to no intervention, placebo acupuncture also reduced anxiety, though not as strongly as actual acupuncture. The researchers concluded that "both auricular acupuncture and placebo procedure were shown to be effective in reducing levels of exam anxiety in medical students."[10]

Acupuncture May Help the Anxiety Associated with In Vitro Fertilization

In a systematic review and meta-analysis published in the *European Journal of Integrative Medicine*, researchers from China reviewed the use of acupuncture to ease the anxiety and/or depression that may occur during *in vitro* fertilization treatments. The researchers located eleven randomized and one quasi-randomized controlled trials with 2,867 participants who met their criteria. All of the studies were published between 2005 and 2020; eleven were conducted at a single center and one was multicentered. While six studies took place in China, the other studies were from Sweden, the United States, Brazil, Iran, Turkey, and Australia/New Zealand. Seven studies used traditional acupuncture; two used auricular acupuncture; two used transcutaneous electrical acupoint stimulation; and one applied electroacupuncture. There were five different types of control groups. Four studies used sham acupuncture; five had no acupuncture; one study used sham and no acupuncture; one study used rest; and the final study used conventional analgesia. While different scales were used to measure anxiety levels, eight studies with 2,219 patients used the Spielberger State-Trait Anxiety Inventory. Five studies noted that there were no adverse effects. The researchers found that eleven studies demonstrated that acupuncture relieved IVF-related anxiety; only one study showed no relief. Yet the researchers cautioned that "there still remains a dearth of evidence on how many patients may benefit from anxiety and depression relief during IVF treatment."[11]

Acupuncture May Help People Dealing with Post-Traumatic Stress Disorder

In a trial published in the journal *Medical Care*, researchers from Bethesda, Maryland, Davenport, Iowa, and Alexandria, Virginia, tested the ability of acupuncture to ameliorate the symptoms of PTSD. The cohort consisted of fifty-five military service members with PTSD. They were randomized to receive the usual PTSD treatment plus eight biweekly sixty-minute sessions of acupuncture ($n = 28$) or the usual treatment alone ($n = 27$). At baseline, 60 percent of the subjects were receiving psychotropic medication, active counseling, or both.

Assessments were conducted at baseline and at four, eight, and twelve weeks post-randomization. Forty-three subjects (78 percent) completed the trial. No trial-related adverse events were reported. The subjects in the acupuncture group experienced significantly greater improvement in their PTSD symptoms than those in the usual treatment group, and these benefits continued for eight weeks after the trial ended. If these findings are confirmed, "acupuncture may offer a unique addition to . . . current PTSD treatment."[12]

References and Further Readings

Amorim, Diogo, Irma Brito, Armando Caseiro et al. "Electroacupuncture and Acupuncture in the Treatment of Anxiety—A Double Blinded Randomized Parallel Clinical Trial." *Complementary Therapies in Clinical Practice* 46 (2022): 101541.

Cui, Jia, Shaobai Wang, Jiehui Ren et al. "Use of Acupuncture in the USA: Changes over a Decade (2002–2012)." *Acupuncture in Medicine* 35, no. 3 (June 2017): 200–7.

Dong, Guo-juan, Di Cao, Yue Dong et al. "Scalp Acupuncture for Sleep Disorder Induced by Pre-Examination Anxiety in Undergraduates." *World Journal of Acupuncture* 28, no. 3 (September 2018): 156–60.

Engel, Charles C., Elizabeth H. Cordova, David M. Benedek et al. "Randomized Effectiveness Trial of a Brief Course of Acupuncture for Posttraumatic Stress Disorder." *Medical Care* 52, No. 12 Supplement 5 (December 2014): S57–S64.

Fan, Jing-qi, Wei-jing Lu, Wei-qiang Tan et al. "Effectiveness of Acupuncture for Anxiety Among Patients with Parkinson Disease: A Randomized Clinical Trial." *JAMA Network Open* 5, no. 9 (2022): e2232133.

Kim, Young-Dae, In Heo, Byung-Cheul Shin et al. "Acupuncture for Posttraumatic Stress Disorder: A Systematic Review of Randomized Controlled Trials and Prospective Clinical Trials." *Evidence-Based Complementary and Alternative Medicine* (2013): Article ID 615857.

Klausenitz, Catharina, Henriette Hacker, Thomas Hesse et al. "Auricular Acupuncture for Exam Anxiety in Medical Students—A Randomized Crossover Investigation." *PLoS ONE* 11, no. 12 (2016): e0168338.

Leung, Brenda, Wendy Takeda, and Victoria Holec. "Pilot Study of Acupuncture to Treat Anxiety in Children and Adolescents." *Journal of Paediatrics and Child Health* 54, no. 8 (August 2018): 881–8.

Mak, Arthur Dun-Ping, Vincent Chi Ho Chung, Suet Ying Yuen et al. "Noneffectiveness of Electroacupuncture for Comorbid Generalized Anxiety Disorder and Irritable Bowel Syndrome." *Journal of Gastroenterology and Hepatology* 34, no. 10 (October 2019): 1736–42.

Wiles, M. D., J. Mamdani, M. Pullman, and C. Andrzejowski. "A Randomised Controlled Trial Examining the Effect of Acupuncture at the EX-HN3 (Yintang)

Point on Pre-Operative Anxiety Levels in Neurosurgical Patients." *Anaesthesia* 72, no. 3 (March 2017): 335–42.

Wunsch, Jakub K., Catharina Klausenitz, Henriette Janner et al. "Auricular Acupuncture for Treatment of Preoperative Anxiety in Patient Scheduled for Ambulatory Gynaecological Surgery: A Prospective Controlled Investigation with a Non-Randomised Arm." *Acupuncture in Medicine* 36, no. 4 (August 2018): 222–7.

Ye, Jia-Yu, Yi-Jing He, Ming-Jie Zhan, and Fan Qu. "Effects of Acupuncture on the Relief of Anxiety and/or Depression During *in vitro* Fertilization: A Systematic Review and Meta-Analysis." *European Journal of Integrative Medicine* 42 (2021): 101287.

Animal Therapy

Introduction

Also known as animal-assisted therapy (AAT), assisted-animal intervention (AAI), and pet therapy, animal therapy is the use of animals as a means to help people deal with and recover from a wide variety of physical and mental health conditions, such as depression, dementia, pain from cancer treatments, postoperative recovery, recovery from a stroke, autism spectrum disorder, attention deficit hyperactivity disorder, schizophrenia, and, of course, anxiety disorders. Although most people are probably familiar with animal therapy with dogs, animal therapy may actually involve a wide variety of animals including cats, horses, birds, dolphins, fish, small pet rodents, and even farm animals. Animal therapy is a complementary treatment and is intended to add but not replace any more conventional treatment for anxiety. The goal of animal therapy is to enhance the treatment already being used.

Animal therapy is based on the belief that there is a strong bond between most people and animals. For many people, interaction with animals is calming. The human/animal bond fosters companionship and reduces stress, loneliness, and fears. That is why animals are often brought in to comfort people when there are natural disasters and school shootings.

It is important to realize that there is a difference between a service animal, such as a service dog, and a therapy animal, such as a therapy dog. A service dog has received extensive training to perform tasks for a person with a disability, such as helping a blind person walk along busy streets and alerting people who are deaf. They may even be trained to protect a person having a seizure and notify a person with diabetes that serum glucose levels are too low. Protected by the Americans with Disabilities Act (ADA), service animals have full public access rights to all public places including stores, restaurants, hotels, and hospitals. They are taught not to interact with anyone but their owner/handler. A therapy dog is trained to provide emotional support to humans. They may be any breed or combination of breeds and any shape or size. Therapy dogs, and other types of therapy animals, are not service animals and are not protected by the ADA.

That is why a business that is not allowed to prohibit a service dog from entering may prohibit a therapy dog. And, a landlord who may not allow pets must allow a service dog.

Regulation, Administration, and Costs

There are no national regulations, and there appear to be few state or local regulations on animal therapy. Though most animal therapy seems to occur on the informal level, there are a number of organizations that train handlers and connect them to healthcare providers. Many handlers are volunteers, who simply love spending time with animals. Before obtaining approval for animal therapy from these groups, both the handler and the animal are required to complete certification requirements. Often, this includes the handler learning how to interact with people and perform the type of therapies they require. The animal needs to pass a physical examination and all immunizations must be current. In addition, to ensure the safety of all the people involved, the handler and animal must complete obedience training. Additional regulation is provided by the American Kennel Club. Dogs certified by certain organizations may have the title AKC Therapy Dog. The organizations they cite are the Alliance of Therapy Dogs, Bright and Beautiful Therapy Dogs, Love on a Leash, Pet Partners, and Therapy Dogs International.

Therapy animals and their handlers work in a wide variety of settings, such as hospitals, long-term care facilities, corporate workplaces, residential treatment centers, grief camps, secondary schools, college and universities, community centers, psychiatric settings, rehabilitation facilities, aquatic centers (dolphins), and in the case of horse therapy (known as equine therapy or hippotherapy) within a horse barn, arena, or ring. The lengths and types of interaction vary. An interaction with a child reading a book to an animal will be far less structured than an equine program in which the child must be carefully monitored.

In the United States, the vast majority of animal therapy providers appear to be owners of dogs who volunteer their time and services. Many join organized therapy dog groups which screen both the human and the dog and provide educational materials as well as liability insurance on the unlikely possibility that a problem arises during their volunteering time. There are animal therapy businesses, both for profit and nonprofit that charge for their services. Charges may start around $25 per visit, but many are more expensive. Clearly, businesses with significant overhead costs, such as those with dolphin or horse therapy, cost more. Depending on the facility and the time involved, sessions may cost up to several hundred dollars. Individual sessions tend to be more expensive than group sessions. It is possible, especially with equine therapy, that some of the costs may be covered by insurance.

Side Effects and Risks

People may be allergic or have some form of sensitivity to the animals that are used in animal therapy. In those instances, animal therapy should always be avoided. Of course, there is also the possibility that an animal may be a carrier of infections and diseases that may spread to a child, a senior, or a person with a compromised immune system. Some people simply do not like animals or certain types of animals. And, not all animals are suitable for animal therapy. The animal must be comfortable with people of all ages and being touched anywhere on the body. They must be obedient and not be bothered by sudden movements or yelling sounds. These situations may only increase levels of anxiety.

Obviously, interacting with a well-trained animal generally has a very low risk. However, interacting with certain animals, such as dolphins or horses, has some inherent risks. For example, while riding a dolphin or horse, one may lose balance and fall. To avoid these problems, only participate in animal therapy that is located in a highly recommended, well-run facility, perhaps even regulated and certified by the state.

Research Findings

Animal Therapy with Dogs Appears to Improve Levels of Anxiety, Well-Being, and Mood in University Students

In a trial published in the *International Journal of Environmental Research and Public Health*, researchers from the Edinburgh, Scotland, examined the ability of dog therapy to improve levels of anxiety, well-being, and mood in university students. The cohort consisted of 132 university students, with a mean age of 21.6 years. Eighty-five were female. All of the students were placed in one of three 20-minute interventions. Forty-five students had a standard therapy session with interaction with a dog and the dog's handler; forty-one students only interacted with a dog, and forty-six students only interacted with a handler. Seven dogs and their handlers from the Canine Concern Scotland Trust participated. The researchers administered pre- and post-intervention questionnaires. After the sessions were completed, the subjects who took part in the handler only session were allowed to attend a session with both a handler and a dog. The researchers found that there was a large reduction in anxiety in the students in the two sessions in which a dog was present; it was significantly greater than the minimal reduction that occurred when only a handler was present. The researchers commented that "animal-assisted interventions, activities and visitation programs can be successfully enjoyed within higher education establishments to enhance student well-being and mental health."[1]

Dog Therapy Appears to Reduce Anxiety in People with Anxiety Disorders

In a trial published in the *Journal of Clinical Medicine*, researchers from Poland evaluated the use of dog therapy to lower the anxiety levels of people with an anxiety disorder. The cohort consisted of fifty-one subjects with a clinical diagnosis of anxiety or mixed depressive-anxiety disorders; they were recruited from patients treated in hospital-based group psychotherapy. The mean age of the group was 33.87 years and 77 percent were female. All of the interventions were performed between noon and 5 pm by a 2.5-year-old female German shepherd and her handler. Each of the subjects either took a fifteen to twenty-minute walk with the dog and her handler ($n = 25$) or they walked with a medical student or doctor ($n = 26$). The two groups were demographically similar. Full data were obtained from twenty-one subjects in the treatment group and twenty-six in the control group. The subjects completed the same comprehensive questionnaires before and after the walks. At the end of the walks, the subjects in the treatment group reported significantly lower anxiety than the subjects in the control group. The researchers concluded that "animal-assisted activity may be an effective adjunctive modality for the treatment of patients with anxiety and mixed depressive-anxiety patients."[2]

Pet Therapy May or May Not Help Hospitalized Children with Anxiety

In a quasi-experimental trial published in the *Journal of Pediatric Nursing*, researchers from Nutley and Morristown, New Jersey, studied the ability of a therapy dog to help hospitalized children with anxiety. The initial cohort consisted of ninety-three children between the ages of six and seventeen years. Fifty children had a visit with the research assistant, a dog and the dog's handler, and forty-three children completed an age-appropriate jigsaw puzzle depicting an underwater scene with the research assistant. Each of the visits was eight to ten minutes. Parents were present for all study-related activities. Using the State-Trait Anxiety Scale for Children, the levels of anxiety experienced by each child were measured before and after the visit. Parents completed a brief questionnaire. While the levels of anxiety in the children decreased after both types of visits, the children in the dog therapy group had a significantly greater decrease in anxiety. And, the parents reported a high level of satisfaction with the dog therapy program, and forty-five parents noted that they also benefited from the visit. The researcher concluded that their "findings provide support for a brief pet therapy visit with a trained dog and handler as a tool to decrease anxiety in hospitalized children while promoting parent satisfaction."[3]

In a trial published in the journal *Anthrozoös*, researchers from Virginia and Ohio investigated the use of dog therapy for anxiety and pain in children admitted to the pediatric unit of the Children's Hospital of Richmond at Virginia Commonwealth University. The cohort consisted of forty children between the ages of eight and seventeen years, with a mean age of 11.83 years. The majority were white and owned a pet. Gender was evenly divided. The children, who were admitted for thirty-one different conditions, were randomly assigned to dog therapy or working on an age-appropriate jigsaw puzzle with the research assistant. The visits took place around mid-morning in the child's hospital room within three days of admission; each visit was held for ten minutes. The therapy was provided by seven volunteers who were members of the hospital's dog therapy program. The dogs were varying sizes, both genders, and a variety of breeds and mixed breeds. Children were permitted to freely interact with the dogs. Using a single-item, eleven-point numeric rating scale, levels of anxiety and pain were measured both before and after the visit. The researcher observed no significant differences in anxiety levels between or within the children in both groups. The brief dog therapy encounter did not appear to have any impact on anxiety. The researcher concluded that their "findings fail to support an effect of AAIs on anxiety and pain in children hospitalized in an acute-care setting."[4]

However, Dog Therapy Seemed to Reduce Anxiety in Hospitalized Adults

In a study published in the journal *Clinical Nursing Research*, Boston area researchers explored the effects of dog therapy on anxiety and other factors on fifty-nine adults hospitalized in one of three inpatient units in a large academic medical center—a twenty-bed surgical oncology unit and two general surgical units with twenty-eight and thirty-six beds. There were thirty-two females and twenty-seven males, and all but four patients were white. They ranged in age from twenty-one to eighty years, and forty-four were pet owners. Included among the measures was the Spielberger State/Trait Anxiety questionnaire. The fifteen-minute visits were conducted on Tuesdays and Thursdays. The researchers observed that fifteen minutes were a sufficient amount of time to reduce subjective levels of anxiety and improve other markers of well-being. Nevertheless, the researchers underscored the need "for a more rigorous research design such as a randomized clinical controlled trial with matching patients by diagnosis and/or surgical procedure."[5]

Equine Therapy Seems to Reduce Anxiety and Stress in Youth

In a randomized, controlled trial published in the journal *Animals*, researchers from New York City, Syracuse, New York and Cleveland, Ohio evaluated the effectiveness of Reining in Anxiety (RiA), a therapeutic equine riding program for youth with mild to moderate anxiety. The program included five aspects of cognitive behavioral therapy—in vivo exposure, cognitive restructuring, youth psychoeducation, relaxation, and caregiver psychoeducation about anxiety. The cohort consisted of thirty-nine youth between the ages of six and seventeen years, mean age 11.5 years, with mild to moderate anxiety. They were active students at the Fieldstone Farm Therapeutic Riding Center in northeast Ohio. Slightly more than half were female, and 79 percent were white. The students were joined by their caregivers. The intervention included ten 45-minute weekly sessions. Each lesson had two to four students. Several anxiety assessments, such as the Screen for Child Anxiety Related Disorders and saliva tests to determine levels of cortisol (marker of anxiety and stress), were administered at weeks one, four, seven, and ten. The researchers learned that the riding program resulted in statistically significant reductions in anxiety. The researchers noted that "RiA may be a promising approach for reducing anxiety and stress among youth and that the intervention can be delivered by adaptive/therapeutic horseback riding instructors in a non-clinic setting."[6]

Animal Therapy with Dogs May Help Nursing Students Who Experience Anxiety Before Important Examinations

In a randomized trial published in the journal *Nurse Education in Practice*, researchers from Lawrence, Kansas, examined the use of dog therapy to reduce anxiety in nursing students before important examinations. The cohort consisted of ninety nursing students; they were predominately female, twenty to twenty-two years old, white, and most owned a dog. Before their medication dosage calculation test, forty-six students were placed in the intervention group and forty-four in the control group. The students in the intervention group had unstructured interaction with trained and certified dogs, their handlers, and one another for thirty-five to forty-five minutes before their exam; the students in the control group only interacted with one another for the same period of time. Multiple anxiety assessments were conducted before, during, and after the trial. The researchers learned that the students who interacted with the dogs had significantly lower levels of anxiety before the examination; however, this interaction had no effect on actual examination scores. So, while the students in the intervention were not as anxious, they did not perform any better than the more anxious students in the control group. The researchers concluded that their findings provide "evidence to the need for nursing programs to support their students with safe coping methods."[7]

Animal Therapy May Also Help Nurses at Work

In a prospective study published in the *Journal of Nursing Administration*, researchers from Illinois examined the use of animal therapy to help ease the anxiety experienced by nurses who deal with chronic stressful situation, high-acuity assignments, and rigorous patient care standards. The cohort consisted of forty-five nurses who ranged in age from twenty-two to sixty-two years, with a mean age of 36.73 years. Almost all of the nurses were female; 53 percent were married, 38 percent were single, and 10 percent were divorced. The four-week intervention was held once weekly for the day and night shifts; most of the nurses spent the required minimum time of ten minutes with a therapy dog. The average time was 11.52 minutes. All of the interventions were held at the same site with the same dogs and handlers. Pre- and post-intervention anxiety levels were measured with the Beck Anxiety Inventory. The researchers found that the levels of anxiety experienced by the nurses were significantly reduced by dog therapy. The researchers noted that their findings "were significant and supportive of such interventions for nurses and direct frontline staff."[8]

Farm Animals May Have a Limited Effect on Anxiety

In a randomized, controlled trial published in the journal *Occupational Therapy on Mental Health*, researchers from Norway evaluated the effect of farm animal therapy on anxiety and depression in psychiatric patients. The initial cohort consisted of ninety adult psychiatric patients with a variety of severe psychiatric diagnoses—fifty-nine women and thirty-one men, with a mean age of 34.7 years. Fourteen were inpatients, and seventy-six were outpatients. More than 50 percent of the patients had been ill over five years, and 72 percent had been connected to psychiatric health institutions for more than three years. As many as 83 percent of the patients received daily medications, mainly antipsychotics, antidepressants, sedatives, and mood stabilizers. Fifteen farmers from fifteen farms were recruited to work with the patients; only two had previously worked with psychiatric patients. For twelve weeks, the patients visited the farms twice weekly, for three hours. They were only permitted to work with the animals. Depending upon the type of farm, this included patting, brushing, washing, saddling, riding horses, moving animals, and feeding animals. Sixty patients had an intervention with farm animals and thirty were in the control group. Thirty-one women and ten men completed the intervention, and seventeen women and eleven men completed their time in the control group. Anxiety was measured using the Spielberger State Anxiety Inventory. At the end of the trial, neither the patients in the intervention group or the control group had reductions in anxiety. At the six-month follow-up, the anxiety levels of the patients in the intervention were significantly lower. For the patients in the control group, there were no significant differences. The researchers commented that "the length of the intervention in our study may have been too short or the frequency too few, to get significant differences between the groups, especially when we take into account the psychiatric diagnoses."[9]

Animal Therapy with Dogs May Not Alleviate Anxiety in Adolescents

In a randomized trial published in the journal *Anxiety, Stress, & Coping*, researchers from Massachusetts and Maine studied the effects of therapy dog interaction on adolescent anxiety during a laboratory-based social evaluative stressor. The initial cohort consisted of seventy-five adolescents between the ages of thirteen and seventeen years with low ($n = 18$), middle ($n = 22$), and high ($n = 35$) levels of anxiety. The majority of the teens were white and female, and most owned at least one pet. Because of protocol deviations, seven subjects were excluded. The remaining sixty-seven teens were then divided into three groups; the teens in one group communicated with a therapy dog but had no physical interaction ($n = 22$); the teens in a second group had verbal and physical interaction with a therapy dog ($n = 25$); and the teens in a third group had no interaction with a therapy dog ($n = 21$). There was only a stuffed toy dog. All of the teens were given a series of tasks to induce stress. Three different measures applied six separate times assessed changes in anxiety. While dog handlers were in the room, they did not talk to the teens. Additional subjects were deleted for the final analyses. The researchers expected to determine that the teens in the two therapy groups would have lower levels of anxiety. In contrast, the dogs had no impact on any of the measures of anxiety. "Contrary to our hypotheses, there was no convincing evidence that the presence of a real dog, with or without the opportunity to touch it, reduced anxiety." And this finding was true for the subjects with all three levels of anxiety.[10]

References and Further Readings

Anderson, Della and Stephanie Brown. "The Effect of Animal-Assisted Therapy on Nursing Student Anxiety: A Randomized Controlled Study." *Nurse Education in Practice* 52 (March 2021): 103042.

Barker, Sandra B., Janet S. Knisely, Christine M. Schubert et al. "The Effect of an Animal-Assisted Intervention on Anxiety and Pain in Hospitalized Children." *Anthrozoös* 28, no. 1 (March 2015): 101–12.

Berget, B., Ø. Ekeberg, I. Pedersen, and B. Braastad. "Animal-Assisted Therapy with Farm Animals for Persons with Psychiatric Disorders: Effects on Anxiety and Depression, a Randomized Controlled Trial." *Occupational Therapy in Mental Health* 27 (2011): 50–64.

Coakley, Amanda Bulette, Christine Donahue Annese, Joanne Hughes Empoliti, and Jane M. Flanagan. "The Experience of Animal Assisted Therapy on Patients in an Acute Care Setting." *Clinical Nursing Research* 30, no. 4: (May 2021): 401–05.

Coto, Jeffrey A., Erika K. Ohlendorf, Andrea E. Cinnamon et al. "A Correlational Study Exploring Nurse Work Anxiety and Animal-Assisted Therapy." *Journal of Nursing Administration* 52, no. 9 (September 2022): 498–502.

Grajfoner, Dasha, Emma Harte, Lauren M. Potter, and Nicola McGuigan. "The Effect of Dog-Assisted Intervention on Student Well-Being, Mood, and Anxiety." *International Journal of Environmental Research and Public Health* 14, no. 5 (2017): 483.

Hinic, Katherine, Mildred Ortu Kowalski, Kristin Holtzman, and Kristi Mobus. "The Effect of Pet Therapy and Comparison Intervention on Anxiety in Hospitalized Children." *Journal of Pediatric Nursing* 46 (2019): 55–61.

Hoagwood, Kimberly, Aviva Vincent, Mary Acri et al. "Reducing Anxiety and Stress Among Youth in a CBT-Based Equine-Assisted Adaptive Riding Program." *Animals* 12, no. 19 (September 20, 2022): 24911.

Mueller, Megan K., Eric C. Anderson, Erin K. King, and Heather L. Urry. "Null Effects of Therapy Dog Interaction on Adolescent Anxiety During Laboratory-Based Social Evaluative Stressor." *Anxiety, Stress, & Coping* 34, no. 4 (2021): 365–80.

Wolyńczyk-Gmaj, Dorota, Aleksandra Ziólkowska, Piotr Rogala et al. "Can Dog-Assisted Intervention Decrease Anxiety Level and Autonomic-Agitation in Patients with Anxiety Disorders?" *Journal of Clinical Medicine* 10 (2021): 5171.

Benzodiazepines

Introduction

Benzodiazepines are a class of medication that slow activity in the brain and nervous system. They are most often used for treating anxiety, insomnia, and mental health disorders. But, they are also used to induce procedural sedation and improve brain-related conditions, such as seizures. In addition, it is not uncommon for them to be used off-label for other problems, such as tics, bipolar disorder, depression, mania, palliative sedation, geriatric agitation, addiction, alcohol withdrawal, acute and chronic pain, traumatic brain injury, and tinnitus.

The nervous system uses chemical and electrical signals to send messages. One class of chemical signals, known as neurotransmitters, includes gamma-aminobutyric (GABA). GABA helps to regulate such actions as movement and anxiety. Benzodiazepines enhance the ability of GABA, at the GABA-A receptor, which then reduces the activity of the brain and nervous system, as well as levels of anxiety.

Benzodiazepines are classified by their strength and duration of action. While the strength and duration of a medication varies from one person to another, some types of benzodiazepines offer shorter, more potent benefits and others are not as effective but the benefits last longer. Short-term, stronger benzodiazepines tend to be used for quick relief, such as presurgical anxiety; long-term, lower-strength benzodiazepines are preferred for chronic problems, such as refractory anxiety disorders.

In the United States, benzodiazepines are commonly prescribed. A 2018 article in the *Journal of Clinical Psychiatry* cited data from the 2015–2016 National Surveys on Drug Use and Health. It found that 12.5 percent of adults in the United States used benzodiazepines.[1] Currently, in the United States, 99 percent of the benzodiazepine prescriptions are for alprazolam (Xanax), clonazepam (Klonopin), diazepam (Valium), and lorazepam (Ativan). These have all been approved by the FDA for anxiety disorders. And, while there are other benzodiazepines, such as chlordiazepoxide (Librium), those are rarely used for anxiety, and there is little recent research. Today, chlordiazepoxide is primarily used for alcohol withdrawal.

Before the discovery of benzodiazepines, physicians generally treated anxiety with barbiturates. But, they had a risk of significant side effects and complications, such as respiratory depression. In 1955, while searching for an alternative to barbiturates, Hoffmann-La Roche chemist Leo Sternbach discovered the first benzodiazepine, chlordiazepoxide. By 1960, the new medication was marketed as Librium. Soon, other companies began creating their own benzodiazepines. Initially, they appeared to be safer than barbiturates. They were thought to be less toxic and have fewer side effects. Benzodiazepines soared in popularity. By the mid to late 1970s, they were a frequently prescribed medication. But, concerns about their side effects and risks eventually emerged. A decade later, clinicians noted that people were dependent on these medications and have been found abusing them.[2] Today, benzodiazepines have a FDA Black Box warning, indicating that there are risk of physical dependence, withdrawal reactions, misuse, abuse, and addiction. Using benzodiazepines with opioids may lead to extreme sedation or even death.

Regulation, Administration, and Costs

In the United States and many other countries, benzodiazepines are classified as controlled substances. Tightly regulated, they are only available by prescription. Benzodiazepines are controlled because they have dangerous side effects, especially when misused, as they often are. While it is normally recommended that people take a low dose of a benzodiazepine for a relatively short period of time, such as two to four weeks, people often take them for many months or years. If a physician refuses to prescribe any future doses or refuses to increase a dose, it is not uncommon for patients to find another medical provider who will prescribe them. When people are desperate, they may obtain these medications illegally.

After administration, alprazolam, clonazepam, diazepam, and lorazepam begin to work within one hour. The half-life of the medications or the time when half of the medication is metabolized or eliminated from the body is eleven to fifteen hours for alprazolam, eighteen to fifty hours for clonazepam, fifty to hundred hours for diazepam, and ten to fourteen hours for lorazepam.

Alprazolam

Alprazolam is sold as a tablet, extended-release tablet, oral disintegrating tablet, and concentrated solution. The tablet, oral disintegrating tablet, and concentrated solution are taken two to four times per day; the extended-release tablet is taken once per day in the morning. For the tablet, oral disintegrating tablet, and concentrated solution, most adults are started on a low dose of 0.25 mg to 0.5 mg three times per day; generally, people should not take more than 6 mg per day in divided doses. For the extended-release tablet, the starting dose is 0.5 mg to 1 mg once daily. This may be increased to 3 mg to 6 mg once daily. Older adults may begin with a dose of 0.25 mg two or three times per day. The dose for children will be determined by a medical provider. Costs vary according to the type of alprazolam. But, without insurance, it is a very expensive medication.

Clonazepam

Clonazepam is sold as a tablet or disintegrating tablet. For anxiety, adults are generally started on 0.25 mg two times per day. The dose is usually not more than 4 mg per day. Dosing for children is determined by a medical provider. Older adults may be started on a lower dose. Without insurance, clonazepam is very expensive.

Diazepam

Diazepam is sold as a tablet or an oral solution that comes with a dropper. Adults take 2 to 10 mg two to four times a day. Older adults begin with 2 to 2.5 mg one to two times a day. The dose for children is determined by a medical provider. Doses for older adults and children may be carefully increased. Diazepam is not recommended for children under the age of six months. Without insurance, diazepam is a very expensive medication.

Lorazepam

Lorazepam is sold as a tablet, oral liquid, or injectable solution, to be administered by a healthcare professional before a procedure. Adults and children twelve years of age and older usually begin with 2 mg to 6 mg per day in divided doses. The maximum dose per day is 10 mg. Older adults begin with 1 to 2 mg per day in divided doses. Children under the age of twelve need to follow the guidance of their medical provider. Without insurance, lorazepam is a moderately priced medication.

Side Effects and Risks

There are many side effects associated with benzodiazepines. These include dizziness, weakness, unsteadiness, depression, loss of orientation, headache, sleep disturbances, behavioral changes such as increased risk taking, confusion, irritability, aggression, excitement, impaired coordination, memory impairment, and ironically, increased anxiety.

Benzodiazepines are addictive. As a result, medical providers tend to use them with caution. It is possible to withdraw from benzodiazepines, but that should be done only with the guidance by a medical provider. Normally, withdrawal involves the slow tapering of dosage. If a benzodiazepine is suddenly completely discontinued after a few months of use, withdrawal symptoms may include a loss of self-worth, agitation, and insomnia. If the benzodiazepine has been used long than a few months, withdrawal symptoms may include seizures, tremors, upset stomach, nightmares, hallucinations, muscle cramping, shortness of breath, sweating, restlessness, irritability, feelings of unreality, vomiting, and sweating. In some instances, people withdrawing from a benzodiazepine may have life-threatening symptoms and may require emergency hospitalization.

And, benzodiazepines are misused by numbers of people every year. The previously cited 2015–2016 National Surveys on Drug Use and Health found that 2.1 per cent of US adults misused benzodiazepines at least once, and 0.2 percent had a benzodiazepine use disorder. Among benzodiazepine users, 17.1 percent misused them and 1.5 percent had benzodiazepine use disorders.[3] Those who misuse benzodiazepines may or may not know that they interact dangerously with alcohol and medications such as opioids, barbiturates, and tranquilizers. When such interactions occur, the side effects are intensified. Benzodiazepine addicts have a higher risk of developing dementia with gradual memory loss and problems associated with language and motor skills.

Since benzodiazepines slow nerve signals, they slow reflexes and induce sedation, making it difficult or even impossible to drive and safely complete certain tasks. When beginning a course of benzodiazepines, it is best not to plan to drive or to take on any potentially dangerous tasks. If benzodiazepines suppress nervous signals too sharply, there may be dangerous results, even death. Medical providers may offer more guidance on the safety concerns of specific benzodiazepines.

Benzodiazepines have a risk of overdose. Symptoms of an overdose include extreme sedation and drowsiness, low rate of breathing, confusion and difficulty thinking, slurred speech, loss of muscle control, and coma. Fortunately, there is a medication called flumazenil that is an antidote; it quickly reverses the effects. However, it must be injected rapidly into a vein.

Benzodiazepines should not be taken at the same time as an antacid or proton pump inhibitor. Antacids and proton pump inhibitors, which are used to treat acid reflux, reduce the rate of benzodiazepine absorption. Further, benzodiazepines should never be used with cannabis. And, unless there are no other options available, women who are pregnant or planning to become pregnant should not take benzodiazepines, as their use is associated with premature delivery and low birth weight. Benzodiazepines may increase the risk of falling in people who have balance issues. Because of these falling concerns as well as the previously noted memory problems, some health professionals will not prescribe benzodiazepines to older people.

Research Findings

In the Short Term, Benzodiazepines Appear to Be Effective for Treating Anxiety in the Elderly, but More Research Is Needed

In a systematic review published in the *Annals of Clinical Psychiatry*, researchers from Akron, Ohio, examined the efficacy and tolerability of using benzodiazepines to treat anxiety disorders in older adults, defined as fifty-five years or older. Only five randomized controlled trials met their inclusion criteria. Four were placebo controlled, and two had an active comparator. The subjects had anxiety disorder as their primary diagnosis, including generalized anxiety disorder and panic disorder. In most of the trials, minorities were underrepresented. The trials used the Hamilton Anxiety Rating Scale as a measurement tool. While the subjects in all five trials experienced significant reductions in anxiety, the quality of data in two of the studies were considered "good" and only "fair" in another trial. Two studies had missing data/data analysis, which prevented a data appraisal. Acknowledging that there are too few available trials to draw definitive conclusions, the researchers commented that the evidence indicated that "benzodiazepines showed good efficacy and tolerability in low doses for short-term use among older adults with anxiety disorders." No study noted any "negative results." The researchers underscored the need for more studies evaluating the use of benzodiazepines "among this vulnerable population."[4]

Despite the Potential Problems, Many Elderly Seem to Become Long-Term Benzodiazepine Users

In a study published in *JAMA Internal Medicine*, researchers from Ann Arbor, Michigan, and Philadelphia, Pennsylvania, wanted to determine what percentage of elders who receive new prescriptions for benzodiazepine proceed to become long-term users of the medication. The cohort consisted of 576 subjects, with a mean age of 78.4 years, who obtained their benzodiazepine prescription from a nonpsychiatric clinician within Pennsylvania's prescription assistance program for low-income older adults. One year later, 152 subjects (26.4 percent) were considered to be long-term users; the subjects in this group had been taking their medication for a mean of 232.7 days. The researchers noted that it is evident that larger numbers of nonpsychiatric clinicians are prescribing psychotropic medications to older adults. That is why, "it is critical to improve access to and education regarding nonpharmacologic treatment so clinicians feel they have treatment alternatives to offer."[5]

Children on Benzodiazepines Have an Increased Risk of Fractures

In a study published in the journal *Pediatrics*, researchers from New York City and New Brunswick and Piscataway, New Jersey, wanted to learn if benzodiazepines and selective serotonin reuptake inhibitors (SSRIs) increased the risk of fractures among children and young adults with anxiety disorders. Using claims from commercially insured children (six to seventeen years) and young adults (eighteen to twenty-four years), the researchers assembled large cohorts of 120,715 children and 179,768 young adults who recently began treatment with benzodiazepines (usually alprazolam or lorazepam) or SSRIs for their anxiety disorder. (Most often, the type of anxiety disorder was not specified. However, when specified, the most common types were generalized anxiety disorder, panic disorder, and adjustment disorder with anxiety.) Because certain fractures are more likely to be caused by falls, the researchers were primarily interested in fractures of the upper and lower limbs, specifically shoulders, upper arms, forearms, wrists, femurs, lower legs, and ankles. The researchers learned that during anxiety disorder treatment, the children taking a benzodiazepine (12,840) had a fracture rate of 33.1 per 1,000 and those on a SSRI (107,875) had a rate of 25.1 per 1,000. Fracture rates were lower among the young adults, and there was minimal difference between the two treatments. Interestingly, 82 percent of the children and 77 percent of the young adults on a benzodiazepine did not refill their prescription. Three months after initiating benzodiazepine treatment, only 8 percent of the children and 11 percent of young adults remained on treatment. During the same time period, more than half of those on a SSRI continued treatment. The researchers concluded that "increased caution in the weeks after benzodiazepine initiation with children with anxiety disorders may be warranted."[6]

Benzodiazepines Appear to Be More Effective Than SSRIs and SNRIs for Generalized Anxiety Disorder

In a comprehensive literature search and meta-analysis published in the journal *Expert Opinion on Pharmacotherapy*, researchers from Boston, Massachusetts, compared the efficacy of benzodiazepines, selective reuptake inhibitors (SSRIs), and selective norepinephrine reuptake inhibitors (SNRIs) for the treatment of generalized anxiety disorder. The researchers located fifty-four articles with data from fifty-six unique randomized, placebo-controlled pharmacotherapy trials that met their criteria. The fifty-six trials had 12,655 subjects with generalized anxiety disorder; 6,464 received active medication and 6,191 received placebos. There were twenty-three benzodiazepine trials with 1,149 subjects, sixteen SSRI trials with 2,712 subjects, and seventeen SNRI trials with 2,603 subjects. While the earlier studies tended to examine benzodiazepines, more recent studies usually addressed SSRIs and SNRIs. Of the fifty-four articles, twelve were thought to have a high risk of bias, nine were given a low risk, and the risk of bias in the remaining thirty-three was unclear. The researchers learned that benzodiazepines, SSRIs, SNRIs were all more effective than placebos in relieving generalized anxiety disorder. Further, in contrast to the current prescribing guidelines, which advises prescribing SSRIs or SNRIs before benzodiazepines, benzodiazepines were more effective for generalized anxiety disorder than the two other types of medications. The researchers commented that as a result of their findings, they recommended that benzodiazepines "should be considered as a viable treatment option for adults with GAD [generalized anxiety disorder], especially for the initial treatment phase." However, since the other two types of medications offered effective anxiety relief, during the first four to eight weeks of treatment, optimal results may possibly be obtained with the combined use of a SSRI or a SNRI with a benzodiazepine. After that period of time, the benzodiazepine dosage may be reduced or tapered.[7]

Despite Being Advised Not to Use Benzodiazepines, Many Women Are Using Them Before, During, and After Pregnancy

In a systematic review and meta-analysis published in the *Journal of Affective Disorders*, researchers from the Netherlands and New York City studied the use of benzodiazepine medication twelve months before pregnancy, during pregnancy, and twelve months after pregnancy. The researchers located thirty-two studies reporting on twenty-eight countries, representing a total of 7,343,571 pregnancies. Sample size per cohort ranged from 50 to 1,886,825. Six studies addressed the year before pregnancy, thirty-two focused on the pregnancy, and four reviewed the year after pregnancy. Most of the studies had a low risk of bias on at least five out of seven quality criteria or 87.5 percent, and there was substantial heterogeneity among the different studies. Prevalence rates were reported over a thirty-seven-year period of time—from 1980 to 2017. The researchers determined that benzodiazepine use increased from preconception to pregnancy, with a subsequent postpartum decrease, which was statistically significant. They found that the worldwide use of benzodiazepine before pregnancy was 0.9 percent and during pregnancy was 1.9 percent, with the highest prevalence of 3.1 percent in the third trimester. The overall prevalence during the year after pregnancy was 0.5 percent. The highest prevalence rates were Eastern Europe (14 percent), followed by Southern Europe (3.8 percent) and Central and South America (2.3 percent). Lowest prevalence rates were found in Asia (0.9 percent) and Northwestern Europe (1.2 percent). North, Central, and South America were in the middle. Lorazepam was the most frequently used benzodiazepine. The researchers concluded that there appeared to be a relatively high rate of benzodiazepine use during pregnancy, especially during the third trimester. "Considering most used or prescribed drugs are considered as high-risk by the Food and Drug Administration with potentially severe adverse outcomes for the (unborn) child, this is a worrying finding." The researchers commented that more research is needed on benzodiazepines and pregnancy, and women and medical providers need to be more aware of this problem.[8]

And, Using Alprazolam During Pregnancy May Cause Serious Problems

In a prospective study published in the journal *Frontiers in Pharmacology*, researchers from Korea evaluated the safety of the use of alprazolam during pregnancy. Their cohort consisted of 725 pregnancies from January 2000 to

December 2019; in this cohort, 96 women were exposed to alprazolam and 629 were not. All of the women were followed up until their delivery. The women in the exposed group were somewhat older than the unexposed group; 29.2 percent of the exposed group were thirty-five years or older, while 19.6 percent of the unexposed group were from that demographic. Unexposed women drank more alcohol; 27.1 percent of the exposed women drank alcohol, as did 39.7 percent of the unexposed women. The daily doses of alprazolam in the exposure group ranged from 0.13 to 0.50 mg, which is lower than the usual doses. On average, the women in the exposure group gave birth at 38.8 weeks and at 39.3 weeks in the non-exposure group. The women in the exposure group had significantly more spontaneous abortions, and their babies had significantly lower birth weights and Apgar scores. Though not statistically significant, when compared to the women in the non-exposure group, the risk of preterm birth in women in the exposure group increased 2.27 fold. The researchers concluded "that alprazolam exposure during pregnancy was significantly associated with adverse pregnancy and neonatal outcomes."[9]

Alprazolam May Be More Effective Than Lorazepam for Anxiety Disorders

In a sixteen-week, double-blind, placebo-controlled trial published in the journal *Pharmacotherapy*, researchers from Los Angeles and Kalamazoo, Michigan, compared the efficacy and safety of alprazolam and lorazepam for 200 adults, mean age of forty-one years, with moderate to moderately severe anxiety. Ninety-two percent were white, and 59 percent were female. Fifty percent were married, and 27 percent were separated or divorced. Eighty subjects were assigned to alprazolam and eighty to lorazepam, with forty taking a placebo. Dosing was flexible and ranged from 1 to 4.5 mg/day for alprazolam and from 2 to 9 mg/day for lorazepam. At the end of the trial, the mean daily dose for alprazolam was 3.3 mg and it was 5.1 mg for lorazepam. Side effects reported by the subjects included insomnia, constipation, nasal congestion, blurred vision, headaches, and unsteadiness. According to the Hamilton Anxiety Rating Scale, both medications were more effective than the placebo in relieving the symptoms of anxiety. On some measures, alprazolam gave significantly more improvement than lorazepam. One-fourth or more of each group did not complete the trial; most of the dropouts occurred after week eight. "The ease with which patients dropped out of the study suggests that they had not become psychologically dependent on the medication."[10]

Alprazolam and Diazepam Seem to Be Equally Effective for Generalized Anxiety Disorder

In a four-week, double-blind trial published in the *Journal of Clinical Pharmacology*, researchers from Montreal, Canada, compared the use of alprazolam and diazepam to treat mild to moderate generalized anxiety. The cohort consisted of eleven men and thirty-seven women, ranging in age from twenty to sixty-seven years, mean 39.5 years, with generalized anxiety disorder and a lack of improvement after a five-day placebo administration. Before entering the trial, twenty-four patients had been treated with oxazepam and thirteen with lorazepam. Eleven had never taken a psychotropic medication. Although the doses could be adjusted, twenty-four patients initially took 0.5 mg alprazolam and twenty-four took 5 mg diazepam. The mean optimal daily dose of alprazolam was 2 mg and that of diazepam was 15.8 mg. The researchers conducted several assessments including the Hamilton Anxiety Rating Scale and the Physician's Global Impression Scale, and the patients completed questionnaires. The final analyses included forty-six patients. Although diazepam appeared to offer faster relief, the patients in both groups improved. It should, however, be added that at baseline, the patients in the diazepam group considered themselves less anxious than those in the alprazolam group. As a result, they may have naturally obtained more immediate relief. The main side effects were drowsiness, tremor, light-headedness, and dry mouth. There was one toxic reaction to alprazolam, which may have been an allergic response. The researchers concluded that both alprazolam and diazepam "appeared to be effective in the treatment of generalized anxiety disorder, and the statistically significant differences between the two drugs were not clinically striking."[11]

Clonazepam Is More Effective for Panic Disorder Than Paroxetine

In a thirty-four-month, prospective, randomized, parallel-group, open-label trial published in the *Journal of Clinical Psychopharmacology*, which was an extension of an earlier eight-week study, researchers based in Brazil compared the efficacy and safety of clonazepam and paroxetine (Paxil), a SSRI, for panic disorder. The total treatment time for both studies was thirty-six months. All of the initial subjects had two or more panic attacks during the month preceding inclusion in the study. The subjects were seen monthly at the clinic, and there were periodic assessments. Subjects with a good outcome during the first eight-week trial continued taking their monotherapy. But, subjects with a partial primary treatment were switched to a combination therapy. So, forty-seven subjects on clonazepam and thirty-seven on paroxetine continued taking their monotherapy. Ten subjects who were on clonazepam and eleven who were on paroxetine were switched to combination therapy. Patients already taking clonazepam were administered 10 mg/day of paroxetine, and patients already taking paroxetine were administered 1 mg/day clonazepam. There were no significant demographic differences between the treatment groups. Most of the subjects were college-educated females who were employed. Over 90 percent had panic disorder and agoraphobia. At the beginning of the long-term study, the mean doses of clonazepam and paroxetine were 1.9 mg/day and 38.4 mg/day, respectively. During the study, the mean dose of clonazepam remained the same, and the mean dose of paroxetine slightly decreased to 38.2 mg/day. Eleven patients failed to complete the study. During the first eight-week trial, the subjects treated with clonazepam had decreases in panic attacks from 5.1 to 0.26 per month, and those on paroxetine had reductions from 5.4 to 0.24 per month. During the long-term treatment, an average of 87 percent of clonazepam-treated patients, 85 percent of paroxetine-treated patients, and 61 percent of combination-treated patients were free of panic attacks. Many of the subjects experienced adverse effects such as drowsiness and fatigue from clonazepam and increased appetite and weight gain from paroxetine. Fortunately, these side effects tended to decline as the months passed. While both treatments similarly reduced the number of panic attacks, the subjects taking clonazepam had significantly fewer adverse events than those treated with paroxetine. All of the adverse events from clonazepam-treated subjects and almost all of those from paroxetine-treated subjects were mild. None of the adverse events was severe. The patients taking the combination therapy improved during the first four months of therapy, but did not reach the levels of improvement of the monotherapy groups. The researchers concluded that "the efficacy of clonazepam and paroxetine for the treatment of panic disorder was maintained over the long-term course." However, "there was a significant advantage with clonazepam over paroxetine with respect to the frequecy and nature of adverse events."[12]

When Combined with Group Therapy, Clonazepam Is a More Effective Treatment for Generalized Social Anxiety Disorder

In a twelve-week, randomized trial published in *European Psychiatry*, researchers from Brazil and New York City wanted to determine if treating generalized anxiety disorder with clonazepam and psychodynamic group therapy or long-term group therapy was better than treating the disorder only with clonazepam. All of the subjects had been dealing with their anxiety disorder for at least two years. Clonazepam was started at a dose of 0.5 mg taken twice daily. Doses were increased up to 1.0 mg taken twice daily in weeks two to twelve. Dose reductions were allowed to increase tolerability. At the end of the trial, clonazepam was gradually discontinued. Half of the subjects participated in two individual evaluation interviews and twelve weekly ninety-minute group sessions. The mean number of patients per group session was nine. Several scales were used to assess anxiety symptoms and other factors such as quality of life. The final analyses included fifty-seven patients. The researchers determined that the patients in the combination group had significantly greater improvement in global functioning than those in the only clonazepam group. Though not statistically significant, they improved in other measures as well. The mean dose of clonazepam for the combination group was 1.29 mg/day and for the clonazepam monotherapy group was 1.48 mg/day. The researchers concluded "that the addition of PGT [psychodynamic group therapy] may be a promising augmentation strategy to clonazepam with some gains in global functioning of patients with GSAD [generalized social anxiety disorder]."[13]

While Diazepam Appears Useful for Generalized Anxiety Disorder, When Beginning a Course of Diazepam the Medication May Impair the Ability to Drive Safely

In a trial published in the *Journal of Clinical Psychopharmacology*, researchers from the Netherlands examined the driving performance of men and women with mild to moderate generalized anxiety disorder who were treated with either diazepam or buspirone, an anxiolytic medication addressed in another entry in this book. The cohort consisted of two groups of twelve outpatients each with equal numbers of men and women. After a wash-out period of one week during which all of the subjects took placebos, each patient was treated either with 5 mg diazepam three times per day for four weeks or with buspirone for the same period of time. On the evening of the seventh day of each treatment week, researchers administered the Hamilton Rating Scale for Anxiety and the ninety-item Symptom Check List. These were followed by an on-the-road driving test that began 1.5 hours after the last drug or placebo was taken. The test consisted of operating an instrumented vehicle over a 100-kilometer highway circuit while attempting to maintain a constant speed and a steady lateral position within the right traffic lane. Following the first week of treatment, diazepam significantly impaired speed control. After the first and second treatment week, two patients in the diazepam group were too sedated to complete their tests. And, for the first three weeks of treatment, diazepam significantly impaired control over the lateral position. Both medications proved to be equally effective for reducing anxiety symptoms. Further, the abrupt discontinuation of diazepam triggered a relapse of "psychic anxiety symptoms" and a partial relapse of "somatic anxiety symptoms." By the fourth week, there was no significant impairment. The researchers concluded that during the first few weeks of treatment with diazepam, driving performance may be notably impaired. In their admittedly small sample, about one-third of the subjects were severely impaired, and "the remainder showed moderate-severe to no negative effects of diazepam on their driving ability." Moreover, "anyone accompanying the driving tests of the four highly sensitive subjects in the diazepam group would judge them to drive extremely unsafely and dangerously."[14]

While High Doses of Diazepam Seem to Be Quite Useful for Anxiety, Lower Doses Do Not Appear to Be Similarly Effective

In a systematic review and meta-analysis published in the journal *Human Psychopharmacology*, researchers from Japan reviewed randomized controlled trials on the use of diazepam for anxiety that were published in Japan and in the Japanese language. They identified seventeen relevant trials in which a total of 2,012 Japanese patients with anxiety disorders were randomly allocated to diazepam, placebo, or an alternative test compound. There were sixteen parallel studies and one crossover study. The initial doses of diazepam ranged from 4.5 mg/day to 9 mg/day; the maximum doses reached ranged from 6 mg/day to 18 mg/day. When adverse events occurred, doses were reduced. Study duration ranged from one to eight weeks. The researchers learned that at higher doses, diazepam was significantly more effective than placebos in treating anxiety disorders. It was particularly effective at the maximum doses of 12 or 18 mg/day, with a treatment duration of two or more weeks. At a dose of 9 mg/day or less, there was no significant difference between diazepam and the placebo. Still, the researchers commented that "caution should be exercised in assessing these results."[15]

Administering Lorazepam to Children the Night Before Reconstructive Burn Surgery Reduces Anxiety

In a prospective, randomized, double-blind trial published in the *Journal of Burn Care & Rehabilitation*, researchers from Cincinnati, Ohio, noted that children often have a high level of anxiety before reconstructive burn surgery. Generally, these children have already had surgeries and are well aware of postoperative pain. Their preoperative anxiety has been found to be associated with postoperative regression, nightmares, separation anxiety, eating problems, and fear of physicians. And, calmer children have a better overall surgical experience. They even require less anesthesia. The cohort consisted of forty-five children who ranged in age from six to eighteen years, with a mean age of 12.5 years. At bedtime on the night before their surgery, while already hospitalized, the children were administered either 0.025 mg/kg of oral lorazepam ($n = 23$) or a placebo ($n = 22$). Before the surgeries, each child's level of anxiety was quantified. Additional assessments were conducted on the day after surgery. The researchers observed a statistically significant difference in preoperative self-rated anxiety between the two groups, with the lorazepam group rating themselves as having less anxiety. Unfortunately, the researchers were unable to detect this difference. Nevertheless, the researchers commented, "that we could not confirm this by our observation does not make the decrease in anxiety experienced by these patients any less real." Since no adverse reactions were observed, the researchers noted that they would recommend this protocol.[16]

Like Diazepam, Lorazepam May Impair the Ability to Drive Safely

In a study published in the *Journal of Analytical Toxicology*, researchers from Seattle, Washington, reviewed positive lorazepam drug-impaired driving cases submitted to the Washington State Toxicology Laboratory. During the six years that they reviewed, there were 170 drivers who tested positive for lorazepam. The mean concentration of lorazepam found in the blood of theses drivers was 0.048 mg/L. Because of multiple arrests, two drivers were counted twice. The researchers found 147 arrests of people in which lorazepam and other drug(s) were detected and 23 arrests of people in which only lorazepam was found. In the instances in which there were additional drugs, the most frequently detected drugs were muscle relaxants or painkillers. Lorazepam concentrations found in drivers with no other drugs present ranged from <0.01 to 0.38 mg/L, with a mean of 0.03 mg/L. These concentrations ranged from the sub-therapeutic levels to concentrations higher than those associated with a 10 mg daily dose. The subjects often had slowed speech that was thick, low, and slurred. Coordination tended to be poor, and the subjects appeared to be lethargic and have problems with a modified finger-to-nose test and the walk-and-turn and one-leg-stand tests. The researchers observed that lorazepam had the potential to significantly impair driving and psychomotor abilities, regardless of the concentrations detected. This is probably a function of the individual's tolerance of the sedating side effects. The researchers concluded that lorazepam "is most frequently taken with other CNS depressants that are likely to have a compounding effect on driving performance." That is why "physicians should take care to stress the risks to patients taking this medication alone, and especially in combination with other drugs."[17]

Acute Administration of Lorazepam in Long-Term Users of Lorazepam May Negatively Impact the Elderly

In a double-blind, placebo-controlled, crossover trial published in the journal *Progress in Neuro-Psychopharmacology & Biological Psychiatry*, researchers from several US locations and the UK evaluated the acute administration of lorazepam in elders who were long-term users of the medication. The initial cohort consisted of 37 psychiatric outpatients, ranging in age from 60 to 91 years, who had been taking lorazepam for anxiety and related conditions for between 3 and 252 months. On two different days, approximately one week apart, the subjects were administered their highest daily dose of lorazepam (0.25 to 3.00 mg) or a placebo. So, the subjects either received a placebo first followed by lorazepam or lorazepam first followed by a placebo. After each administration, there was a five-hour assessment of memory, psychomotor speed, and subjective mood status. Blood samples were collected at baseline and during the testing. Thirty-one subjects completed the trial. Five of the six non-completing subjects were too physically or mentally fatigued to finish the entire assessment. As might be expected, plasma levels of lorazepam increased in the subjects who were administered lorazepam and did not increase in those taking the placebo. The researchers learned that the subjects taking lorazepam had a significant decline in total recall and psychomotor performance when tested one hour and 2.5 hours after administration. At the same time, while the lorazepam administration did not appear to have a mood-altering effect for the entire cohort, a subgroup analysis found that the eleven subjects who had a diagnosis of generalized anxiety disorder were calmer and more tranquil. The researchers concluded that "the reduced recall and psychomotor slowing that we observed, along with an absence of significant therapeutic benefits, following acute lorazepam administration in elderly long-term users reinforces the importance of cognitive toxicity as a clinical factor in benzodiazepine use, especially in this population."[18]

References and Further Readings

Bais, Babette, Nina M. Molenaar, Hilmar H. Bijma et al. "Prevalence of Benzodiazepines and Benzodiazepine-Related Drugs Exposure Before, During and After Pregnancy: A Systematic Review and Meta-Analysis." *Journal of Affective Disorders* 269 (May 15, 2020): 18–27.

Blanco, Carlos, Beth Han, Christopher M. Jones et al. "Prevalence and Correlates of Benzodiazepine Use, Misuse, and Use Disorders Among Adults in the United States." *Journal of Clinical Psychiatry* 79, no. 6 (October 16, 2018): 18m12174.

Bushnell, Great A., Tobias Gerhard, Stephen Crystal, and Mark Offson. "Benzodiazepine Treatment and Fracture Risk in Young Persons with Anxiety Disorders." *Pediatrics* 146, no. 1 (July 2020): 20193478.

Clarkson, Jayne E., Ann Marie Gordon, and Barry K. Logan. "Lorazepam and Driving Impairment." *Journal of Analytical Toxicology* 28 (September 2004): 475–80.

Cohn, J. B. and C. S. Wilcox. "Long-Term Comparison of Alprazolam, Lorazepam and Placebo in Patients with an Anxiety Disorder." *Pharmacotherapy* 4, no. 2 (March–April 1984): 93–8.

Elie, Robert and Yves Lamontagne. "Alprazolam and Diazepam in. the Treatment of Generalized Anxiety." *Journal of Clinical Psychopharmacology* 4, no. 3 (June 1984): 125–9.

Gerlach, Lauren B., Donovan T. Maust, Shirley H. Leong et al. "Factors Associated with Long-Term Benzodiazepine Use Among Older Adults." *JAMA Internal Medicine* 178, no. 11 (2018): 1560–2.

Gomez, Angelina F., Abigail L. Barthel, and Stefan G. Hofmann. "Comparing the Efficacy of Benzodiazepines and Serotonergic Anti-Depressants for Adults with Generalized Anxiety Disorder: A Meta-Analytic Review." *Expert Opinion on Pharmacotherapy* 19, no. 8 (June 2018): 883–94.

Gupta, Aarti, Gargi Bhattacharya, Syeda Arshiya Farheen et al. "Systematic Review of Benzodiazepines for Anxiety Disorders in Late Life." *Annals of Clinical Psychiatry* 32, no. 2 (May 2020): 114–26.

Inada, Toshiya, Shoko Nozaki, Ataru Inagaki, and Toshiaki A. Furukawa. "Efficacy of Diazepam as an Anti-Anxiety Agent: Meta-Analysis of Double-Blind, Randomized Controlled Trials Carried Out in Japan." *Human Psychopharmacology* 18, no. 6 (August 2003): 483–7.

Knijnik, Daniela Z., Carlos Blanco, Giovanni Abrahãon Salum et al. "A Pilot Study of Clonazepam Versus Psychodynamic Group Therapy Plus Clonazepam in the Treatment of Generalized Social Anxiety Disorder." *European Psychiatry* 23, no. 8 (December 2008): 567–74.

Lee, Hyunji, Jae-Whoan Koh, Young-Ah Kim et al. "Pregnancy and Neonatal Outcomes After Exposure to Alprazolam in Pregnancy." *Frontiers in Pharmacology* 13 (April 2022): Article 854562.

McCall, J. E., C. G. Fischer, G. Warden et al. "Lorazepam Given the Night Before Surgery Reduces Preoperative Anxiety in Children Undergoing Reconstructive Burn Surgery." *Journal of Burn Care & Rehabilitation* 20, no. 2 (March–April 1999): 151–4.

Nardi, Antonio E., Rafael C. Freire, Marina D. Mochcovitch et al. "A Randomized, Naturalistic, Parallel-Group Study for the Long-Term Treatment of Panic Disorder with Clonazepam or Paroxetine." *Journal of Clinical Psychopharmacology* 32, no. 1 (February 2012): 120–6.

Pomara, Nunzio, Sang Han Lee, Davide Bruno et al. "Adverse Performance Effects of Acute Lorazepam Administration in Elderly Long-Term Users: Pharmacokinetic and Clinical Predictors." *Progress in Neuro-Psychopharmacology & Biological Psychiatry* 56 (2015): 129–35.

Van Laar, M. W., E. R. Volkerts, and A. P. P. van Willigenburg. "Therapeutic Effects and Effects on Actual Driving Performance of Chronically Administered Buspirone and Diazepam in Anxious Outpatients." *Journal of Clinical Psychopharmacology* 12, no. 2 (April 1992): 86–95.

Wick, Jeannette Y. "The History of Benzodiazepines." *The Consultant Pharmacist* 28, no. 9 (September 2013): 538–48.

Beta-Blockers

Introduction

Developed in the mid-twentieth century, beta-blockers are a group of medications that are used to treat high blood pressure, abnormal heart rhythm, heart failure, chest pain, and other heart issues. Currently, in the United States, they are used by about thirty million adults. Though not approved for anxiety by the US Food and Drug Administration, they are also sometimes used "off-label" for that disorder.

Beta-blockers are believed to calm several problems associated with anxiety, including a fast heart rate, high blood pressure, a shaky voice and hands, sweating, and dizziness. By altering the body's response to anxiety, beta-blockers may soften the intensity of the symptoms and lessen the physical effects. In addition, there is evidence that some beta-blockers may alter how the body remembers and responds to fearful memories. If that is true, beta-blockers may be useful for post-traumatic stress disorder and phobias.

Also referred to as beta-adrenoceptor antagonists or beta-adrenergic blocking agents, beta-blockers inhibit the effects of epinephrine or adrenaline on beta receptors. (A beta receptor is the site on a cell, as in the heart, which upon interaction with epinephrine or nonepinephrine, controls heartbeat and heart contractability, vasodilation, smooth muscle inhibition, and other physiological processes.) This prevents adrenaline from making the heart pump harder or faster. Epinephrine is a hormone and neurotransmitter that plays a crucial role in the body's fight or flight response, which may lead to anxiety. Lowering the effects of epinephrine on the body may reduce the intensity of anxiety. There are two main types of beta-blockers. Nonselective beta-blockers stop epinephrine from binding to beta receptors throughout the body; selective beta-blockers prevent epinephrine from binding to beta receptors in the heart. In the United States, the most common beta-blockers are acebutolol (Sectral), bisoprolol (Zebeta), carvedilol (Coreg), propranolol (Inderal), atenolol (Tenormin), and metoprolol (Lopressor). Propranolol and atenolol are the two beta-blockers that are more likely to be prescribed for anxiety. And, because they only deal with the physical effects of anxiety and do not address any underlying chemical imbalance or psychological underpinnings, they are best used for people who experience anxiety in specific situations, such as performance anxiety.

Beta-blockers work differently than most anti-anxiety medications. Since they are fast acting, they are good for people who need quick relief, and they work well for acute short-term anxiety. Beta-blockers may be particularly helpful for people who have intolerable side effects from other anti-anxiety medications and for those who have the symptoms of anxiety and high blood pressure.

Regulation, Administration, and Costs

Like all prescriptive medication, beta-blockers are regulated by the FDA. For anxiety, the typical dose of propranolol is a 40 mg tablet taken up to three times per day and for atenolol it is 50 to 100 mg per day as a single dose. But, a medical provider may suggest beginning with a lower dose. These drugs, which are probably covered by insurance, are inexpensive, as low as a few dollars per month.

Side Effects and Risks

Side effects of beta-blockers include rashes and other skin reactions, bradycardia or slowed heart rate, increased risk of anesthesia complications, fatigue, cold hands and feet, headache, dizziness or light-headedness, dry mouth or eyes, insomnia, nightmares, or other sleep changes, nausea, depression, shortness of breath, low blood pressure, gastrointestinal problems, and impotence. More serious side effects include very slow or irregular heartbeat, low blood sugar, asthma attack, swelling and fluid retention and weight gain.

People with certain medical conditions should not take beta-blockers. These include cardiogenic shock, bronchial asthma, low blood sugar, final-stage heart failure, very low blood pressure, very slow heart rate, some heart blockages, hypotension, and sinus bradycardia. Beta-blockers may modify the symptoms of hypoglycemia in people with diabetes, making it more difficult to determine the correct dosage of insulin. Beta-blockers may interact with other medications used to treat heart conditions and antidepressants.

Beta-blockers are generally considered safe for pregnant women and children. But, some are believed to be better choices than others. Healthcare providers should be aware of the most recent research and recommendations. As for nursing moms, it is known that beta-blockers are found in breast milk; atenolol, acebutolol, and nadolol are present in high amounts. Since they have only small amounts in breast milk, propranolol, labetalol, and metoprolol are better options.

Research Findings

Atenolol Seems Useful for the Symptoms of Anxiety

In a retrospective, observational investigation published in the journal *Military Medicine,* researchers from Japan and Irvine, California, examined the effectiveness of atenolol for anxiety disorders. After identifying ninety-two male and female patients from outpatient Navy and Marine mental health clinics in Okinawa, Japan, who had received an atenolol prescription for anxiety and/or post-traumatic stress disorder symptoms between November 2017 and September 2019, the researchers collected information on the general beneficial and adverse effects of atenolol and the preference of atenolol to propranolol. Prescribed doses ranged from 25 to 200 mg per day. The researchers learned that seventy-nine subjects (86 percent) reported having a positive response to atenolol, which they were continuing to use. Eighty-three patients either denied having adverse effects or noted that they were tolerable. Both males and females benefited equally. Among subjects with a PTSD diagnosis, 87 percent noted benefits, and among those with a diagnosis of another specified trauma or other stressor, twelve out of twelve improved. When the PTSD, trauma, or other stressor patients were combined, 90 percent benefited. Overall, 85 percent of the patients with an anxiety disorder reported benefit. And, the twelve subjects who had previously taken propranolol for anxiety found that they preferred atenolol; atenolol had fewer adverse effects, was easier to take, and was more effective for symptom relief. The researchers commented that the majority of the subjects "reported a beneficial effect of atenolol to help alleviate their anxiety-related symptoms."[1]

In a prospective, randomized, double-blind study published in the *European Journal of Clinical Pharmacology,* researchers from the UK compared the use of atenolol and a placebo for the treatment of anxiety. The initial cohort consisted of seventy-one men and women in the atenolol group and sixty-seven men and women in the placebo group. The subjects were all patients, between the ages of eighteen and fifty years, who had presented with primary anxiety of two weeks to six months' duration. They received either 50 mg of atenolol per day or a matching placebo. Patients were evaluated after two and four weeks of treatment when the treatment ended. There were twenty-four withdrawals in the atenolol group and twenty in the placebo group. Four patients were excluded for violating the protocol. Thus, forty-five patients from each group completed the trial. While both atenolol and the placebo improved the symptoms of anxiety, the researchers determined that when compared with the control group, the improvement in the treatment group was significantly greater for atenolol at two and four weeks. After twenty-eight days, both affective and somatic features of anxiety improved with atenolol, with significant improvement for affective symptoms.[2]

Propranolol May Lower Anxiety Levels Among Ophthalmology Residents Performing Surgery

In a ten-week, randomized, double-blind, crossover trial published in the journal *Transactions of the American Ophthalmology Society,* researchers from Illinois wanted to learn if propranolol would decrease tremor and anxiety levels in five third-year ophthalmology residents performing surgery. One hour before performing ophthalmic microsurgery, the residents, who were all healthy men under the age of thirty years, took a capsule containing either 40 mg propranolol or a placebo. Before the actual trial, all of the residents had been administered a test dose of propranolol without incident. At the end of each surgery, the resident and attending surgeon completed a questionnaire. The resident surgeon in each case answered a question on anxiety. In the seventy-three surgeries included in this trial, forty doses of propranolol and thirty-three doses of placebo were administered. The resident surgeons found that propranolol had a highly significant effect in decreasing anxiety and tremor, and there were no reported side effects. Still, the researchers noted that "caution must be exercised in extrapolating these results in a small group of young, healthy men to others."[3]

Propranolol May Help Overcome Stage Fright

An article published in *The American Journal of Medicine* described two trials that evaluated the use of beta-blockers to prevent stage fright in a total of twenty-nine subjects. These trials were carried out in the Music Department of the University of Nebraska and in the Julliard Theatre at the Julliard School. The University of Nebraska study was double-blind and crossover in design and primarily included thirteen musical performance students from local colleges and universities. Propranolol and a placebo were given 1.5 hours before recitals on two consecutive days. The second study had a similar double-blind, crossover format, and the sixteen subjects, who were members of the New York Philharmonic Orchestra, took propranolol or a placebo 1.5 hours before a recital. Stage fright symptoms were assessed by a questionnaire and the State-Trait Anxiety Inventory, and the quality of the music performance was evaluated by experienced music critics. In the Nebraska study, the performers favored propranolol. However, there were too many errors for a meaningful evaluation by the music faculty. In the New York study, there was an overwhelming preference for propranolol. The propranolol was able to eliminate the physical impediments to performance; "this effect was achieved not by giving the performer any increased ability or by tranquilization, but by removing physical impediments."[4]

Propranolol May Well Be Useful for Post-Traumatic Stress Disorder

In a trial published in the journal *Biological Psychiatry*, researchers from France, Canada, and California investigated the use of propranolol to reduce the symptoms of PTSD. The cohort consisted of nineteen trauma victims recruited in a French emergency room shortly after motor vehicle accidents or physical assaults. All of the subjects, who were between the ages of twenty-one and thirty years, had tachycardia of at least ninety beats per minute after twenty minutes of rest in a lying position. Between two and twenty hours after the trauma, eleven subjects agreed to take 40 mg of propranolol three times per day for seven days, followed by a taper period of eight to twelve days; eight subjects refused to take the medication but agreed to participate in the study. The two groups did not differ on demographics, exposure characteristics, severity of physical injury, or peritraumatic emotional responses. Two months after the trauma, one of the eleven subjects in the propranolol group and three of the eight subjects in the nontreatment group had symptoms of PTSD. The nontreatment subjects also had more pronounced symptoms. The researchers noted that "administering propranolol to young healthy individuals with tachycardia is effective in mitigating PTSD symptoms and perhaps in preventing PTSD."[5]

In a prospective, observational, single large academic center study published in the *Journal of Cardiothoracic and Vascular Anesthesia*, researchers from Italy examined the ability of propranolol to prevent the future development of PTSD in patients having cardiac surgery. The cohort consisted of 121 consecutive patients scheduled for elective cardiac surgery with cardiopulmonary bypass. Some of the patients were treated preoperatively, postoperatively, and at discharge with the beta-blockers carvedilol, atenolol, or metoprolol at standard dosages. Six months after the surgery, patients were contacted by phone and then mailed a modified version of the Posttraumatic Stress Symptom Inventory-10. Of the seventy-one patients who completed and mailed the questionnaire, fourteen (19.7 percent) had a diagnosis of PTSD. Seven of the thirteen female patients who were not treated with beta-blockers received a diagnosis of PTSD compared with zero out of the twelve patients who were treated with beta-blockers. When compared to female patients who were treated with beta-blockers, female patients who were not treated with beta-blockers during the perioperative periods reported dramatic increases in PTSD symptoms. The researchers concluded "that the use of beta-blockers might protect against the development of PTSD in women after cardiac surgery."[6]

But Another Study Had Different Results for Propranolol and PTSD

In a trial published in the *Journal of Child and Adolescent Psychopharmacology*, researchers from Galveston, Texas, examined whether acute treatment with propranolol prevented PTSD, anxiety, and depression in children hospitalized in the pediatric intensive care unit with large burns. The cohort consisted of 202 children, who were all survivors of pediatric burns; 89 had been treated with acute propranolol and 113 had not been treated with propranolol. The mean age at the time of the burn was 7.3 years, and the mean age at recruitment was 12.8 years. There were 135 males and 67 females, and the groups were overwhelmingly Hispanic, with a few Caucasians and African Americans. The groups were comparable in the age at the time of the burn, age at the time of recruitment, number of postburn years, burn size, and days treated after burn injury. On average, it had been 5.9 years since the children had burns that covered an average of 56.4 percent of the surface of their bodies. The mean dose of propranolol was 3.64 mg/kg per day, and the mean duration of propranolol inpatient treatment days was 26.5. The researchers learned that 3.5 percent of the children who received propranolol and 7.2 percent of those who did not receive propranolol had at least some degree of PTSD. While that was a clear difference, it was not statistically significant. The researchers concluded that there is a need for additional research on "the long-term benefits of propranolol in the prevention of trauma symptoms."[7]

Propranolol May Not Be Useful for Dental Anxiety

In a randomized, parallel, placebo-controlled, two-group trial published in the journal *Frontiers of Psychiatry*, researchers from the Netherlands, the UK, and Ireland tested the ability of perioperative propranolol to ease anxiety during dental extractions in patients with dental anxiety or dental phobia. The cohort consisted of fifty-two patients with high levels of fear who were about to have a minimum of two teeth removed at least one month apart. On their first visit, one hour before the procedure, the subjects received either two 40 mg capsules of oral propranolol ($n = 19$) or an identical in appearance placebo ($n = 17$). Next, they were asked to remember their memory of a distressing event that initiated or exacerbated their dental anxiety. After their surgery, the subjects received another 40 mg capsule of propranolol. No propranolol was administered before the second extraction, but the subjects were again asked to recall what triggered the distressing dental anxiety feelings. The researchers found no statistically significant differences in dental anxiety and intraoperative state anxiety reduction between the propranolol and placebo groups. The researchers concluded "that fear memory reactivation and administration of perioperative propranolol may not reduce dental anxiety in patients with high levels of fear of dental extractions."[8]

Acebutolol and Atenolol Do Not Appear to Reduce Anxiety in Volunteers with Induced Anxiety

In a double-blind, crossover trial published in the journal *Psychopharmacology*, researchers from the UK studied the ability of the beta-blockers acebutolol and atenolol to reduce anxiety in healthy volunteers with induced anxiety. Twelve healthy male volunteers, between the ages of nineteen and thirty-one years, self-administered acebutolol (400 mg per day), atenolol (100 mg per day), or a placebo. Each treatment was administered for four days and on each of the last three days the subjects had an anxiety-induction procedure involving both easy and difficult versions of the Stroop test and syntactic reasoning. Measures of anxiety were taken during a difficult task and after a period of quiet relaxation.

The researchers learned that the procedures used to induce anxiety did indeed "robustly" create differential levels of anxiety. Neither acebutolol or atenolol reduced anxiety nor did they cause any cognitive impairment. The researchers concluded that "acebutolol and atenolol, at steady-state plasma levels, do not appear to act as anxiolytics."[9]

Propranolol May Not Be Very Useful for the Symptoms of Anxiety

In a systematic review and meta-analysis published in the *Journal of Psychopharmacology*, researchers from the Netherlands and the UK reviewed randomly controlled trials on the ability of oral propranolol to alleviate the symptoms of anxiety or an anxiety disorder. They located eight trials that met their criteria; these studies addressed panic disorder with or without agoraphobia ($n = 130$), specific phobias ($n = 37$), social phobia ($n = 16$), and PTSD ($n = 19$). Unfortunately, the researchers noted that their studies were not well designed. Still, the researchers found no statistical difference in the use of propranolol and benzodiazepines for anxiety and panic attack frequency. Four trials, which had a moderate risk of bias, failed to show evidence of the therapeutic benefit of propranolol in patients with dental phobia, animal-type specific phobia, and social phobia. No randomized controlled trials were available on the effects of propranolol on the treatment of any other anxiety disorder, and no evidence was found for the effects of propranolol on PTSD symptom severity. The researchers concluded that "the quality of evidence for the efficacy of propranolol at present is insufficient to support the routine use of propranolol in the treatment of any of the anxiety disorders."[10]

Propranolol May Not Be Useful for Short-Term Anxiety Associated with Intellectual Stress

In a double-blind crossover trial published in the *British Journal of Clinical Pharmacology*, researchers from the UK tested the effects of 80 mg propranolol and 1 or 2.5 mg lorazepam (Ativan) on experimentally induced anxiety and performance in student volunteers. The cohort consisted of eleven female and six male students, with a mean age of twenty-two years, from a school of pharmacy in London. One student was eliminated because she suffered from occasional bouts with asthma. The students took either propranolol or lorazepam or matching placebos before being tested with a number of different demanding tests, specifically digit-performance substitution, symbol copying, and verbal learning. Although the performance tests raised levels of anxiety, neither medication altered the students' self-perceptions and ratings of levels of anxiety. "The results suggest that if administered acutely, neither drug is beneficial in the treatment of short-term anxiety associated with intellectual stress."[11]

References and Further Readings

Armstrong, Cody and Michelle R. Kapolowicz. "A Preliminary Investigation on the Effects of Atenolol for Treating Symptoms of Anxiety." *Military Medicine* 185 (November/December 2020): e1954–e1960.

Brantigan, C. O., T. A. Brantigan, and N. Joseph. "Effect of Beta Blockade and Beta Stimulation on Stage Fright." *The American Journal of Medicine* 72 (January 1982): 88–94.

Elman, Michael J., Joel Sugar, Richard Fiscella et al. "The Effect of Propranolol Versus Placebo on Resident Surgical Performance." *Transactions of the American Ophthalmology Society* 96 (1998): 283–91.

File, Sandra E. and R. G. Lister. "A Comparison of the Effects of Lorazepam and Those of Propranolol on Experimentally-Induced Anxiety and Performance." *British Journal of Clinical Pharmacology* 19 (1985): 445–51.

Kilminster, S. G., M. J. Lewis, and D. M. Jones. "Anxiolytic Effects of Acebutolol and Atenolol in Healthy Volunteers with Induced Anxiety." *Psychopharmacology* 95 (1998): 245–9.

Rosenberg, Laura, Marta Rosenberg, Sherri Sharp et al. "Does Acute Propranolol Treatment Prevent Posttraumatic Stress Disorder, Anxiety, and Depression in Children with Burns." *Journal of Child and Adolescent Psychopharmacology* 28, no. 2 (March 2018): 117–23.

Saul, P., B. P. Jones, K. G. Edwards, and J. A. Tweed. "Randomized Comparison of Atenolol and Placebo in the Treatment of Anxiety: A Double-Blind Study." *European Journal of Clinical Pharmacology* 28 (Supplement) (1985): 109–10.

Steenen, Serge Al. Arjen J. van Wijk, Geert JMG van der Heijden at al. "Propranolol for the Treatment of Anxiety Disorders: Systematic Review and Meta-Analysis." *Journal of Psychopharmacology* 30, no. 2 (February 2016): 128–39.

Steenan, Serge A., Naichuan Su, Roos van Westrhenen et al. "Perioperative Propranolol Against Dental Anxiety: A Randomized Controlled Trial." *Frontiers in Psychiatry* 13 (February 2022): Article 842353.

Tarsitani, Lorenzo, Vincenzo De Santis, Martino Mistrette et al. "Treatment with Beta-blockers and Incidence of Post-Traumatic Stress Disorder After Cardiac Surgery: A

Prospective Observational Study." *Journal of Cardiothoracic and Vascular Anesthesia* 26, no. 2 (April 2012): 265–9.

Valva, Guillaume, François Ducrocq, Karine Jezequel et al. "Immediate Treatment with Propranolol Decreases Posttraumatic Stress Disorder Two Months After Trauma." *Biological Psychiatry* 54, no. 9 (November 1, 2003): 947–9.

Buspirone

Introduction

In a class of medications known as anxiolytics, buspirone is a prescription drug used to treat anxiety disorders or the short-term treatment of the symptoms of anxiety. Pronounced as "byoo spye rone," buspirone affects the serotonin and dopamine neurotransmitters in the brain, increasing the action of serotonin receptors, which helps reduce anxiety. Buspirone has a unique structure and pharmacological profile. Unlike many drugs used to treat anxiety, it does not exhibit anticonvulsant, sedative, hypnotic, or muscle-relaxant properties.

First synthesized in 1968, buspirone was patented in 1975. Originally developed as an antipsychotic medication, it was found to be ineffective for psychosis. Today, buspirone is primarily used to treat anxiety disorders, specifically generalized anxiety disorder (GAD). It is most often used as a second-line agent after selective serotonin reuptake inhibitors (SSRIs) when a patient does not respond to or is unable to tolerate side effects of SSRIs. Patients taking buspirone do not become physically dependent and do not have problems with withdrawal.

Regulation, Administration, and Costs

Like all prescription medicine in the United States, buspirone requires the approval of the US Food and Drug Administration (FDA). Buspirone was approved in 1986 to treat anxiety disorders or for the short-term relief of the symptoms of anxiety.

Buspirone is sold as an oral tablet that ranges in doses from 5 to 30 mg. It is usually taken two or three times each day. The maximum daily dose is 60 mg. Because food may affect how buspirone is absorbed, the tablets must be taken either consistently with or without food. Most people begin with a lower dose that may be increased. People on buspirone should avoid eating grapefruit or drinking grapefruit juice; consuming these foods may increase the risk of side effects. Occasionally, buspirone is used without FDA approval, a practice known as off-label prescribing, for pediatric anxiety or for other forms of anxiety.

Buspirone usually costs no more than about $10 per month. It should be covered, at least in part, by insurers. At present, buspirone is not sold in any brand-name form.

Side Effects and Risks

Buspirone has been associated with a long list of side effects and risks. These include dizziness, nausea, diarrhea, headache, confusion, fatigue, nervousness, difficulty falling asleep and staying asleep, sleepiness, abnormal dreams, nervousness, ataxia (impaired balance), paresthesia ("pins and needles"), feelings of anger or hostility, light-headedness, blurred vision, chest pain, nasal congestion, sore throat, musculoskeletal pain, tinnitus, tremor, weakness, numbness, changes in weight or appetite, and increased sweating. Potentially more serious side effects and risks include rash, hives, itching, swelling of the face, eyes, mouth, throat, or lips, fast or irregular heartbeat, blurred vision, uncontrolled shaking of a part of the body, agitation, fever, severe muscle stiffness, or twitching, seizures, central nervous system depression, hallucinations, agitation, trouble breathing, serotonin syndrome, and loss of coordination. Symptoms of an overdose include nausea, vomiting, dizziness, drowsiness, blurred vision, and upset stomach. Avoid the use of monoamine oxidase inhibitors (MAOIs) within fourteen days before or after buspirone therapy. It may increase the risk of serotonin syndrome and/or elevated blood pressure. Sexual side effects are rarely seen with buspirone. In fact, there is some evidence that when buspirone is taken in combination with a selective serotonin reuptake inhibitor medication, it may help reduce the sexual side effects associated with that medication.

It is not known whether it is safe to take buspirone while pregnant or breastfeeding. However, animal studies have found that buspirone passes into breast milk and may or may not affect an infant or young child who is breastfeeding.

People with liver or kidney problems should discuss these issues with their medical providers before taking buspirone. The drug is broken down in the liver and expelled through the kidneys. People with liver or kidney problems may build up higher levels of buspirone in their bodies. Treating anxiety problems with another medication may be a better choice.

Research Findings

Buspirone Is Useful for Generalized Anxiety Disorder

In a placebo-controlled, double-blind, parallel group multicenter trial published in the journal *Psychopharmacology*, researchers from the UK and France compared the use of buspirone and hydroxyzine, an antihistamine used to treat anxiety and allergic conditions, for people with GAD. The initial cohort consisted of 244 men and women who were treated at sixty-two centers—forty-eight in France and fourteen in the UK—by primary care physicians interested in psychiatric disorders. Seventy percent of the patients were female, and the average age was forty-one years. For four weeks, they were randomly placed on buspirone (5 mg morning and mid-day and 10 mg evening), hydroxyzine (12.5 mg morning and mid-day, and 25 mg evening), or three capsules per day of a placebo. There were eighty-two, eighty-one, and eighty-one subjects in each of the groups, respectively. Levels of anxiety were assessed on days –7, 0, 7, 14, 21, 28, and 35. Before the trial, there were no significant differences between the groups. In the three groups, thirty-one of the buspirone subjects, thirty-two of the hydroxyzine subjects, and twenty-three of the placebo subjects reported one or more side effects, such as somnolence, headache, and migraine. The researchers found that the subjects in both intervention groups improved, and both buspirone and hydroxyzine were superior to placebo. A sub-analysis suggested that buspirone was better for patients with both anxiety and depressive symptoms.[1]

In a randomized, single-blind trial published in the journal *Psychiatry and Clinical Neuroscience*, researchers from Iran and Australia tested the efficacy and safety of buspirone and sertraline (Zoloft) for treating older men and women with GAD. The trial was conducted at an outpatient psychiatry clinic in the northeast section of Iran. The cohort consisted of forty-six subjects who were over the age of sixty years and met the criteria for GAD. For eight weeks, twenty-five subjects were assigned to treatment with buspirone (10 to 15 mg per day) and twenty-one to sertraline (50 to 100 mg per day). Both buspirone and sertraline effectively reduced levels of GAD in the subjects; they both had clinically significant improvement. The mean difference in the Hamilton Rating Scale for Anxiety (HRSA) score at the beginning of the study to that after eight weeks was greater in the buspirone group, but that difference was not significant. There were no clinically significant adverse events, and no one withdrew from the trial. The researchers concluded that "further studies with larger sample size, evaluating the effect of medical illness, cognitive impairment, depression, and combined therapy with support and psychotherapy are recommended."[2]

In a randomized, double-masked, comparative trial published in the journal *Clinical Therapeutics*, researchers from Beverly Hills, California, compared the administration of doses of buspirone twice per day to the administration of these same total dose three times per day to treat men and women between the ages of eighteen and sixty-five years with GAD. They wanted to determine if one type of administration was better than the other. Did one type of administration offer more relief from the symptoms of GAD? Did one have fewer adverse events? Obviously, it is easier to take two pills per day than three, but not at the expense of efficacy and safety. For eight weeks, a total of 137 subjects received buspirone, titrated from 15 mg per day to 30 mg per day; there were sixty-nine subjects in the two times per day group and sixty-eight in the three times per day group. At baseline, there were no significant demographic differences between the subjects in the two groups or in their anxiety scores. By the end of the first week of treatment, the subjects in both groups had significant reductions in their levels of anxiety. The most common reported adverse events were headache, dizziness, and nausea. The researchers concluded that the two types of administration were equally safe and effective. So, it may well be desirable to prescribe the twice daily administration of buspirone.[3]

In a double-blind, placebo-controlled ten-week trial published in *Psychopharmacology*, researchers from Germany compared the use of buspirone to lorazepam, a benzodiazepine, for treating generalized anxiety disorder. The initial cohort consisted of 125 psychiatric outpatients with GAD. The patients were randomized to receive 15 mg per day of buspirone ($n = 58$), 3 mg per day of lorazepam ($n = 57$), or a placebo ($n = 10$) for four weeks. During weeks five and six, the medications were tapered. That was followed by a four-week placebo period, when the active drugs were replaced with a placebo. Assessment of anxiety symptoms was based on clinical interviews conducted with each subject during their visits with specially trained general practitioners or internists. Physical examinations and blood tests were also administered.

During the course of the trial, twenty-six subjects left; of these, twelve took buspirone, ten took lorazepam, and four took the placebo. Most left during the placebo control period. Dizziness, headache, gastrointestinal upset, sedation, and drowsiness were the most reported side effects. While buspirone was found to have potent antianxiety properties, lorazepam appeared to be slightly better in reducing the symptoms of anxiety. Yet, during the placebo period, the buspirone-treated subjects tended to remain stable, while the lorazepam subjects had an "appreciable increase in anxiety." The buspirone-treated subjects required only two to four weeks of treatment "in order to become and remain improved for at least some period of time."[4]

Buspirone May Be Useful for Anxiety in Youth with High-Functioning Autism Spectrum Disorder

In a retrospective chart review published in the *Journal of Child and Adolescent Psychopharmacology*, researchers from Boston, Massachusetts, evaluated the ability of buspirone to treat anxiety in youth with high-functioning autism spectrum disorder (HF-ASD), a medical problem commonly seen with this disorder. The cohort consisted of thirty-one youth, between the ages of eight and seventeen years, who were treated at the Massachusetts General Hospital Outpatient Child Psychiatric Clinic with buspirone for at least eight weeks. All of the care providers were board-certified child and adolescent psychiatrists. The patients, who were mostly male, received an average daily dose of 41.6 mg for an average duration of 271.9 days. Anxiety symptoms were initially rated as markedly severe in twenty-two patients and moderate in the remaining nine. Eighteen youth improved at least markedly and nine improved moderately; four had no change in the severity of their symptoms. Thus, 50 percent of the patients had a "robust response" to the buspirone therapy. Though no one had a worsening of symptoms, side effects resulted in the discontinuation of buspirone in two patients. The researchers commented that "treatment with buspirone was overall well tolerated and was associated with clinically significant improvement in symptoms of anxiety in youth with ASD [autism spectrum disorder]."[5]

Even Though Buspirone Improves the Symptoms of Anxiety, It May or May Not Be Appropriate for People Dealing with Parkinson's Disease

In a trial published in the journal *Parkinsonism and Related Disorders*, researchers from Rochester, New York, noted that approximately 30 percent of people who have been diagnosed with Parkinson's disease have anxiety. Yet, more than half of the people with Parkinson's who have anxiety do not receive a pharmacological treatment. That is why these researchers wanted to learn if buspirone would be an effective medication for these patients. The initial cohort consisted of twenty-one subjects who were enrolled at a single movement disorders center from October 18, 2016, to June 18, 2018. They were men and women with idiopathic

Parkinson's disease and clinically significant anxiety without significant cognitive impairment. They had a mean age of 65.5 years, and 76.5 percent were male. For twelve weeks, seventeen subjects were placed on buspirone, 7.5 mg twice daily, which could be increased up to 30 mg twice daily; four subjects took placebos. Of the seventeen subjects on buspirone, fourteen (82 percent) had an experienced an adverse event. Nine of these subjects experienced adverse events consistent with worsened motor function, the most frequent of which was freezing of gait. Seven failed to complete the study, five due to intolerability. At the same time, it is notable that the twelve subjects taking buspirone who completed the trial had improvements in multiple measures of anxiety. Among the completers, the mean total daily dose was 26 mg. While acknowledging that a high number of the subjects were unable to complete the trial, the researchers noted that "among those who did tolerate the medication, it was associated with an improvement in anxiety." They suggested that future research should try to determine predictors of buspirone intolerability and attempt to find alternative anxiety treatments for people with Parkinson's disease.[6]

Buspirone May or May Not Help People with Panic Disorder

In a controlled, multicenter trial published in the *British Journal of Psychiatry*, researchers from France examined the ability of buspirone to enhance the benefits of cognitive behavior therapy (CBT) for people with panic disorder with agoraphobia. The cohort consisted of seventy-seven patients—forty-five women and thirty-two men; thirty-seven were placed on CBT plus buspirone and forty had CBT and a placebo. Twenty-five of the subjects in the CBT and buspirone group and twenty-four in the CBT and placebo group had not previously taken a medication for their symptoms. Forty-eight subjects (twenty-three women and twenty-five men) completed the sixteen sessions of CBT; 57 percent of those on CBT and buspirone and 67 percent of those on CBT and placebo. There was high compliance with the medication; those on buspirone took 91.9 percent of their medicine and those on placebo took 88.9 percent. Buspirone was administered during the study and tapered off when the sixteen sessions were completed. The researchers found that the subjects in both groups demonstrated improvements in panic attacks, depression, and agoraphobia. Generalized anxiety improved only in the CBT and buspirone groups. Between-group comparisons found buspirone to also have an effect on agoraphobia. While the subjects clearly benefited from both CBT and buspirone, those who had the combination seemed to obtain even better results.[7]

In a trial published in the *Journal of Clinical Psychopharmacology*, researchers from Philadelphia, Pennsylvania, and Boston, Massachusetts, wanted to determine if the combination of buspirone and imipramine, a tricyclic antidepressant, would be useful for patients with panic disorder who were discontinuing their long-term use of benzodiazepine. The cohort consisted of forty patients who were taking stable doses of a benzodiazepine; they were demographically similar. Forty-eight percent were female, 45 percent were married, and 85 percent had at least a high school education. Without altering their benzodiazepine medication, for four weeks, the subjects were assigned to double-blind treatment with buspirone (5 mg), imipramine (25 mg), or a placebo. They were expected to take six pills per day. Sedation and dry mouth were the only listed adverse events. During the next six weeks, their benzodiazepine was tapered and discontinued. At that point, the subjects returned to the care of their primary care physicians and came for follow-ups with the researchers. The researchers noted that before the tapering began, all three treatments reduced anxiety and depressive symptoms. But, unfortunately, that did not translate into successful taper outcome. Still, there were some encouraging findings. Unsuccessful taper patients did reduce their benzodiazepine intake significantly. In fact, 38 percent of the unsuccessful taper patients were eventually able to become benzodiazepine free after twelve months. In addition, treatment during tapering had no statistically significant beneficial effect on benzodiazepine taper outcome. Yet, successful taper panic disorder patients who were off benzodiazepine three months post taper were still off after twelve months. All patients off benzodiazepine at twelve months had significantly lower anxiety levels than the patients still on benzodiazepine. Even those patients who were unsuccessful in their tapering attempts had significant reductions in their daily benzodiazepine intake. The researchers commented that "pretreatment and concurrent treatment during BZ [benzodiazepine] taper with imipramine or buspirone neither decreased BZ withdrawal symptoms nor increased taper success rates in long-term BZ users with a PD [panic disorder] diagnosis."[8]

Buspirone May Be Useful for Adolescents with Obsessive-Compulsive Disorder

In a case report published in the journal *European Child & Adolescent Psychiatry*, researchers from Denmark described six adolescent patients with obsessive-compulsive disorder. They noted that the usual pharmaceutical treatment for this problem is a selective serotonin reuptake inhibitor. However, since five of the six patients did not respond adequately to at least three months of this protocol (the other had only two months), the researchers added a daily dose of 20 mg buspirone to the treatment. In three of the cases, the researchers found that the addition of buspirone to the SSRI treatment resulted in a "dramatic" reduction of OCD symptoms. Two patients had only minor improvement, and one showed no significant reduction of symptoms. There were no reported side effects caused by this combined pharmacological treatment nor did any teen need to discontinue treatment. The researchers commented that "in severe and treatment refractory OCD, buspirone might well be a safe and efficacious possibility as an addiction to SSRI treatment and as an augmenting factor." However, they underscored the need for future research with "a higher number of childhood and adolescent OCD patients."[9]

References and Further Readings

Ceranoglu, T. A., Janet Wazniak, Ronna Fried et al. "A Retrospective Chart Review of Buspirone for the Treatment of Anxiety in Psychiatrically Referred Youth with High-Functioning Autism Spectrum Disorder." *Journal of Child and Adolescent Psychopharmacology* 29, no. 1 (2019): 28–33.

Cottraux, Jean, Ivan-Druon Note, Charley Cungi et al. "A Controlled Study of Cognitive Behavior Therapy with Buspirone or Placebo in Panic Disorder with Agoraphobia." *British Journal of Psychiatry* 167 (1995): 635–41.

Laakmann, G., C. Schüle, G. Lorkowski et al. "Buspirone and Lorazepam in the Treatment of Generalized Anxiety Disorder in Outpatients." *Psychopharmacology* 136 (1998): 357–66.

Lader, M. and J. C. Scotto. "A Multicentre Double-Blind Comparison of Hydroxyzine, Buspirone and Placebo in Patients with Generalized Anxiety Disorder." *Psychopharmacology* 139, no. 4 (October 1998): 402–6.

Mokhber, Naghmeh, Mahmoud Reza Azarpazhooh, Mohammad Khajehdaluee et al. "Randomized, Single-Blind, Trial of Sertralinne and Buspirone for Treatment of Elderly Patients with Generalized Anxiety Disorder." *Psychiatry and Clinical Neuroscience* 64 (2010): 128–33.

Rynn, Moira, Felipe Garcia-Espana, David Greenblatt et al. "Imipramine and Buspirone in Patients with Panic Disorder Who Are Discontinuing Long-Term Benzodiazepine Therapy." *Journal of Clinical Psychopharmacology* 23, no. 5 (October 2003): 505–8.

Schneider, Ruth B., Peggy Auinger, Chistopher G. Tarolli et al. "A Trial of Buspirone Parkinson's Disease: Safety and Tolerability." *Parkinsonism and Related Disorders* 81 (2020): 69–74.

Sramek, John J., Edyta J. Frackiewicz, and Neal R. Cutler. "Efficacy and Safety of Two Dosing Regimes of Buspirone in the Treatment of Outpatients with Persistent Anxiety." *Clinical Therapeutics* 19, no. 3 (1997): 498–506.

Thomsen, P. H. and H. U. Mikkelsen. "The Addition of Buspirone to SSRI in the Treatment of Adolescent Obsessive-Compulsive Disorder: A Study of Six Cases." *European Child & Adolescent Psychiatry* 8 (1999): 143–8.

Cannabis and CBD

Introduction

Cannabis is a plant, *Cannabis sativa*, that contains compounds that many people believe make it useful as a medicinal drug for the treatment of a wide variety of medical problems, such as chronic pain, nausea and vomiting from chemotherapy treatment, some of the symptoms of multiple sclerosis, low appetite, Tourette's syndrome, depression, and anxiety. (*Cannabis sativa* is a plant species that includes both cannabis and hemp plants. In a way, they are like siblings in the same family.) Cannabis contains more than one hundred active ingredients known as cannabinoids. The most abundant ingredient is delta-9-tetrahydrocannabiol (THC). That is followed by cannabidiol (CBD). Though the words "cannabis" and "marijuana" tend to be used interchangeably, marijuana actually refers to the parts of the cannabis plant that contain higher amounts of THC, or the substance that makes people "high." Hemp contains higher amounts of CBD, which is not psychoactive and does not give a high feeling.

The human body naturally produces some cannabinoids; they function like neurotransmitters, sending messages throughout the nervous system and into the brain areas that play a role in memory, thinking, concentration, movement, coordination, pleasure, and sensory and time perception. Although the exact mechanism is unknown, it is believed that chemicals from the cannabis plant interact with receptors in the body's endocannabinoid system (ECS) to promote relaxation. (ECS is a biological system in the body that helps regulate and balance key bodily functions.)

While many think of cannabis as a relatively new part of the landscape, cannabis seeds have actually been available for thousands of years. In an article published in the journal *Dialogues in Clinical Neuroscience*, the author noted that cannabis was first "attested to" around 12,000 years ago near the Altai Mountains in Central Asia. Since then, cannabis seeds have been part of the migration of nomadic people. In fact, there are records of the medicinal use of cannabis in ancient China, Egypt, and Greece and later in the Roman Empire. Decades ago,

CBD and THC were isolated from each other. However, because CBD was not psychoactive, it was frequently eclipsed by interest in and concern about THC.[1]

While statistics on CBD use vary, it is estimated that around one-third of American adults have used CBD at least once. An estimated sixty-four million have tried CBD in the last twenty-four months. Of those who use CBD, 22 percent say that it helped them supplement or replace prescription or over-the-counter medications. In 2019, the top states for CBD sales were California, Florida, and New York. The most frequent reasons for using CBD are pain, anxiety, and insomnia.[2]

According to the National Center for Drug Abuse Statistics, about fifty-five million Americans currently use marijuana. That is about 16.9 percent of the population. About 45 percent of Americans have tried marijuana at least once. Fifty-five million Americans reported using marijuana within the past year. That means that there are about 50.68 percent more marijuana users than tobacco smokers. In 2017, 24 percent of 12th graders used marijuana during the previous year. Why is marijuana becoming so popular in the United States? The National Center for Drug Abuse Statistics maintains that many people believe that marijuana is "less risky" than tobacco, alcohol, and painkillers. Further, 56 percent of Americans think using marijuana is "socially acceptable."[3]

Regulation, Administration, and Costs

Under federal law, CBD derived from cannabis is considered a Schedule 1 drug and is illegal. However, because hemp is not a controlled substance, CBD derived from a hemp source that contains less than 0.3 percent THC by dry weight is not illegal. However, the ability to legally purchase CBD products varies from state to state. Marijuana, which contains THC, is a Schedule 1 drug that is illegal. With the exception of federal government-approved research studies, the federal government prohibits the manufacture, distribution, dispensation, and possession of marijuana. But, as is well-known, many states have legalized the processing and sale of medical and/or recreational marijuana. So, though the federal laws remain unchanged, in certain states, it is relatively easy for adults to purchase marijuana.

While the Food and Drug Administration (FDA) has not approved cannabis for any medical use, it has approved a few drugs that contain individual cannabinoids. For example, Epidiolex, which contains a purified form of CBD, is a treatment for seizures in a rare form of epilepsy. And, Marinol and Syndros, which contain a synthetic form of THC, treat nausea and vomiting caused by chemotherapy for cancer.

CBD is available in a variety of forms—oils, capsules, tablets, gummies, topicals, and salves—and it may be infused into food, drinks, and beauty products. There are three main types, and the specific type should be noted on the label. Full-spectrum CBD contains all parts of the cannabis plant; broad-spectrum CBD contains most of the compounds of the cannabis plant, and it may have trace amounts of THC. And isolate CBD only contains CBD with no other cannabinoids or THC. These products may not produce a notable effect. Marijuana is primarily sold as "weed" that is smoked or as edibles in gummies, extracts, flowers, and drinks or mixed into salad dressings, candies, seltzers, cakes, cookies, chocolate bars, potato chips, complete meals and other foods. Smoked marijuana quickly travels to the lungs and enters the bloodstream. So, the effects are felt rapidly. Edibles are processed through the stomach and liver.

Marijuana is less often sold as tinctures, topicals, and vaporizers. While prices of CBD and marijuana vary widely, they tend to be expensive. And, the better-quality products tend to be quite expensive. It is always best to ask knowledgeable healthcare professionals for recommendations. And, in those states where marijuana is legal, people working at dispensaries are often well-versed on the topic. Again, try to select a recommended dispensary.

Side Effects and Risks

Probably the most notable concern about CBD is the potential for product adulteration. A quick google search of CBD on the internet yields hundred if not thousands of small, medium, and large producers and manufacturers. It is hard to know which products are purer and safer than others. A few years ago, *JAMA Network Open* published a study in which researchers from Maryland, Mississippi, North Carolina, and Canada examined the content of 105 CBD products; forty-five were purchased from retail stores and sixty were bought online. Of the eighty-nine products that listed the total amount of CBD on the label, sixteen were "overlabeled," fifty-two were "underlabeled," and only twenty-one were labeled accurately. THC was detected in thirty-seven products, although all contained less than 0.3 percent. Of these thirty-seven, four were labeled THC free, fourteen indicated that they contained less than 0.3 percent THC, and nineteen did not reference THC. Twenty-nine products made therapeutic claims, fifteen products made cosmetic claims, and only forty-nine products noted that they were not Food and Drug Administration approved.[4]

Though CBD is usually well tolerated, it may cause a few side effects. These include dry mouth, diarrhea, reduced appetite, drowsiness, and fatigue. It may also interact with other medications, such as blood thinners.

While there is a concern about purity in illegally purchased marijuana, that is far less of a problem in those states where marijuana is legal and regulated. Nevertheless, marijuana comes with a whole set of side effects and risks. These include short-term effects, such as altered senses, changes in mood, impaired body movement, difficulty thinking and problem-solving, weakened memory, hallucinations, delusions, breathing problems, increased heart rate, intense nausea and vomiting, and psychosis. Long-term effects include lung and other respiratory problems (from inhaled marijuana) and alterations in the brain and brain development. Because the effects of edible marijuana take longer to appear, people may easily consume more than they intend. Children, adolescents, and young adults are at increased risk for these problems. The use of marijuana during pregnancy may alter the physical and mental development of the fetus. Other problems associated with marijuana include lower life satisfaction, poorer physical and mental health, relationship problems, less academic and career success, and more job absences, accidents, and injuries.

Research Findings

Evidence Is Emerging That CBD Is Useful for Anxiety

In a retrospective chart review published in *The Permanente Journal*, researchers from Colorado examined the usefulness of CBD for anxiety and sleep problems in adult patients at a integrative medical and psychiatric clinic in Fort Collins, Colorado. The cohort consisted of seventy-two patients, with an average age of thirty-four years, who were treated for at least one month with CBD as an adjunct to their current medications. Forty-seven of these patients had an anxiety disorder. Nearly all of the patients were treated with 25 mg/day in capsule form. A small group of patients were treated with 50 mg/day or 75 mg/day. One patient, with a severe psychiatric history, was treated with 175 mg/day. Using the Hamilton Anxiety Rating Scale, assessments of anxiety levels were determined every month. The researchers learned that the levels of anxiety in almost 80 percent of the patients improved, and these improvements were sustained over time. Only about one-fifth of the patients reported a worsening of their symptoms. The CBD was well tolerated, and a few patients had side effects, especially fatigue. No patient discontinued treatment because of tolerability problems. The researchers concluded that the "current understanding of the physiology and neurologic pathways points to a benefit with anxiety-related issues."[5]

CBD May Well Be Useful for Treatment-Resistant Anxiety in Young People

In an open-label, single-arm trial published in the *Journal of Clinical Psychiatry*, researchers from Australia tested the usefulness of CBD for younger people with treatment-resistant anxiety. The initial cohort consisted of thirty-one people between the ages of twelve to twenty-five years who did not respond to antidepressant medication and/or cognitive-behavioral therapy. There was no control group and patients, investigators, and clinicians were not blinded to the intervention. All of the subjects took CBD. After enrollment, the subjects received the study medication for twelve weeks in the form of 200 mg oral tablets that were increased as needed, and they attended study visits at weeks four, eight, twelve, and twenty-six. They also continued their usual treatment. Levels of anxiety were measured with the Overall Anxiety Severity and Impairment Scale. The final analyses included thirty subjects. By the end of the trial, twenty-six subjects had improved, and of those who had improved, sixteen had substantially improved. Almost all of the subjects reported mild or moderate side effects, such as fatigue, low mood, increased or decreased appetite, drowsiness, nausea, diarrhea, dry mouth, insomnia, and hot flashes or cold chills; these resolved spontaneously. The researchers concluded that "CBD can reduce anxiety severity and has an adequate safety profile in young people with treatment-resistant anxiety disorders."[6]

Expectations That CBD Will Be Effective in Healthy Adults Appears to Alter Levels of Acute Stress and Anxiety, Even When No CBD Is Present

In a randomized, crossover trial published in the journal *Psychopharmacology*, researchers from Nova Scotia, Canada, evaluated the ability of the belief that CBD will be effective (CBD expectancy) to relieve stress and anxiety in a group of healthy adults, at least nineteen years old. The initial cohort consisted of forty-three adults, twenty men and twenty-three women, who were regular users of cannabis but had abstained from cannabis for at least seventy-two hours before testing. They all attended two experimental sessions in which they self-administered CBD-free hempseed oil sublingually. During one session, the subjects were purposely told that the oil contained CBD, and in the other session they were told their oil had no CBD. Following administration, the subjects were evaluated with the Maastricht Acute Stress Test. While the researchers found no overall systematic changes in subjective stress and anxiety, those subjects who believed that CBD would reduce stress and anxiety had significantly diminished levels of anxiety. "Overall, findings suggested that expectation likely plays some role in the purported stress- and anxiety-reducing effects of CBD."[7]

Delta 9-THC May Be Useful as a Treatment for Chronic PTSD

In a three-week, open-label, adjusted doses pilot trial published in the journal *Clinical Drug Investigation*, researchers from Israel studied the use of Delta 9-THC, the most abundant form of THC, for chronic PTSD. The researchers noted that many patients with chronic PTSD obtain only partial relief from the available treatments. That is why they use marijuana. The researchers wanted to learn if this use was safe and well tolerated. The cohort consisted of ten patients, seven males and three females, mean age of 52.3 years, with chronic PTSD; on average, they were taking four different medications. They were all diagnosed with PTSD at least one year before entering the study, and it had been at least three years since their traumatic event. The patients were initially told to take 2.5 mg THC twice each day. If the subjects tolerated this well for two days, the dose was increased to 5 mg twice each day. All of the patients reached this dose. There were four reported cases of side effects—dry mouth in two patients, headache in one patient, and dizziness in another patient; all of these side effects were mild and continued throughout the trial. The researchers determined that the subjects experienced a statistically significant reduction in the severity of several PTSD symptoms, and they concluded that their findings "provided preliminary evidence on the safety and tolerance of Delta 9-THC as an added-on treatment for chronic PTSD, and the results support further studies regarding the therapeutic effect of Delta 9-THC in chronic and acute PTSD."[8]

Medical Cannabis May or May Not Help People with PTSD

In a study published in the *Journal of Affective Disorders*, researchers from Pullman, Washington, and Philadelphia, Pennsylvania, obtained data from 404 anonymous medical cannabis users who self-described in a cannabis app as having PTSD. There were 220 women, 176 men, and eight "other." The app tracked changes in symptoms—anxiety, intrusive thoughts, flashbacks, and irritability—obtained from different strains and doses of cannabis. The sample studied collectively used the app 11,797 times over thirty-one months to track symptoms immediately before and after using cannabis. The researchers only included the results of inhaled cannabis and only sessions in which the subjects re-rated their symptoms within four hours of cannabis use when the symptoms should have reappeared. The researchers determined that the symptoms of anxiety were reduced in 93 percent of the tracked sessions. Women reported more anxiety-reducing sessions than men, but men had less anxiety at baseline. Overall, there was a 57 percent reduction in the severity of anxiety. However, the improvement experienced by the different users varied markedly, "indicating that cannabis may not uniformly reduce PTSD symptoms for everyone." So, while there is evidence that cannabis provides temporary relief from anxiety, the degree of relief experienced varies from person to person. And, cannabis did not appear to provide long-term anxiety relief, "as baseline symptoms were maintained over time and dose used for anxiety increased over time, which is indicative of development of tolerance."[9]

In a randomized, double-blind, placebo-controlled crossover trial published in the online journal *PLoS ONE*, researchers from several locations in the United States but based in Philadelphia, Pennsylvania, noted that veterans in the United States are increasingly using cannabis to self-treat PTSD. So, they decided to test the use of three different smoked cannabis preparations and a placebo for treating the symptoms of PTSD in military veterans who were active users of cannabis. In the first stage of the trial, there were two crossover phases with seventy-six US military veterans and four treatment groups—High THC, High CBD, THC and CBD, and placebo. After a two-week wash-out period, the second stage included seventy-four subjects in three active treatment groups— High THC, High CBD, and THC and CBD. At the end of the first stage, all of the groups, including the placebo group, had statistically significant reductions in PTSD severity. Interestingly, nearly half of those using the placebo thought they were using cannabis. At the end of the second stage, the subjects using THC and CBD used significantly more cannabis than the subjects in the High THC group, and they had greater reductions than those smoking High CBD. Adverse events tended to be mild to moderate and did not significantly differ by treatment. Still, a total of thirteen subjects ended the study early because of adverse events. The most common adverse events were cough, throat irritation, and anxiety. The researchers concluded that they "failed to find a significant group difference between smoke cannabis preparations containing High CBD, High THC, and THC and CBD against placebo in regard to their impact on PTSD symptoms."[10]

Reductions in Cannabis Use Are Associated with Improvements in Anxiety

In a study published in the *Journal of Substance Abuse Treatment*, researchers from California and South Carolina examined the relationship between reductions in cannabis use and changes in anxiety, depression, sleep quality, and quality of life. In this study, the researchers used longitudinal data originally from a randomized, double-blind, placebo- controlled trial on cannabis use disorder medication. The trial, which included 302 adults between the ages of eighteen and fifty years, was implemented at six sites across the United States. The researchers divided the total number of adults into those who reduced their use of cannabis ($n = 152$) and those who increased their use ($n = 150$). Levels of anxiety were measured with the Hospital Anxiety and Depression Scale. Though the two groups did not differ in age, gender, educational achievement, and employment, there were more Black subjects and fewer "other" in the reduction group. A notable 35.8 percent of the total sample indicated clinically significant anxiety. From the collected data, the researchers observed that the reduction in cannabis use was associated with reductions in levels of anxiety. As a result, the researchers advised clinicians who treat patients with cannabis use disorder and anxiety "focus on use reduction or abstinence goals."[11]

People with Social Anxiety Disorder Have an Increased Risk of Using Marijuana

In a trial published in the journal *Addictive Behaviors*, researchers from Tallahassee, Florida, and Burlington, Vermont, studied the association between social anxiety and marijuana use in 159 undergraduates enrolled in an introductory psychology course; they had a mean age of 18.74 years, and 54.7 percent were female. The vast majority were white. The subjects completed multiple questionnaires about their marijuana and alcohol use as well as the

Liebowitz Social Anxiety Scale. The researchers learned that 58.4 percent had used marijuana during the past three months, 52.2 percent had used it during the past month, and 13.8 percent used it daily. As the researchers had predicted, social anxiety was incrementally related to marijuana problems but not to the frequency of marijuana use. To the researchers, it appeared that "coping motives play an important role in the co-occurrence of these two problems." Future research needs to determine why some socially anxious people start using marijuana but others do not.[12]

Cannabis Use May or May Not Be Associated with Slightly Elevated Levels of Anxiety

In a meta-analysis published in the *Journal of Epidemiology & Community Health*, a researcher from the UK reviewed the association between cannabis use in the general population and elevated anxiety symptoms. The researcher located ten studies that met the criteria. Four of the studies took place in the United States, three in Europe, and the others were from Colombia, Australia, and New Zealand. Seven studies had adolescents at baseline and three studies had adults. Sample sizes ranged from 338 to 34,653, with a total number of 58,538 subjects. Follow-up periods ranged from one to fifteen years, and five studies were considered high quality. The researcher found that the odds of developing anxiety symptoms were 1.15 times higher for more frequent cannabis users than less frequent users or nonusers. However, when only the high-quality studies were included, the difference was not significant. The researchers concluded "that cannabis use is a relatively minor risk factor for later anxiety in the general population."[13]

References and Further Readingses

Berger, Maximus, Emily Li, Simon Rice et al. "Cannabidiol for Treatment-Resistant Anxiety Disorder in Young People: An Open-Label Trial." *Journal of Clinical Psychiatry* 83, no. 5 (August 2022): 21m14130.

Bonn-Miller, Marcel O., Sus Sisley, Paula Riggs et al. "The Short-Term Impact of Smoke Cannabis Preparations Versus Placebo on PTSD Symptoms: A Randomized Cross-Over Clinical Trial." *PLoS ONE* 16, no. 3 (2021): e02.

Buckner, Julia D., Marcel O. Bonn-Miller, Michael J. Zvolensky, and Norman B. Schmidt. "Marijuana Use Motives and Social Anxiety Among Marijuana-Using Young. Adults." *Addictive Behaviors* 32 (2007): 2238–52.

Crocq, Marc-Antoine. "History of Cannabis and the Endocannabinoid System."
    Dialogues in Clinical Neuroscience 22, no. 3 (September 2020): 223–8.

Hser, Yih-Ing, Larissa J. Mooney, David Huang et al. "Reductions in Cannabis Use Are
    Associated with Improvements in Anxiety, Depression, and Sleep Quality, But Not
    Quality of Life." *Journal of Substance Abuse Treatment* 81 (October 2017): 53–8.

LaFrance, Emily M., Nicholas C. Glodosky, Marcel Bonn-Miller, and Carrie Cuttler.
    "Short and Long-Term Effects of Cannabis on Symptoms of Post-Traumatic Stress
    Disorder." *Journal of Effective Disorders* 274 (2020): 298–304.

Roitmaan, Pablo, Raphael Mechoulam, Rena Cooper-Kazaz, Arieh Shalev. "Preliminary,
    Open-Label, Pilot Study of Add-On Oral Delta 9-Tetrahydrocannabinol in Chronic
    Post-Traumatic Stress Disorder." *Clinical Drug Investigation* 34 (2014): 587–91.

Shannon, Scott, Nicole Lewis, Heather Lee, and Shannon Hughes. "Cannabidiol in
    Anxiety and Sleep: A Large Case Series." *The Permanente Journal* 23 (2019): 18–41.

Spindle, Tory R, Dennis J. Sholler, Edward J. Cone et al. *JAMA Network Open* 5, no. 7
    (2022): e2223019.

Spinella, Toni, Sherry H. Stewart, Julia Naugler et al. "Evaluating Cannabidiol (CBD)
    Expectancy Effects on Acute Stress and Anxiety in Health Adults: A Randomized
    Crossover Study." *Psychopharmacology* 238 (2021): 1965–77.

Twomey, Conal D. "Association of Cannabis Use with the Development of Elevated
    Anxiety Symptoms in the General Population: A Meta-Analysis." *Journal of
    Epidemiology & Community Health* 71, no. 8 (August 2017): 811–16.

Cognitive Behavioral Therapy

Introduction

Cognitive behavioral therapy (CBT) is a type of talk therapy in which patients work in a specific format with a mental health counselor, such as a psychotherapist, to solve a problem. During a limited number of structured sessions, the therapist helps patients gain an increased awareness of inaccurate or negative thinking. In so doing, patients develop a clearer view of their challenges and a better understanding of appropriate responses, and they learn to replace their negative and disturbing feelings, thoughts, and behavior patterns with more objective, realistic ones. And, time is devoted to practicing the newly learned skills and applying them to real-world situations.

CBT is used to treat a wide variety of psychiatric disorders including anxiety. Because it enables people to gain a relatively quick comprehension of their problems, it is frequently a preferred method of treatment, especially by those who do not wish to devote the time and financial resources to ongoing psychotherapy, which may continue for indefinite periods of time. Still, CBT is not a quick fix. It requires real work and a good deal of self-evaluation and commitment to change.

First emerging during the 1960s, CBT was founded by the psychiatrist Aaron Beck. He believed that certain types of thinking, "automatic negative thoughts," contributed to emotional problems. While earlier behavior therapies tended to focus on associations, reinforcements, and punishments, CBT emphasizes how thoughts and feelings influence behaviors. Today, CBT is a widely used form of therapy that appears to be useful for all forms of anxiety. Because of its focus on specific goals and results, it tends to appeal to a wide range of people.

Regulation, Administration, and Costs

A wide variety of professionals may be trained in CBT. These include psychiatrists, psychologists, licensed professional counselors, licensed social workers, licensed family and marriage therapists, psychiatric nurses, and other licensed professionals with mental health training. The actual regulation of these professionals varies according to their training and state where they practice. Thus, a psychiatrist, who is a physician who specializes in psychiatric issues, will be regulated and licensed in a different way than a licensed social worker or a psychiatric nurse.

CBT may be conducted in private, one-on-one meetings with a therapist or in groups, with family members or with other people who have similar issues. Meetings may be held in different settings, such as an office or community center. There are even online resources and online groups. Normally, the discussions will focus on specific problems, such as anxiety or even a type of anxiety, such as social anxiety disorder, and will employ a goal-oriented approach. During the therapy process, people may be asked to do "homework," including journaling and reading additional materials, which may help support the sessions. They may be asked to chronicle feelings and emotions and to read more about their specific form of anxiety. The actual therapy process tends to follow a format which begins with identifying thoughts, emotions, and beliefs about certain concerns. Then, with the assistance of the therapist, the patient generates a list of potential solutions and evaluates the strengths and weaknesses of each possibility. Once a decision is made on how to move forward, the patient pinpoints and reshapes his or her negative and inaccurate thinking, thus implementing the solution. Typically, CBT includes between five and twenty sessions. The actual length tends to be related to the duration and severity of the problem, and, of course, a patient's willingness to change.

Costs for CBT vary according to a number of factors. Obviously, a private session with a psychiatrist is more expensive than a group session in a community center with a licensed mental health professional. Some programs, especially support groups run by volunteers, may be free to community members. Treatment in larger expensive cities will cost more than less affluent areas of the country. In most cases, people should expect to spend at least $100 to $200 per session. CBT may or may not be covered, at least in part, by health insurers. If finances are a determining factor, as they are for most people, it is best to check before beginning treatment.

Side Effects and Risks

While there are no significant side effects or risks to CBT, since it requires people to explore painful feelings, emotions, and experiences, it may make some people feel uncomfortable and vulnerable. It is not uncommon for people to become upset or angry during sessions, sometimes yelling and/or crying and feeling quite drained. These risks tend to be minimized when working with highly trained and skilled therapists. Be sure to visit a therapist who is licensed to practice and has experience in CBT and the anxiety condition being addressed.

Research Findings

CBT Seems Useful for Several Types of Anxiety

In a meta-analysis published in the journal *Depression and Anxiety*, researchers from Boston, Massachusetts, Austin and Dallas, Texas, and University, Mississippi examined the use of CBT for several types of anxiety—acute stress disorder, generalized anxiety disorder (GAD), obsessive-compulsive disorder (OCD), panic disorder (PD), post-traumatic stress disorder (PTSD), and social anxiety disorder (SAD). Their cohort consisted of forty-one studies with a total of 2,835 patients; all of the studies randomized CBT to a psychological placebo or a pill placebo. PTSD was the most commonly represented disorder with fourteen studies and 1,252 patients, and twenty-nine studies compared CBT to a psychological placebo with supportive counseling being the most common comparison treatment. Thirty-four studies examined individual CBT and seven had group CBT. Mean treatment duration was eleven sessions, and the average age of the subjects was thirty-six years; 58.9 percent were female, and 73 percent were white. Of the thirty-five studies that included information about the use of psychiatric medications, eighteen studies excluded patients on these medications, fifteen studies included patients on stable doses, and two studies excluded only patients on certain medication such as SSRIs. For the later two groups, nine studies reported data on the number of patients taking psychiatric medications. On average, 34.2 percent of those samples took psychiatric medications. Patients participating in CBT had significantly higher dropout rates than those using placebos. The researchers learned that CBT was associated with significantly greater benefit for anxiety disorders than placebos, and these effects extended beyond the symptoms of the disorder being treated. The researchers concluded that their "results provide strong evidence that CBT is an efficacious treatment for anxiety and related disorders in adults, and its effects meaningfully exceed that of placebo."[1]

In a systematic review and meta-analysis published in the journal *JAMA Pediatrics*, researchers from Rochester, Minnesota, compared the effectiveness and safety of CBT and pharmacotherapy for childhood anxiety disorders. The cohort consisted of 115 randomized and nonrandomized studies which included 7,719 patients. Of these 4,290 (55.6 percent) were female, and the mean age of the children was 9.2 years. Seventy studies (60.7 percent) included patients with separation anxiety disorder, seventy-two (62.6 percent) had generalized anxiety disorder, eighty-two (71.3 percent) had social anxiety disorder, fifty-two (45.2 percent) had a specific phobia, thirty-six (31.3 percent) had panic disorder, sixty-seven (58.3 percent) had patients with no comorbidity, and forty-six (40.0 percent) had children with anxiety and a disorder such as autism. The medications used were SSRIs, SNRIs, tricyclic antidepressants, and benzodiazepines. The overall risk of bias was moderate to high. While adverse effects were reported with most drugs, CBT was associated with fewer dropouts than pill placebos. When compared to wait-listing and no treatment, CBT significantly decreased primary anxiety symptoms and improved response and remission. And, combining SSRIs with CBT "reduced primary anxiety symptoms and improved treatment response and remission" better than using each alone.[2]

Telephone-Delivered CBT May or May Not Be Better than Telephone-Delivered Nondirective Supportive Therapy for Rural Older Adults with Generalized Anxiety Disorder

In a randomized clinical trial published in *JAMA Psychiatry*, researchers from Winston-Salem, North Carolina, compared the use of telephone-delivered CBT to telephone-delivered nondirective supportive therapy (NST) for rural older adults with generalized anxiety disorder. The initial cohort consisted of 141 adults sixty years and older with a principal or coprincipal diagnosis of GAD; they all lived in one of forty-one rural counties in North Carolina with populations of fewer than 20,000 people. Seventy subjects were in the CBT group and seventy-one in the NST group. The subjects received one of the two treatments from one of three therapists, and assessments were completed either by phone or mail. Telephone-delivered CBT consisted of nine to eleven fifty-minute weekly sessions focused on the recognition of anxiety symptoms, relaxation, cognitive restructuring, the use of coping statements, problem solving, worry control, behavioral activation, exposure therapy, and relapse prevention with options on sleep and pain. The telephone-delivered NST consisted of ten weekly fifty-minute sessions which provided a supportive atmosphere for the participants to share their feelings. No direct coping suggestions were offered. Several different anxiety and other assessments were conducted by phone or mail at baseline and at two-and-four-month follow-ups. The researchers learned that both treatments reduced symptoms of anxiety, worry, depression, and GAD. But, CBT was superior to NST in reducing worry, depression, and GAD. And, telephone-delivered therapy appeared to be well received, and the attrition rate was 11.3 percent, which is relatively low. Reduction of anxiety symptoms was similar in both groups.[3]

CBT Seems Useful for Anxiety and Depression in Children and Adolescents with OCD

In a trial published in the journal *Psychiatry Research*, researchers from Los Angeles, California, evaluated the ability of CBT to help anxiety and depression in children with OCD. The cohort consisted of 137 children and adolescents with OCD between the ages of seven and seventeen years, with 57 percent female and 78 percent Caucasian; they were recruited from a university-based clinic. Over half of the sample met the criteria for a comorbid psychiatric disorder. The children and teens received twelve sessions of CBT and were assessed by independent evaluators who were all masters- or doctoral-level psychologists with extensive experience in pediatric OCD and related conditions. The sessions included psychoeducation, exposure, and cognitive restructuring. Multiple assessments were conducted including the Yale-Brown Obsessive Compulsive Scale and the Multidimensional Anxiety Scale for Children. The researchers determined that youth anxiety and depression symptoms significantly declined during the course of CBT. The degree of anxiety decreased with every CBT session. The subjects who responded to CBT demonstrated a steeper slope of improvement than their non-responding counterparts, and those youth who achieved reliable clinical change were the most likely to have elevated symptoms at pretreatment. The researchers concluded "that youth with a primary diagnosis of OCD experienced reductions in anxiety and depression symptoms over the course of CBT treatment."[4]

Some Youth with Anxiety Disorders May Have Long-Term Benefits from CBT

In a trial published in the *Journal of Anxiety Disorders*, researchers from Norway wanted to learn if there were long-term benefits of individual and group CBT delivered in community-based mental health clinics. The cohort consisted of

139 youth who ranged in age at recruitment from eight to fifteen years; they came from seven different clinics. The youth were diagnosed with separation anxiety disorder, social anxiety disorder, and/or generalized anxiety disorder. The youth had either ten individual sixty-minute CBT sessions or ten group ninety-minute CBT sessions. Some of the youth had two booster sessions. Seventeen therapists delivered their sessions as part of their routine caseloads. All of the therapists received CBT training in the *FRIENDS for life* protocol, and they were supervised throughout the treatments. A variety of assessments were conducted by sixteen assessors, who were clinicians employed by the clinics. When follow-ups were held an average of 3.9 years later, the subjects ranged in age from eleven to twenty-one years, with a mean age of 15.5 years. At that time, 27.3 percent of the subjects reported having additional treatment for anxiety. A notable 53 percent no longer met the criteria for having an anxiety disorder, and 63 percent did not meet the criteria for their principal anxiety diagnosis. No statistically significant differences were observed between the sixty-minute individual and ninety-minute group sessions. The subjects with social anxiety disorder were significantly less likely to have lost their principal diagnosis. The researchers commented that these youth may "need more extensive treatment." The researchers concluded that their "findings provide encouragement for the wider use and implementation of CBT in community mental health clinics."[5]

CBT Seems to Be About as Effective as Mindfulness-Based Therapy for Anxiety Symptoms

In a systematic review and meta-analysis of randomized controlled trials published in the journal *Annals of Palliative Medicine*, researchers from China compared the effectiveness of CBT to the usefulness of mindfulness to treat the symptoms of anxiety. Their cohort included 11 studies with 819 subjects; 407 subjects were in the CBT group and 422 were in the mindfulness group. Sample sizes were between 26 and 148 subjects; 61.3 percent were female. Duration of interventions ranged from eight to eighteen weeks. The studies were conducted in Canada, the United States, Denmark, the Netherlands, the United Kingdom, Australia, and China. Seven trials were at low risk for performance bias; of the nine studies that reported dropout rates, four were below 20 percent and five were over 20 percent. The researchers found that both CBT and mindfulness yielded "promising results in alleviating anxiety." After each session, there were no significant differences between the two intervention groups. However, for those subjects who had anxiety symptoms below the threshold for diagnostic criteria, mindfulness was favored over CBT. The researchers concluded that more rigorous studies comparing CBT and mindfulness are needed, "including more information on patient demographics, follow-up results, process evaluation, and treatment compliance."[6]

CBT Appears to Have Long-Term Benefits for People with Panic Disorder

In a prospective study published in the journal *BMC Psychiatry*, researchers from Norway examined the ability of CBT to help people dealing with panic disorder. The cohort consisted of sixty-eight patients who received CBT treatment for panic disorder and agoraphobia between 1989 and 2008. Treatments were delivered in groups of six to ten participants; the groups met for eleven weekly four-hour sessions. Evaluations were conducted by personal interviews at pretreatment, the first and last sessions, and at three months, one year, and twelve to thirty-one years later; the mean follow-up time was 23.8 years. Among the assessments used was the Phobic Avoidance Rating Scale (PARS), an observer rated scale that measures the degree of avoidance. The researchers observed a 50 percent reduction in PARS scores in 82 percent of the patients at the end of the treatment and a 98 percent reduction by the twenty-four-year follow-up. Ninety-five percent of the patients reported high to very high satisfaction with CBT. The researchers commented that their "results correspond well with previous short-term studies on the treatment of panic disorder and agoraphobia."[7]

Remote CBT May Also Help People with Panic Disorder

In a systematic review and meta-analysis published in the *Journal of Anxiety Disorders*, researchers from Australia investigated the ability of remote CBT to treat the symptoms of panic disorder. The researchers located twenty-one studies, with 1,604 subjects, 71 percent female, that met their criteria. The treatment groups included 1,286 subjects, and there were 318 in the control groups. Fourteen of the twenty-one studies, with 817 subjects, were randomized controlled studies, and seven were open trials or nonrandomized controlled trials. Remote CBT treatments were both high and low in levels of intensity. While high intensity treatments tended to be face-to-face between the clinician and subjects, low intensity treatments usually involved the patient engaging with pre-prepared material and devoid of simultaneous communication. The studies were conducted in Australia, Europe, North America, and Japan. The researchers learned that remote high and low intensity treatments for CBT were effective treatments for panic disorder. And, they concluded "that remote treatments may be able to be disseminated based on treatment preference."[8]

Guided Internet-Based CBT May Benefit People with Social Anxiety Disorder

In a trial published in the journal *Internet Interventions*, researchers from Norway, Sweden, and Denmark examined the use of guided internet-based CBT as a treatment for social anxiety disorder. The researchers noted that a clinic in Bergen, Norway, began offering guided internet-based CBT for social anxiety disorder in 2013. From 2014 to 2017, 169 patients, who were referred by general practitioners, were included in the study; of these, 145 started treatment. The patients had been dealing with the symptoms of social anxiety disorder for an average of fourteen years. The guided internet-based CBT program had nine online text-based modules that included psychoeducation, working with autonomic thought, behavioral experiment, shifting focus, and relapse prevention. The patients were expected to spend an average of seven to ten days per module. And, though the treatment continued for up to fourteen weeks; they only finished a mean of 5.3 out of nine modules. At least once per week, each patient received about ten to fifteen minutes of therapist guidance through a secure email system. Periodic social anxiety-related evaluations were conducted. Among the 145 patients who started treatment, a total of 113 (77.9 percent) responded to the post-treatment assessment and 52 (35.9 percent) responded to the six-month follow-up. The researchers learned that all tested variables demonstrated significant improvement during treatment. Statistically significant individual variations were seen. The patients with the higher levels of pretreatment symptoms experienced the most improvement. However, it is notable that 16.6 percent of the patients had a significant deterioration. The researchers concluded that guided internet-based CBT for social anxiety disorder "is an effective treatment for the majority of patients undergoing routine care."[9]

There Are Credible Reports of Negative Side Effects of CBT

In a study published in the journal *Cognitive Therapy and Research*, researchers from Berlin, Germany, and Singapore interviewed 100 CBT therapists from three clinics to discuss their experiences with CBT-related side effects and unwanted events. (Side effects were defined as negative reactions to appropriately delivered therapy, and unwanted events were defined as the consequences of inadequate treatment.) The mean age of the therapists was 32.2 years; 78 percent were female, and 96 percent had a university degree in psychology. They had an average of 5.1 years of professional experience. The therapists reported side effects in forty-three patients and 372 unwanted events in ninety-eight patients. The most frequent side effects were "negative wellbeing/distress, deterioration of symptoms, and strains in family relations." Fourteen percent of the side effects were rated as mild, 45.6 percent as moderate, 35.1 percent as severe, and 5.3 percent as very severe. As for duration, 31.6 percent lasted for hours, 31.6 percent lasted for days, 21.1 percent for weeks, 5.3 percent for months, and 8.8 percent were expected to be persistent. The most frequent unwanted events were "negative wellbeing/distress" and "deterioration of existing symptoms." The least frequent were "change in life circumstances and emergence of new symptoms." The unwanted events lasted only hours for 15.9 percent, days for 14.0 percent, weeks for 26.1 percent, months for 22.0 percent, and 16.7 percent were expected to be persistent. Why is this information important? People should realize that "psychotherapy is not harmless." Furthermore, therapists may use this information "when informing their patients about the treatment and also for risk monitoring in the course of treatment."[10]

References and Further Readings

Bilet, Truls, Torbjørn Olsen, John Roger Andersen, and Egil W. Martinsen. "Cognitive Behavioral Group Therapy for Panic Disorder in a General Cohort Setting: A Prospective Cohort Study with 12 to 31 Years Follow-Up." *BMC Psychiatry* 20 (2020): 259.

Brenes, Gretchen A., Suzanne C. Danhauer, Mary F. Lyles et al. "Telephone-Delivered Cognitive Behavioral Therapy and Telephone-Delivered Nondirective Supportive Therapy for Rural Older Adults with Generalized Anxiety Disorder: A Randomized Clinical Trial." *JAMA Psychiatry* 72, no. 10 (October 2015): 1012–20.

Carpenter, Joseph K., Leigh A. Andrews, Sara M. Witcraft et al. "Cognitive Behavioral Therapy for Anxiety and Related Disorders: A Meta-Analysis of Randomized Placebo-Controlled Trials." *Depression and Anxiety* 35, no. 6 (June 2018): 502–14.

Efron, Gene and Bethany M. Wooten. "Remote Cognitive Behavioral Therapy for Panic Disorder: A Meta-Analysis." *Journal of Anxiety Disorders* 79 021): 102385.

Kodal, Arne, Krister Fjermestad, Ingvar Bjelland et al. "Long-Term Effectiveness of
    Cognitive Behavioral Therapy for Youth with Anxiety Disorders." *Journal of Anxiety
    Disorders* 53 (2018):58–67.
Li, Jingjing, Zhu Cai, Xiaoming Li et al. "Mindfulness-Based Therapy Versus Cognitive
    Behavioral Therapy for People with Anxiety Systems: A Systematic Review and
    Meta-Analysis of Random Controlled Trials." *Annals of Palliative Medicine* 10, no. 7
    (July 2021): 7596–612.
Nordgreen, Tine, Rolf Gjestad, Gerhard Andersson et al. "The Effectiveness of Guided-
    Internet Based Cognitive Behavioral Therapy for Social Anxiety Disorder in a
    Routine Care Setting." *Internet Interventions* 13 (2018): 24–9.
Rozenman, Michelle, John Piacentini, Joseph O'Neill et al. "Improvement in Anxiety
    and Depression Symptoms Following Cognitive Behavior Therapy for Pediatric
    Obsessive Compulsive Disorder." *Psychiatry Research* 276 (2019): 115–23.
Schermuly-Haupt, Marie-Louise, Michael Linden, and A. John Rush. "Unwanted Events
    and Side Effects in Cognitive Behavioral Therapy." *Cognitive Therapy and Research*
    42, no. 3 (June 2018): 219–29.
Wang, Z., S. P. H. Whiteside, L. Sim et al. "Comparative Effectiveness and Safety
    of Cognitive Behavioral Therapy and Pharmacotherapy for Childhood Anxiety
    Disorders: A Systematic Review and Meta-Analysis." *JAMA Pediatrics* 171, no. 11
    (November 2017): 1049–56.

Exercise

Introduction

Exercise is a planned, structured, repetitive physical activity for the purpose of enjoyment and/or supporting health. It is any movement that works the body at a greater intensity than usual, raises heart rate, and works muscles. Whether it is a lighter form of exercise, such as walking, or a more challenging type of exercise, such as vigorous uphill cycling, regular exercise offers a myriad of physical and psychological benefits, such as enhancing physical fitness and reducing anxiety.

There are two broad categories of exercise—aerobic and anaerobic. Aerobic exercise, such as walking and running, improves how the body uses oxygen. It takes place over average levels of intensity and longer periods of time. Aerobic exercise usually begins with a warm-up period that soon becomes at least twenty or more minutes of exercise and ends with a period for cooling time. However, it is not uncommon for people to simply begin exercising and eliminate the warming up and cooling down periods. Anaerobic exercise focuses on building power, strength, and muscle mass. It includes high-intensity brief movements, such as weightlifting, sprinting, and isometrics. Anaerobic exercises do not use oxygen for energy, and they appear to offer fewer anti-anxiety health benefits.

While it is known that people with anxiety tend to be more sedentary and less active than those without this disorder, it is also believed that exercise, especially aerobic exercise, may be one of the best nonmedical ways to improve anxiety. Though more rigorous exercise is probably the better choice, any form of exercise is preferable to no exercise. People have experienced improvement in their anxiety symptoms from a wide variety of exercises ranging from something as low key as tai chi to high-intensity interval training. Even walking around the house is better than sitting indefinitely at the computer or in front of the television. At the very least, it may divert thoughts away from anxiety and decrease muscle tension. But, it has been shown that increasing the heart rate alters brain chemistry, increasing the availability of anti-anxiety neurochemicals, such as serotonins and gamma aminobutyric acid (GABA).

Since regular exercise is important, it is always best to select an exercise that one enjoys. That way, people are less likely to find excuses not to exercise. If possible, exercise with a friend or in a class; that enables people to benefit from social support. And, unless there is inclement weather or an air-quality alert, exercising outside or in a green space is almost always preferable.

Regulation, Administration, and Costs

There are no state or federal regulations regarding exercise. In the vast majority of instances, as long as one is exercising in a safe and unobtrusive manner, people are free to exercise wherever and whenever they wish. Of course, one should always use common sense. Do not attempt to exercise in a crowded subway car or on a busy street; whenever possible, select a less traveled side street, walkway, sidewalk, or hiking path. Many people run or walk around their neighborhoods, or if they have the space and financial resources, buy exercise equipment for their home. Administrative issues are involved only when one joins an exercise class or a gym. Then, one pays the required fees and follows the prevailing rules. As for costs, many types of exercise expenses are minimal. Thus, a good pair of supportive pair sneakers should be used for walking or running, and ice skates are needed for ice skating. Biking requires a little larger investment. But, unless one joins a more expensive gym or program, fees are probably reasonable.

Side Effects and Risks

When exercising, the primary concern is to prevent injury to muscles, bones, or joints. Though not as common, cardiac risks are also possible. There are some ways to reduce these risks, such as gradually easing into a new exercise program, and making time for warm-up and cool-down sessions. Still, people who regularly exercise can expect at least a few, hopefully minor, injuries to occur. As in many other aspects of life, there is a risk-benefit ratio here. Of course, there are risks, but they are clearly outweighed by the benefits. Regular exercise appears to not only alleviate anxiety but also reduce the risks associated with so many other health concerns, such as cardiovascular disease and cancer.

Research Findings

Exercise Training Appears to Help the Symptoms of Generalized Anxiety Disorder

In a trial published in the journal *Psychotherapy and Psychosomatics*, researchers from Georgia and South Carolina tested the ability of resistance training or aerobic exercise to calm the anxiety of sedentary women. The cohort consisted thirty sedentary women, between the ages of eighteen and thirty-seven years, who had been diagnosed with primary generalized anxiety disorder. They were randomly and equally assigned to six weeks of twice weekly resistance training or six weeks of twice weekly aerobic exercise training, or a wait list. The subjects did not report any adverse events, and all of the subjects completed the trial. Symptoms were evaluated with the Penn State Worry Questionnaire. At the end of the trial, remission rates were 60 percent for the resistance training group, 40 percent for the aerobic training group, and 30 percent for those on the wait list. The researchers noted that "exercise training is a feasible, safe and well-tolerated short-term treatment option or potential adjuvant therapy for sedentary women diagnosed with GAD [generalized anxiety disorder]."[1]

Exercise Seems to Help Obsessive-Compulsive Disorder

In a trial published in the *Journal of Anxiety Disorders*, researchers from Providence, Rhode Island, investigated acute changes in obsessive-compulsive disorder symptoms after twelve weeks of moderate-intensity exercise sessions. The cohort consisted of fifteen men and women with a mean age of 41.9 years; eight were female. The subjects had all been treated for OCD for at least three months. In the beginning, the exercise sessions lasted twenty minutes; by week twelve, they were forty minutes in length. The subjects were able to use several types of exercise equipment, including treadmills, recumbent bicycles, and elliptical machines. Before and after each sessions, the subjects rated their mood, anxiety, obsessions, and compulsions. Also, the subjects were told to engage in two or three additional sessions of moderate-intensity aerobic exercise during the week and to complete a weekly log of these activities. The researchers found that the subjects consistently reported significant reductions in negative mood, anxiety, obsessions, and compulsions at the end of each session, And, while these changes remained fairly stable over the course of the trial, the magnitude of the acute change in levels of self-reported obsessions and compulsions lessened over the duration of the intervention. "Results of this study point toward the promising effect of single sessions of exercise in aiding patients with OCD to experience significant improvements in mood, anxiety, obsessions and compulsions."[2]

Both Aerobic Exercise and Acute Resistance Training Reduced Levels of State Anxiety

In an eight-week trial published in the *Journal of Sports Medicine and Physical Fitness*, researchers from Bloomington, Indiana, compared the ability of aerobic exercise and acute resistance training to reduce state anxiety. The cohort consisted of forty-two college students, with a mean age of 21.8 years, who had enrolled in step aerobic or resistance classes; there were twenty-six females and sixteen males. State anxiety was assessed before and after exercise with a section of Spielberger's 16 State-Trait Anxiety Inventory; these assessments were conducted at weeks one, four, and eight of each program. The students participated in their preferred form of exercise—step aerobic or resistance. The aerobic sessions involved a five-minute warm-up, a forty-five-minute step aerobic workout, and a five-minute cooldown. During the resistance training classes, the subjects completed eight to ten repetitions of each activity followed by a one- to two-minute rest period. During each session, six to eight exercises were completed. The researchers determined that both types of exercise significantly reduced state anxiety, and improvement was evident during the first week of both programs. The researchers concluded that their results, "if confirmed by subsequent replications, would have practical implications in the prescription of physical activity for purposes of enhancing mental health."[3]

People Being Treated for Their Anxiety with Cognitive Behavior Therapy May or May Not Obtain Additional Benefits from a Walking Program

In a trial published in the *Journal of Anxiety Disorders*, researchers from Australia wanted to learn if people being treated for their generalized anxiety disorder, panic disorder, or social phobia with cognitive behavioral therapy (CBT) would benefit from the addition of a walking program. Six groups, with a total of thirty-eight subjects with a mean age of 38.7 years, were assigned to participate in CBT and a home-based walking program and five groups, with a total of thirty-six subjects with a mean age of 39.4 years, were assigned to CBT and educational meetings. The goal of the walking program was to reach at least thirty minutes of brisk walking or other exercise five or more times per week. The educational meetings focused on healthy eating. At baseline, the groups had similar demographic characteristics and anxiety scores. The programs for panic disorder and generalized anxiety disorder continued for eight weeks; the programs for social phobia were ten weeks. The subjects completed an activity questionnaire and assessments were conducted with the Depression Anxiety Stress Scale. The researchers determined that the subjects with social phobia, who had the best CBT attendance rates, benefited the most from the intervention. At the same time, the results for those with generalized anxiety disorder and panic disorder were "questionable." The researchers wondered if this difference was the result of the longer duration of the panic disorder intervention. Still, those who made the most improvements in their levels of physical activity achieved the best results. The researchers commented that because there are so few studies on the use of exercise to treat anxiety disorders, "the potential of exercise interventions as adjunct to GCBT [group cognitive behavior therapy] for anxiety disorder needs to be further explored."[4]

Exercise May Be Useful for Post-Traumatic Stress Disorder

In a randomized trial published in the journal *Military Medicine*, researchers from Missouri noted that large numbers of post-deployment US veterans are diagnosed with post-traumatic stress disorder. So, according to these researchers, there is an "urgent" need for more effective treatments for this disorder. Would a six-week therapeutic horseback riding offer such an effective treatment? The cohort consisted of twenty-nine veterans with PTSD or PTSD and traumatic brain injury. Initially, fifteen subjects were assigned to a riding group and fourteen to a wait-list control group. The subjects in the wait-list group began riding after the subjects in the first group completed their six weeks.; by then the group had thirteen subjects. And, another set of data were completed for them. An occupational therapist assessed each subject and matched them with the most appropriate horse. Unless canceled for bad weather, the sessions were held weekly. They included grooming and interacting with the horse before applying riding tackle and riding. There were no adverse events during any riding session. Demographic and health information was obtained from the subjects, and PTSD symptoms and other related problems were measured multiple times. The searchers learned that during the study, while the veterans were riding, they experienced statistically significant decreases in their PTSD symptoms.

However, the decline was not uniform for all veterans. Those who rode more sessions had larger declines than those who rode fewer sessions. Overall, they had an 81.8 percent likelihood of PTSD improvement. The researchers noted that their findings "suggest that riding is a constructive activity for reducing PTSD symptoms in our participants and that riding for longer periods of time has a strong influence than riding for shorter periods of time." While the researchers noted that the riding program is not a replacement for traditional PTSD treatment, "as a complementary therapy, riding centers may be a readily accessible resource to veterans in rural areas."[5]

Exercise Seems to Be Useful for Anxiety in People Living with HIV

In a cross-sectional trial published in the journal *AIDS CARE*, researchers from Germany, Australia, and Brazil noted that people living with the HIV virus have a higher prevalence of anxiety and depression than those living without this problem. As a result, they wanted to learn if recreational exercise would help alleviate some of this distress. The cohort consisted of 450 people living with HIV; they were recruited from German institutions involved in the care of people with HIV/AIDS. The subjects ranged in age from nineteen to seventy-five years, with a median age of forty-four years; 7.3 percent were female. They completed questionnaires on a number of factors, including exercising and anxiety. The subjects were categorized into recreational exercisers and sedentary. The researchers learned that in the exercising group of subjects, which had 260 subjects, the prevalence of anxiety was 12.7 percent; in the sedentary group, which had 190 subjects, the prevalence of anxiety was 21.6 percent. The difference between the groups was significant. The researchers concluded that "recreational exercise is associated with a lower risk for anxiety."[6]

There May or May Not Be an Association Between Physical Fitness in Women with Fibromyalgia and Level of Anxiety

In a population-based, cross-sectional study published in the journal *Quality of Life Research*, researchers from Spain and the Netherlands evaluated the association between physical fitness and anxiety in women with fibromyalgia. The cohort consisted of 439 women with fibromyalgia from southern Spain; the women had a mean age of 52.2 years. Levels of anxiety were measured with the State-Trait Anxiety Inventory and the anxiety subscale of the Fibromyalgia Impact Questionnaire. Forty-three percent of the subjects had moderate levels of anxiety, and 28 percent had severe anxiety. Physical fitness was measured with the Senior Fitness Test battery and handgrip strength test. The researchers learned that the levels of fitness were inversely related to the symptoms of anxiety; the better the fitness, the lower the levels of anxiety. Among the fitness components, upper body flexibility had the strongest association with anxiety. In fact, "upper body flexibility was an independent indicator of anxiety levels."[7]

However, another group of researchers found different results. In a randomized controlled trial published in the journal *Archives of Physical Medicine and Rehabilitation*, researchers from Spain evaluated the ability of exercise therapy in chest-high warm water to ease some of the symptoms associated with fibromyalgia, such as anxiety. The initial cohort consisted of sixty middle-aged women with fibromyalgia and twenty-five healthy women. The women with fibromyalgia were placed in an exercise group or a control group. So, there were three groups—the women with fibromyalgia who exercised, the women with fibromyalgia who did not participate in the exercise program, and the healthy controls. At baseline, the women had similar demographic characteristics. The water program, which was held three times per week for sixteen weeks, included strength training, aerobic training, and relaxation exercises. Among the many measures administered was the State Anxiety Inventory. When compared to the healthy women, the researchers learned that the women with fibromyalgia showed significant deficiencies. Still, the women who exercised experienced improvements in many areas of their lives, except anxiety. The researchers commented that they "did not find any differences in anxiety levels after treatment."[8]

Exercise May Be Useful for State Anxiety in Breast Cancer Survivors

In a pilot trial published in the journal *Oncology Nursing Forum*, researchers from Victoria, Canada, wanted to learn if exercise would help breast cancer survivors deal with their state anxiety. The initial cohort consisted of twenty-five breast cancer survivors and twenty-five aged-matched women without a cancer diagnosis who were recruited from the Victoria, Canada, area. The mean age of the survivors was fifty-nine years, and the mean age of the healthy women was fifty-six years. Forty percent of all the women had a bachelor's degree, and around 80 percent were married or living with a partner. More than half of the women participated in American College of Sports Medicine recommended levels of weekly physical activity. Each subject was asked to complete both light and moderate exercises on two separate days. Before and after the exercises, anxiety levels were measured with the State Anxiety Inventory. The researchers learned that acute exercise reduced state anxiety levels in both the cancer survivors and those without a cancer diagnosis. And, they noted that their findings "generally support the authors' hypothesis that acute exercise would decrease state anxiety levels for breast cancer survivors and those without a cancer diagnosis and supports additional investigation in this area."[9]

Exercise May Help People with Chronic Low Back Pain and Anxiety

In a study published in the journal *Complementary Therapies in Clinical Practice*, researchers from Croatia, Italy, and Israel examined the use of yoga to reduce the anxiety associated with chronic low back pain (CLBP). The cohort consisted of sixteen males and fourteen females with a mean age of 34.2 years, who had CLBP and mild to moderate anxiety. They were randomly divided into a fifteen-person yoga and education group and a fifteen-person control group; at baseline, the groups were not statistically different. The subjects in the yoga group attended seventy-five-minute yoga training classes two times per week for eight weeks. The classes were managed by a yoga teacher with extensive experience in posture and back problems. The members of the control group only received a pamphlet that offered information on biomechanical aspects of the vertebral spine, as well as the ergonomic use of the spine. In addition, twice each week they received a newsletter. Before and after the intervention, a psychological assessment was performed on all of the subjects, and a questionnaire evaluated their pain. The researchers determined that at the end of the intervention there were statistically significant differences between the groups in levels of anxiety. And, they concluded that "yoga combined with education has a favorable effect, compared to an informational pamphlet alone on individuals with CLBP."[10]

References and Further Readings

Abrantes, Ana M., David R. Strong, Amy Cohn et al. "Acute Changes in Obsessions and Compulsions Following Moderate-Intensity Aerobic Exercise Among Patients with Obsessive-Compulsive Disorder." *Journal of Anxiety Disorders* 23, no. 7 (October 2009): 923–7.

Blacklock, Rachel, Ryan Rhodes. Chris Blanchard, and Catherine Gaul. "Effects of Exercise Intensity and Self-Efficacy on State Anxiety with Breast Cancer Survivors." *Oncology Nursing Forum* 37, no. 2 (March 2010):206–12.

Córdoba-Torrecilla, S., V. A. Aparicio, A. Soriano-Maldonado et al. "Physical Fitness Is Associated with Anxiety Levels in Women with Fibromyalgia: The Al-Ándalus Project." *Quality of Life Research* 25 (2016): 1053–8.

Field, Tiffany, Miguel Diego, and Maria Hernandez-Reif. "Tai Chi/Yoga Effects on Anxiety, Heartrate, EEF and Math Computations." *Complementary Therapies in Clinical Practice* 16 (2010): 235–8.

Hale, B. S. and J. S. Raglin. "State Anxiety Responses to Acute Resistance Training and Step Aerobic Exercise Across Weeks of Training." *Journal of Sports Medicine and Physical Fitness* 42, no. 1 (March 2002): 108–12.

Herring, Matthew P., Marni L. Jacob, Cynthia Suveg et al. "Feasibility of Exercise Training for Short-Term Treatment of Generalized Anxiety Disorder: A Randomized Controlled Trial." *Psychology and Psychosomatics* 81, no. 1 (December 2011): 21–8.

Johnson, Rebecca A., David L. Albright, James R. Marzolf et al. "Effects of Therapeutic Horseback Riding on Post-Traumatic Stress Disorder in Military Veterans." *Military Medical Research* 5 (2018): 3.

Kuvačić, Goran, Patrizia Fratini, Johnny Padulo, and Antonio Dello Iacono. "Effectiveness of Yoga and Educational Intervention on Disability, Anxiety, Depression, and Pain in People with CLBP: A Randomized Controlled Trial." *Complementary Therapies in Clinical Practice* 31 (2018): 262–7.

Merom, Dafna, Philayrath Phongsavan, Renate Wagner et al. "Promoting Walking as an Adjunct Intervention to Group Cognitive Behavioral Therapy for Anxiety Disorders—A Pilot Group Randomized Trial." *Journal of Anxiety Disorders* 22 (2008): 959–68.

Munguía-Izquierdo, Diego and Alejandro Legaz-Arrese. "Assessment of the Effects of Aquatic Therapy on Global Symptomatology in Patients with Fibromyalgia Syndrome: A Randomized Controlled Trial." *Archives of Physical Medicine Rehabilitation* 89, no. 12 (December 2009) 2250–7.

Pérez-Chaparro, Camillo, Maria Kangas, Phillip Zech et al. "Recreational Exercise Is Associated with Lower Prevalence of Depression and Anxiety and Better Quality of Life in German People Living with HIV." *AIDS Care* 34, no. 2 (2022): 182–7.

Gabapentin

Introduction

Gabapentin is an anticonvulsant medication that helps to control certain types of seizures, and it also functions as a muscle relaxer and antispasmodic drug. Some forms of gabapentin may treat people with restless legs syndrome and nerve pain, such as postherpetic neuralgia or the burning or stabbing nerve pain that is a common complication of shingles. And, gabapentin had been successfully used for hot flashes.

First discovered in the 1970s, gabapentin was approved by the US Food and Drug Administration (FDA) in 1993 and had been available generically in the United States since 2004. Although it was originally intended to be a muscle relaxer and antispasmodic medication, it became evident that gabapentin was useful for seizures. Although approved for seizures and some other medical problems, gabapentin is used off-label for anxiety disorders. While some providers may recommend gabapentin as a first line of treatment for anxiety, most providers are far more likely to suggest another medication, such as a selective serotonin reuptake inhibitor (SSRI). On the other hand, SSRIs tend to require six to eight weeks to take effect. So, gabapentin may be the preferred medication when a more timely relief of anxiety is needed. With gabapentin, some people feel relief fairly quickly. However, it may take one to four weeks for patients to experience the full benefits. From the limited research that is available, gabapentin seems most useful for generalized anxiety disorder, social anxiety disorder, and post-traumatic stress disorder.

Researchers have determined that gabapentin appears to work by altering activity in the brain and influencing the chemicals in the brain known as neurotransmitters, which send messages between nerve cells. It calms and reduces the excitability of nerve cells, lowering the incidence and intensity of seizures and markedly reducing anxiety.

Regulation, Administration, and Costs

As with all prescription medications, gabapentin is regulated by the Food and Drug Administration. Sold as brand-name products, including Horizant, Gralise, and Neurontin, or as a generic drug, gabapentin is available as a capsule, tablet, extended-release tablet, or liquid. The correct dosage of gabapentin is dependent on a number of factors, including the type and brand of gabapentin, the strength of the product, and the kidney function, weight, age, and general health of the patient. The number of daily doses and whether or not the doses should be taken with food should be determined by a healthcare provider. It is important not to exceed the recommended dose or to take two doses of gabapentin at the same time. Gabapentin is generally started with one dose of 300 mg per day and may be increased to three times per day. Though the starting dose is lower than that usually prescribed for seizures, the dose is frequently increased. Normally, providers recommend beginning the first dose in the evening. Gabapentin is inexpensive and should be covered, at least in part, by health insurance.

Side Effects and Risks

Gabapentin has a host of different potential side effects. The most serious concerns are breathing problems and suicidal thoughts or behaviors. Suicidal thoughts and behaviors may appear more often in people with psychiatric problems. About 10 percent of people taking gabapentin have dizziness, sleepiness, water retention, and problems walking. Children and older adults are at increased risk for these.

Other possible side effects include back or chest pain, constipation, diarrhea, vomiting, gastrointestinal upset, increased appetite and weight gain, blurry vision, bruising, mood changes, chills, cough, fatigue, fever, cold or flu-like symptoms, hoarseness or dry mouth, memory loss, mouth ulcers, shortness of breath, sore throat, swollen glands, trembling, urinary problems, weakness, and uncontrolled eye rolling. Some of the more common side effects in children are depression and other mood changes, behavioral problems, school performance issues, hyperactivity, and a problem with concentration. Ironically, it may also cause anxiety in some children, especially those who have a predisposition for anxiety. Of course, when that occurs, it should be reported to the prescribing provider.

In addition, there is the chance of an overdose. Symptoms of an overdose include sleepiness, lethargy, double vision, seizures, difficulty swallowing and breathing, hoarseness, slurred speech, diarrhea, and coma. And, gabapentin may react with other medications, vitamins, and herbal supplements. Before taking gabapentin, people should provide their medical provider with a complete list of their medications and supplements.

Women who are pregnant or planning to become pregnant should be aware that the intake of gabapentin during pregnancy may increase the risk of the fetus developing a cardiac malformation. After childbirth, gabapentin passes into breast milk. Since children under the age of three years should not take gabapentin, it may not be safe for infants and toddlers to drink breast milk with gabapentin.

Because gabapentin may cause drowsiness, people should exercise caution while driving or using machinery. Also, since antacids lower the body's ability to absorb gabapentin, these medications should be taken at least two hours apart. People on gabapentin should avoid or limit alcohol, which may trigger increases in sleepiness or dizziness.

Research Findings

Gabapentin May Be Useful for Women with Breast Cancer-Related Anxiety

In an eight-week, randomized, double-blinded, controlled trial published in the journal *Breast Cancer Research and Treatment*, researchers from Rochester, New York, and Palo Alto, California, investigated the use of gabapentin for women with anxiety after treatment for breast cancer. The cohort consisted of 420 breast cancer patients who had completed all chemotherapy cycles and had two or more hot flashes per day for at least seven days prior to enrollment. The women were divided into three groups: 139 women took 300 mg gabapentin, 144 took 900 mg gabapentin, and 137 took a placebo. After four and eight weeks of treatment, the women taking either dose of gabapentin had significantly lower levels of anxiety than the women taking the placebo. At four weeks, but not eight weeks, the extent of improvement appeared to be a function of the degree of anxiety at baseline; those with the highest levels of anxiety at baseline had the most improvement. The 300 mg dose appeared to be optimal, except for those with the highest levels of anxiety; for them, both doses had similar effects. "Given its similar pharmacology efficacy in the treatment of hot flashes, and low cost, gabapentin may provide a low cost and parsimonious alternative treatment choice for clinicians seeking drug treatments for breast cancer survivors presenting in primary care practices with anxiety symptoms."[1]

Gabapentin May Be Useful for Those Who Experience Public Speaking-Related Anxiety

In a double-blind trial published in the *Journal of Psychopharmacology*, researchers based in Brazil evaluated the effectiveness of 400 mg and 800 mg of gabapentin on anxiety related to simulated public speaking. The cohort consisted of thirty-two normal, active male university students between the ages of seventeen and thirty years. Before beginning their simulated public speaking, ten subjects took 800 mg of gabapentin, eleven subjects took 400 mg of gabapentin, and eleven subjects took a placebo. Measures of variables, such as excitement, tension, sweating, trembling, and palpitations, as well as physiological changes, such as heart rate and blood pressure, were taken at various points in the trial. The researchers learned that the highest rates of anxiety were felt during the anticipation and speech phases of the trial, and 800 mg of gabapentin attenuated the anxiety. Why is this so important? "Public speaking is recognized as an anxiogenic situation for most people and is one of the most intense and prevalent fears among college students."[2]

Gabapentin May or May Not Be Useful for Surgery-Related Anxiety

In a single-center, blinded, randomized controlled trial published in the *Canadian Journal of Anesthesi*, researchers from Canada examined the use of gabapentin to reduce preoperative anxiety and pain in highly anxious patients. The initial cohort consisted of fifty female patients who all had a score of at least five out of ten on a numeric rating scale of anxiety. As a result, they were considered to have moderate to high levels of anxiety. Upon arrival at the hospital on the day of their major surgery, the subjects were given pre-drug administration questionnaires. Twenty-five women then received 1,200 mg of gabapentin and twenty-five took a placebo. Two hours later, the questionnaires were readministered. Forty-four women completed the entire in-hospital protocol. The researchers determined that anxiety scores were lower in the gabapentin group than in the placebo group; the administration of gabapentin produced a clinically significant reduction in anxiety in these female patients with preoperative anxiety, but they also had an increased level of sedation before entering the operating room, and they were more somnolent one hour after surgery. So, while gabapentin reduced anxiety, its associated sedative properties may delay postoperative discharge.[3]

However, a few years earlier, some of these same researchers from Canada had different results when they tested the use of 600 mg of gabapentin before total hip arthroplasty. In a double-blind, randomized trial published in *Pain Medicine*, seventy patients were randomly assigned to one of three treatment groups before/after anesthesia—placebo/placebo ($n = 24$), gabapentin/placebo ($n = 22$), and placebo/gabapentin ($n = 24$). The subjects in the second group received 600 mg gabapentin two hours before surgery; the other subjects took placebos. The patients were asked to rate their levels of anxiety prior to the administration of the preoperative medications and two hours later. The researchers learned that the administration of 600 mg of gabapentin prior to surgery did not reduce preoperative levels of anxiety. "These results demonstrated that anxiety scores were not different after treatment with GBP [gabapentin] or placebo, regardless of baseline level of anxiety."[4]

In a randomized, placebo-controlled trial published in the *Indian Journal of Anesthesia*, researchers compared the preoperative use of gabapentin, alprazolam (Xanax), and a placebo on preoperative anxiety and postoperative pain and morphine use. The cohort consisted of seventy-five patients scheduled for abdominal hysterectomies under general anesthesia. On the night before surgery and two hours before surgery, the patients took 600 mg of gabapentin or 0.5 mg alprazolam or a placebo. The preoperative anxiety levels of the patients were assessed the night before surgery and again in the preoperative holding area. Before administration of the drugs, anxiety scores between the three groups were comparable. After the administration of the drugs, levels of anxiety were only significantly lower in the alprazolam group. So, the patients in the gabapentin group did not demonstrate a significant reduction in anxiety. The researchers concluded that gabapentin 600 mg "does not have significant anxiolytic effect compared to alprazolam 0.5 mg."[5]

Gabapentin Seems to Help People with Social Phobia

In a randomized, double-blind, placebo-controlled, parallel-group trial published in the *Journal of Clinical Psychopharmacology*, researchers from Ann Arbor, Michigan, Durham, North Carolina, Middleton, Wisconsin, and Raleigh, North Carolina, studied the efficacy and safety of gabapentin for relieving the symptoms of social phobia, which is also known as social anxiety. The researchers noted that the severity of symptoms in this group was probably higher than in some other treatment studies. The initial cohort consisted of sixty-nine people with social phobia; they were divided into two groups. For fourteen weeks, the subjects in one group took between 300 and 3,600 mg per day of gabapentin; the medication was dispensed in 300 mg capsules. The subjects in the other group took a placebo. The subjects in each group were demographically comparable, and there were only low levels of comorbid psychiatric diagnoses. The maximum dose of gabapentin (3,600 mg or twelve capsules) was achieved by 56 percent of the subjects on gabapentin, and 60 percent of the subjects on the placebo reached their maximum dose. The overall rate of withdrawal averaged two subjects per visit per treatment group. The researchers determined that compared to the placebo, gabapentin significantly reduced the symptoms of social phobia. Interestingly, while both men and women seemed to experience about the same degree of improvement on gabapentin, on the placebo, women exhibited a sizable benefit and men had essentially none. The researchers speculated that women with social phobia may be "more responsive to the nonspecific benefits of being involved in a clinical trial." And, they concluded that "gabapentin offers a favorable risk-benefit ratio for the treatment of patients with social phobia."[6]

In a letter to the editor published in the *Primary Care Companion to the Journal of Clinical Psychiatry,* researchers from Norfolk, Virginia, described a small randomized, double-blind, crossover, five-to-six-month trial they conducted on the use of gabapentin and tiagabine, another medication for seizures, for social anxiety. The cohort consisted of eight adults, five men, between the ages of twenty-one to thirty-nine years. Seven subjects had severe levels of social anxiety, and one subject was in the moderate range. Assigned to take either gabapentin or tiagabine, the subjects began with low doses and were titrated to higher doses, up to 1,800 mg for gabapentin. The researchers found that all of the seven subjects with severe social anxiety responded well to both anticonvulsant medications, and two subjects, one for either medication, reached remission. Four subjects, two on either medication, had clinically significant change. The subjects reported few side effects; sedation and mild dizziness were the most common. Only one person stopped gabapentin because of sedation. The researchers noted that their study added to the existing database that these anticonvulsant medications are useful for the treatment of social anxiety.[7]

Gabapentin May Help People with Severe Symptoms of Panic Disorder

In a randomized, double-blind, placebo-controlled, parallel-group trial published in the *Journal of Clinical Psychopharmacology*, researchers based in Ann Arbor, Michigan, examined the efficacy and safety of using gabapentin to treat the symptoms of panic disorder with or without agoraphobia. During the three weeks prior to screening, all of the subjects had at least one weekly panic attack. For eight weeks, 103 subjects received either gabapentin, dosed between 600 and 3,600 mg per day, or a placebo. At baseline, the subjects in both groups were comparable in demographic and illness characteristics. Doses were increased as long as the symptoms persisted and no limiting events were observed. At the end of the trial, the treatment was tapered over a one-week period of time. Because of adverse effects, about 12 percent of the gabapentin-treated subjects withdrew from the trial, as did 4 percent of the placebo subjects. While the researchers found that gabapentin was no more useful in calming the symptoms of panic disorder in the total cohort, it was an effective treatment for those with severe cases. There was also a high placebo response, especially for those subjects who were less severely ill at baseline. "This suggests that if gabapentin were confirmed to be efficacious for the treatment of panic disorder, it would have a favorable risk-benefit profile."[8]

Gabapentin May Help People with Post-Traumatic Stress Disorder

In a study published in the journal *Annals of Clinical Psychiatry*, researchers from Charleston, South Carolina, wanted to determine if gabapentin would be useful for people with post-traumatic stress disorder. The cohort consisted of thirty consecutive patients treated with gabapentin in a Department of Veterans Affairs PTSD outpatient clinic. The clinic employed a multidisciplinary approach including assessments by psychiatrist, psychologists, nurses, and social workers. Patients were evaluated by the degree of improvement from 0 (zero), meaning no improvement, to 3, meaning marked improvement. Data were obtained from record reviews. Sixty-six percent of the patients had comorbid major depression, and 83 percent were taking an antidepressant. All of the patients had symptoms of insomnia and nightmares that led to treatment with gabapentin. Twenty-three of the patients had moderate or targeted improvement of symptoms. Gabapentin appeared to be well tolerated, and there were no significant documented drug interactions. The average dose of gabapentin in subjects with no or mild clinical effects was notably lower than in subjects with moderate or marked improvement, suggesting a dose-effect relationship. The researchers concluded that "gabapentin may be a useful adjunct in the treatment of chronic PTSD."[9]

Gabapentin Makes Fluoxetine a More Effective Treatment for Obsessive-Compulsive Disorder

In a randomized, open-label trial published in the journal *European Archives of Psychiatry and Clinical Neuroscience*, researchers from Turkey compared the efficacy of fluoxetine (Prozac) alone and with the co-administration of gabapentin and fluoxetine in patients with obsessive-compulsive disorder. The cohort consisted of forty patients, between the ages of eighteen and sixty years, who were diagnosed with OCD; they were all recruited from a psychiatric outpatient clinic. For eight weeks, eleven women and nine men were treated with fluoxetine alone, and the other ten women and ten men were treated with gabapentin and fluoxetine. Twenty mg of fluoxetine was taken in a single morning dose, and 150 mg gabapentin was taken four times each day. If the patients did not respond to the medication by week four, fluoxetine was increased to 40 or 60 mg per day, and gabapentin was increased to 900 mg per day. The subjects were evaluated with various tools, such as the Yale-Brown Obsessive Compulsive Scale, which had questions on the degree of obsessions and the severity of compulsions. Assessments were conducted at baseline and at the end of weeks two, four, and eight. Twelve patients taking fluoxetine alone reported adverse effects, such as an increase in anxiety symptoms, headaches, nausea, and insomnia, and fifteen patients on both medications reported side effects such as sedation, dizziness, dry mouth, and gastrointestinal discomfort. The researchers learned that the patients in both groups had improvements in their OCD symptoms. However, in their second week of treatment, the patients in the combination group had a significantly greater decrease of their OCD symptoms than the patients in the fluoxetine-alone group. The researchers concluded that "the co-administration of fluoxetine and gabapentin, in this preliminary study, gives hope for planning controlled studies in the pharmacotherapy of treatment resistant OCD cases."[10]

References and Further Readings

Clarke, Hance, Joseph Kay, Beverley A. Orser et al. "Gabapentin Does Not Reduce Preoperative Anxiety When Given Prior to Total Hip Arthroplasty." *Pain Medicine* 11 (2010): 966–71.

Clarke, Hance, Kyle R. Kirkham, Beverley A. Orser et al. "Gabapentin Reduces Preoperative Anxiety and Pain Catastrophizing in High Anxious Patients Prior to Major Surgery: A Blinded Randomized Placebo-Controlled Trial." *Canadian Journal of Anesthesia* 60 (2013): 432–43.

de-Paris, Fernanda, Marcia K. Sant' Anna, Monica R. M. Vianna et al. "Effects of Gabapentin on Anxiety Induced by Simulated Public Speaking." *Journal of Psychopharmacology* 17, no. 2 (2003): 184–8.

Hamner, Mark B., Peter S. Brodrick, and Lawrence A. Labbate. "Gabapentin in PTSD: A Retrospective, Clinical Series of Adjunctive Therapy." *Annals of Clinical Psychiatry* 13, no. 3 (September 2001): 141–6.

Joseph, Tim Thomas, Handattu Mahabaleswara Krishna, and Shyamsunder Kamath. "Premedication with Gabapentin, Alprazolam or a Placebo for Abdominal Hysterectomy: Effect on Pre-Operative Anxiety, Post-Operative Pain and Morphine Consumption." *Indian Journal of Anaesthesia* 58, no. 6 (November–December 2014): 693–9.

Lavigne, Jill E., Karen Mustian, Jennifer L. Matthews et al. "A Randomized, Controlled, Double-Blinded Clinical Trial of Gabapentin 300 mg versus 900 mg versus Placebo for Anxiety Symptoms in Breast Cancer Survivors." *Breast Cancer Research and Treatment* 136, no. 2 (November 2012): 479–86.

Pande, Atul C., Jonathan R. T. Davidson, James W. Jefferson et al. "Treatment of Social Phobia with Gabapentin: A Placebo-Controlled Study." *Journal of Clinical Psychopharmacology* 19, no. 4 (August 1999): 341–8.

Pande, Atul C., Mark H. Pollack, Jerri Crockatt et al. "Placebo-Controlled Study of Gabapentin Treatment of Panic Disorder." *Journal of Clinical Psychopharmacology* 20, no. 4 (2000): 467–71.

Urbano, Maria R., David R. Spiegel, Nena Laguerta et al. "Gabapentin and Tiagabine for Social Anxiety: A Randomized Double-Blind, Crossover Study of 8 Adults." *Primary Care Companion to the Journal of Clinical Psychiatry* 11, no. 3 (2009): 123.

Herbal Medicine

Introduction

Also known as botanical medicine or phytomedicine, herbal medicine is the use of plant seeds, berries, roots, leaves, bark, or flowers to treat medical problems. Over the millenniums, it has been used for a wide range of medical concerns including allergies, asthma, eczema, premenstrual syndrome, menopausal symptoms, rheumatoid arthritis, fibromyalgia, migraine, chronic fatigue, irritable bowel, cancer, depression, and, of course, anxiety.

Even before recorded history, plants were used for medicinal purposes. Indigenous cultures, such as Native Americans, used herbs in their healing rituals, and herbs were and are an integral component of traditional Chinese medicine and Ayurveda. It is known that ancient Chinese and Egyptian writings describe the use of herbs as early as 3000 BC.

Decades ago, herbal medicine was replaced by drugs, which tended to be far more costly and more profitable for their manufacturers. Still, the World Health Organization has estimated that 80 percent of people worldwide, or about four billion people, rely on herbal medicine for some part of their health care. In some overpopulated poorer countries, the rural communities may have little to no access to modern medicine. So, the population relies almost entirely on herbal products. In the United States, 30 percent of the population uses herbal remedies. In recent years, the use of herbal supplements has grown over 380 percent.[1]

While scientists have discovered how some herbs work, in many cases they are not sure what component of an herb treats specific medical problems. It is known that herbs tend to contain many ingredients that probably function synergistically to produce a beneficial effect. And, of course, herbs are impacted by the environment and conditions in which they are grown. Before trying prescription medication, with their frequent higher prices and undesirable side effects, it is not uncommon for people dealing with anxiety to try different types of herbal medicine. While there are a myriad of different herbs that are said to be useful for anxiety, many of them have little scientific research to support their claims. The herbs selected for this entry—chamomile, kava kava, lavender, passionflower, saffron, and St. John's wort—have all have been reviewed in at least a few scientific journals.

Regulation, Administration, and Costs

The US Dietary Supplement Health and Education Act of 1994 classified herbal medicine as dietary supplements. That means that while the US Food and Drug Administration requires companies to submit safety data about any new ingredient not sold in the United States as a dietary supplement before 1994, the FDA is not authorized to review dietary supplements for safety and effectiveness before they are marketed. However, the act does require supplements to be made with good manufacturing practices.

A wide variety of herbal medicine is sold in retail stores and online. These products tend to be available in many forms, such as capsules, tablets, liquids, gels, lotions, creams, tinctures, extracts, dried plants and powders, teas, and essential oils. The following lists specific details on each of the herbs:

Chamomile

Chamomile is most often sold in tea bags, capsules, and tincture. There are no dosing recommendations for chamomile. It is inexpensive.

Kava Kava

Kava kava or kava is most often sold as tea bags, capsules, tincture, and extract. Though dosage recommendations vary, it is suggested that it is best not to exceed 250 mg per day. Kava kava is moderately priced.

Lavender

Lavender is most often sold as a tea and essential oil. One to two teaspoons of lavender are recommended as a tea, and one to several drops are recommended as an oil. It is inexpensive.

Passionflower

Passionflower is most often sold in capsules or as a tea. There are no reliable dosing recommendations. Passionflower ranges from inexpensive to moderately priced.

Saffron

Saffron is most often sold in capsules. Up to 1.5 grams per day are believed to be safe. Because it is extremely labor-intensive to harvest, pure saffron is very expensive.

St. John's Wort

St. John's wort tends to be sold as an extract or in capsules. The usual recommended dose is 300 mg three times per day. St. John's wort is moderately priced.

With herbal medicine, it is always best to start with a low dose and slowly increase. Do not exceed the recommendations on the label.

Side Effects and Risks

It is important to realize that herbal products may contain contaminants or substances not mentioned on the label. And, though some herbal products are standardized, meaning that they are guaranteed to contain the specific amount noted on the label, it is not legally required. Herbal products frequently contain varying amounts, and manufacturers interpret the standardizing process in different ways. Further, herbal products purchased in stores or online may be unlike those that are tested in research studies. In 2023, the FDA launched the "Dietary Supplement Ingredient Directory." At this website, members of the public are able to determine what ingredients have been used in products marketed as dietary supplements. In addition, they may read what the FDA has said about those ingredients and any action the FDA may have taken against specific ingredients.[2]

Since herbal medicines lack regulations or standards for preparing or packaging, their doses and strengths may not be consistent. In addition, they have been associated, especially in higher doses, with side effects. There are side effects and risks related to the specific herbs discussed addressed in this entry. They are as follows:

Chamomile

Chamomile is probably safe in the amounts used in tea and for the short-term oral intake. Though uncommon, side effects include nausea, dizziness, and allergic reactions. Allergic reactions are more common in people who are allergic to related plants, such as ragweed, chrysanthemums, marigolds, and daisies. Since it may increase the risk of bleeding, people taking warfarin, a blood-thinning medication, should not use chamomile, and because chamomile may increase concentrations of serum cyclosporine, a drug to prevent transplant rejection, people taking cyclosporine should not consume chamomile. It is not known if chamomile is safe to take during pregnancy or breastfeeding.

Kava Kava

The use of kava kava has been linked to liver injury that may be serious or even fatal. Other problems with this herb include digestive upset, headaches, and dizziness. It may alter the ability to drive safely or use machinery. Long-term high dose use may cause kava dermopathy or dry, flaky skin and yellow discoloration. Kaka kava should not be used during pregnancy or breastfeeding.

Lavender

Lavender use may cause constipation, diarrhea, or headaches. When applied to the skin, it may cause irritation. It is probably safe when inhaled.

Passionflower

Passionflower may cause drowsiness, confusion, and uncoordinated movements in some people. High doses may be very unsafe. It is not known if passionflower is safe to use during pregnancy.

Saffron

Common side effects of saffron include drowsiness, digestive issues, nausea, and vomiting. People may have allergic reactions to saffron, and higher doses may be poisonous.

St. John's Wort

This herb may weaken the effects of many medications, including antidepressants, birth control pills, cyclosporine, some heart medicines such as digoxin and ivabradine, some HIV drugs such as indinavir and nevirapine, some cancer medicine such as irinotecan and imatinib, warfarin, and certain statins such as simvastatin. St. John's wort may cause increased sensitivity to sunlight, especially when taken in high doses. It is not known if it is safe to use topically or while pregnant or breastfeeding. Additional side effects of St. John's wort include insomnia, anxiety, dry mouth, dizziness, gastrointestinal symptoms, fatigue, headache, and sexual dysfunction.

Research Findings

Long-Term Chamomile Treatment Appears Useful for Generalized Anxiety Disorder

In a study published in the journal *Phytomedicine*, researchers from New York City and Philadelphia, Pennsylvania, investigated the long-term use of chamomile for moderate-to-severe generalized anxiety disorder. During the first phase of the trial, researchers recruited 179 patients with generalized anxiety disorder from primary care practices and local communities. The subjects received twelve weeks of 1,500 mg per day of chamomile therapy. Ninety-three subjects participated in this trial; they had a mean age of 47.3 years, sixty-five (69.9 percent) were women, and seventy-three (78.5 percent) were white. The vast majority, 86 percent, had moderate anxiety; the remainder had moderately severe to severe anxiety. The subjects were placed in a twenty-six-week randomized, double-blind, placebo-controlled trial to continue taking 1,500 mg per day of chamomile ($n = 46$) or begin a placebo ($n = 47$). Using measurement tools, the subjects were assessed for generalized anxiety disorder relapse at weeks fourteen, sixteen, twenty, twenty-eight, and thirty-eight. Overall, the subjects were 95.7 percent compliant in the chamomile group and 97.8 percent compliant in the placebo group. During phase two of the trial, seven subjects in the chamomile group and twelve in the placebo group relapsed; the mean time for relapse was 11.4 weeks in the chamomile group and 6.3 weeks in the placebo group. Though this difference was clinically important, it did not reach statistical significance. However, there were other notable outcomes. Compared to the subjects taking the placebo, those on chamomile had a smaller increase in anxiety symptoms, and they had an overall better psychological well-being. And, the long-term use of 1,500 mg per day of chamomile appeared to be safe. The most frequent adverse event was nausea, but that occurred in only three subjects in the chamomile group. The researchers concluded that their "promising long-term results need to be confirmed in a well-powered multicenter clinical trial."[3]

Chamomile Tea May Be Useful for Anxiety in Women Giving Birth to a Live Child for the First Time

In a randomized trial published in the *International Journal of Biology, Pharmacy and Allied Sciences*, researchers from Iran tested the ability of chamomile essential oil to reduce the level of anxiety in nulliparous women (women giving birth to their first live child). The cohort consisted of 130 nulliparous women: 65 were placed in the intervention group and 65 in the control group. At baseline, there were no significant differences between the women in both groups. After completing a questionnaire and measuring anxiety levels, the researchers determined that the women in both groups had moderate levels of anxiety. Then, from a distance of 7 to 10 cm, the women in the intervention group inhaled two drops of chamomile essential oil, and the women in the control group inhaled distilled water. This process was repeated periodically until the end of labor. During the last stage of labor, most of the women in the intervention group had mild anxiety and a smaller number had moderate anxiety. Meanwhile, during the same time, most of the women in the control group had severe anxiety and a smaller number had moderate anxiety. No one had mild anxiety. The researchers advised the increased use of chamomile essential oil during labor. "Since it is a low-cost and low-complication procedure, and due to availability in Iran, its use is recommended to pregnant women in order to reduce anxiety during childbirth."[4]

Aromatherapy Massage with Chamomile and Lavender Oil Eases the Anxiety and Sleep Quality of Patients with Burns, but So Does Massage Without These Oils

In a quasi-experimental trial published in the journal *Burns*, researchers from Iran wanted to determine if aromatherapy massage with chamomile and lavender oils would help adult burn patients deal with anxiety. Levels of anxiety were assessed with the Persian version of Spielberger's State Anxiety Index. The initial cohort consisted of 105 patients, mostly male; they were placed in one of three groups with similar demographic characteristics, and they tended to have moderate-to-high levels of state anxiety (anxiety caused by an anxiety-provoking situation). Thirty-five subjects had aromatherapy massage with chamomile and lavender oils, thirty-five had massage with baby oil, a placebo oil, and thirty-five were controls. The intervention subjects received three twenty-minute massages in a single week; each massage was given between 6:00 and 8:00 pm. The control subjects received daily routine care. The amounts of oil and massage technique were the same for the two massage groups. The final analyses included thirty-four subjects in the intervention group, thirty-three in the placebo group, and thirty-three in the control group. The researchers learned that the subjects in the two massage groups experienced reductions in anxiety. "The use of aromatherapy massage with lavender and chamomile oil and also massage by itself (using baby oil) was effective in reducing the anxiety of burn survivors."[5]

Kava Kava May or May Not Help Generalized Anxiety Disorder

In a five-week, randomized, prospective, placebo-controlled, double-blind trial published in the journal *Psychopharmacology*, researchers from Germany tested the ability of WS° 1490, a kava kava extract, to ease "moderately severe anxiety disorders of non-psychotic origin." The cohort consisted of forty subjects; there were twenty-five males and fifteen females with an average age of forty years. The most frequent cause of anxiety was generalized anxiety disorder; thirteen subjects had that disorder. That was followed by social phobia and simple phobia. Twenty subjects were placed in the treatment group and twenty in the placebo group. Though the kava kava dose began at 50 mg per day, it was quickly raised to 300 mg per day. At baseline, the groups had similar demographic characteristics, and they all had taken a benzodiazepine for at least forty-five weeks. During the first two weeks of the trial, the benzodiazepine medication was first tapered and then stopped. Because of benzodiazepine withdrawal problems, three subjects failed to complete the trial, and there were fifteen reported adverse events. Assessments were conducted with the Hamilton Anxiety Scale and a subjective well-being scale. The researchers learned that the subjects taking kava kava began to improve during their first week of supplementation, and by the end of the trial, their improvement was significantly better than those taking the placebo. The researchers concluded that "WS° 1490 can thus be recommended as an efficacious and safe replacement for benzodiazepines in the treatment of anxiety disorders."[6]

In a sixteen-week, randomized, two-arm, double-blind, multisite, placebo-controlled study published in the *Australian & New Zealand Journal of Psychiatry*, researchers from Australia and Canada examined the efficacy and safety of the longer term use of kava kava for generalized anxiety disorder. The initial cohort consisted of 171 non-medicated subjects with generalized anxiety disorder; eighty-six subjects were placed on kava kava (standardized to 120 mg of kavalactones twice/day) and eighty-five took a placebo. At baseline, the groups had similar demographic characteristics. During the trial, thirty-six subjects in the kava kava group and twenty-three in the placebo group had memory problems, and thirteen in the kava group and four in the placebo group had tremors or shakiness. By the end of the study, almost one-quarter of those in the kava kava group had abnormal liver function tests, while those in the placebo group had a third that rate. Unfortunately, only forty-six subjects in the kava kava group and forty-five in the placebo group completed the trial. Still, the results were notable. The kava kava supplement was less effective than the placebo in improving the symptoms of generalized anxiety disorder. While 43 percent of the subjects in the placebo group responded, only 28 percent of those in the kava kava group responded. The researchers concluded that kava kava was "not effective as a psychotropic medication for diagnosed GAD."[7]

Current Evidence Supports the Use of Kava Kava Only for Anxiety and St. John's Wort Only for Depression

In a systematic review published in the *Journal of Alternative and Complementary Medicine*, researchers from Australia noted that kava kava and St. John's wort are both commonly used for the treatment of anxiety and depression. Hoping to determine if those herbs are actually useful for those medical problems, they conducted a comprehensive review of relevant studies. The researchers found that almost all of the studies found that kava kava alleviated the symptoms of generalized anxiety disorder. However, they could not find any evidence that it was useful for obsessive-compulsive disorder, post-traumatic stress disorder, specific phobias, or depression. As for safety, kava has been linked to liver damage. That is why a number of countries have banned or issued warnings about the herb. The authors advised the removal of kava kava from over-the-counter use so that it may be standardized and better controlled by health professionals. While St. John's wort is one of the most widely used antidepressant agents, the researchers found conflicting results. Still, they noted that it appears to be helpful for mild to moderate depression but not for other depressive disorders, such as seasonal affective disorder and other mood disorders. They concluded that "current evidence for herbal medicine in the treatment of depression and anxiety only supports the use of *Hypericum perforatum* (St. John's wort) for depression and *Piper methysticum* (kava kava) for generalized anxiety."[8]

Lavender May Help Anxiety in Postmenopausal Women

In a triple-blind, randomized, controlled trial published in the journal *Complementary Therapies in Clinical Practice*, researchers from Iran studied the use of lavender and bitter orange for anxiety in postmenopausal women. The cohort consisted of 156 postmenopausal women between the ages of forty-nine and sixty years. They were divided into three groups of fifty-two. For eight weeks, one group of women took 500 mg lavender, twice daily; one took 500 mg per day of bitter orange, twice daily; and the third group took a 500 mg starch placebo, twice daily. A socio-demographic questionnaire and the Spielberger's State-Trait Anxiety Inventory were completed at baseline and at the end of the trial. The women in all three groups had similar demographic characteristics, except the women in the placebo group were the youngest. The researchers learned that 83.7 percent of the women in the lavender group, 83.4 percent of the women in the bitter orange group, and 43.8 percent of the women in the control group had "good" improvements in anxiety. At the same time, 73.5 percent of the women in the lavender group, 79.2 percent of the women in the bitter orange group, and 31.3 percent of the women in the control group reported the "highest satisfaction." The researchers concluded that lavender and bitter orange "can be used to decrease anxiety in postmenopausal women."[9]

Any Type of Lavender Seems to Be Useful for Anxiety

In a systematic review and meta-analysis published in the journal *Asian Nursing Research*, researchers from Korea examined the use of lavender for the ability to relieve anxiety, depression, and physiological factors. The lavender was administered by inhalation, massage, or in an oral preparation. The studies included thirty-eight randomized controlled trials for their qualitative analyses and thirty-seven for their quantitative synthesis. Seventeen trials were from Iran, eight from Turkey, four from Germany, three from Taiwan, two from Korea, and one each from Greece, India, Thailand, and the United States. For anxiety, a total of 3,906 subjects were randomized and 3,825 were analyzed. The subjects with anxiety included patients undergoing surgery or an invasive procedure, critically ill patients with cardiac diseases or in intensive care units, healthy students dealing with stressful situations, pregnant or postpartum women, and people with anxiety and/or depressive disorders. The subjects in the control groups received standard care, placebo, or no treatment. The researchers learned that lavender was better than controls in reducing self-rated anxiety in diverse populations. While inhalation, massage, and oral administration were all effective means of anxiety reduction, lavender aromatherapy seemed to be the most useful.[10]

Passionflower Appears Useful for Generalized Anxiety Disorder

In a randomized, double-blind, controlled trial published in the *Journal of Clinical Pharmacy and Therapeutics*, researchers from Iran evaluated the ability of passionflower and oxazepam, a benzodiazepine, to ease the symptoms of generalized anxiety disorder. The initial cohort consisted of twenty women and sixteen men between the ages of nineteen and forty-seven years who had been diagnosed with generalized anxiety disorder. For four weeks, eighteen patients were assigned to take forty-five drops of passionflower extract per day plus placebo tablets and eighteen were assigned to take 30 mg oxazepam per day plus placebo drops. Both groups had similar demographic characteristics. Patients were assessed by a psychiatrist at the beginning of the trial and days four, seven, fourteen, twenty-one, and twenty-eight. Thirty-two patients completed the trial. The researchers determined that the levels of anxiety began to drop on day seven in the passionflower group and on day four in the oxazepam group. Although the patients in the oxazepam group experienced more "impairment of job performance," the two groups had no significant difference in side effects. The vast majority of patients had no side effects. The researchers concluded that passionflower extract "is potentially a significant improvement over benzodiazepines in the management of GAD."[11]

Passionflower and Midazolam Reduce Anxiety in Patients Undergoing Dental Extraction

In a randomized, controlled, double-blind, crossover trial published in the journal *Medicina Oral Patologia Oral y Cirugia Bucal*, researchers from Brazil compared the use of passionflower and midazolam, a benzodiazepine, for anxiety in patients undergoing two dental extractions of impacted mandibular third molars, scheduled at least fifteen to thirty days apart. The cohort consisted of forty patients; twenty-seven were female. Thirty minutes before each of the surgeries the patients received either 260 mg of passionflower or 15 mg of midazolam. When the second extraction was conducted, the patients received the alternate medication. Anxiety levels were measured during an initial consultation, during the surgeries, and during follow-up visits. The researchers learned that while passionflower and midazolam appeared to be equally effective in reducing anxiety levels, the patients overwhelmingly preferred midazolam, probably because it has amnesia properties; the patients did not remember the surgical procedure. The researchers concluded that passionflower "showed an anxiolytic effect similar to midazolam and was safe and effective for conscious sedation in adult patients."[12]

Saffron May or May Not Be Useful for Anxiety

In a randomized, double-blind, single-center, placebo-controlled trial published in the *Journal of Complementary and Integrative Medicine*, researchers from Iran, China, and the UK examined the use of saffron extract for mild to moderate anxiety and depression. The cohort consisted of sixty patients between the ages of eighteen and seventy years; they were placed in one of two groups which had similar demographic profiles. For twelve weeks, the patients took either a 50 mg saffron capsule or a placebo capsule, twice daily. Patients were interviewed by a single psychiatrist at baseline and at weeks three, six, and twelve. Assessments were conducted with the Beck Anxiety Inventory and the Beck Depression Inventory. Fifty-four patients completed the trial. By the end of the trial, the differences in anxiety and depression between the two groups were statistically significant. The researchers advised the need for future studies "to investigate the exact constituent of saffron as effective agent, and the dosage required for optimum effect on anxiety and depression."[13]

In an eight-week, randomized, double-blind, placebo-controlled trial published in the *Journal of Affective Disorders*, researchers from Australia and Spain evaluated saffron for its ability to ease mild-to-moderate levels of anxiety or depression. The initial cohort consisted of eighty adolescents between the ages of thirteen and sixteen years; they were divided into two groups of forty. At baseline, both groups had similar demographic characteristics. The teens in one group took 14 mg of a standardized saffron extract (affron®) twice daily, and the teens in the other group took an identical in appearance placebo. Thirty-six teens in the saffron group and thirty-two in the placebo group completed the trial. Anxiety and depression assessments were conducted with the Revised

Child Anxiety and Depression Scale. Only one serious adverse effect occurred—nausea and stomach ache—which was reported by a subject who withdrew from the placebo group. The researchers determined that the teens believed that saffron had improved their symptoms of anxiety and depression; it was particularly helpful for separation anxiety, depression, and social phobia. From the perspective of the adolescents, their saffron treatment was associated with a decrease in internalizing symptoms of 33 percent, compared to 17 percent improvement with the placebo. Moreover, 37 percent of the teens experienced at least a 50 percent response from the saffron treatment, compared to only 11 percent from the placebo. "However, these beneficial effects were inconsistently corroborated by parental observations."[14]

In a twelve-week, randomized, double-blind, placebo-controlled trial published in the *Journal of Alternative and Complementary Medicine*, researchers from Iran tested the ability of saffron to help men and women undergoing coronary artery bypass grafting (CABG) with anxiety, depression, and cognition. The initial cohort consisted of seventy-six patients; at baseline, they had similar demographic characteristics. From two days before their surgeries to twelve weeks after, thirty-eight patients took 15 mg of saffron twice daily and the remaining thirty-eight took placebos. Anxiety was assessed with the Hospital Anxiety and Depression Scale. Regrettably, only twenty-three patients taking saffron and twenty-three patients taking the placebo met their first post-baseline visit, and only eighteen patients taking saffron and nineteen patients taking the placebo completed the trial. The researchers failed to find any evidence that saffron supplementation had any impact on levels of anxiety. "The results of this trial do not support the hypothesis of the potential benefits of saffron in treatment of CABG-related neuropsychiatric conditions."[15]

St. John's Wort Does Not Seem Useful for Social Phobia

In a randomized, double-blind, placebo-controlled, parallel-group, pilot trial published in the *Journal of Clinical Psychopharmacology*, researchers from Middleton, Wisconsin, studied the usefulness of St. John's wort for social phobia. The cohort consisted of nineteen men and twenty-one women with a mean age of 37.46 and a primary diagnosis of social phobia, a disorder that has lasted for at least twelve months. For twelve weeks, twenty subjects took daily doses of St. John's wort that began at 300 mg and could be increased up to 1,800 by the end of week six, and twenty subjects took a placebo. Subjects were assessed in person by the study psychiatrist at baseline and the end of weeks four, eight, and twelve. Thirty-one adverse events were reported by fourteen subjects in the St. John's wort group, and thirty-one were noted by thirteen subjects in the placebo group. The most common adverse events were gastrointestinal upset, upper respiratory infection, and dizziness. None of the subjects discontinued because of adverse events. Seventeen subjects in the St. John's wort group and thirteen in the placebo group completed the trial. Anxiety levels were measured with the Liebowitz Social Anxiety Scale; the researchers found that weeks of St. John's supplement failed to reduce levels of anxiety. By the end of the trial, neither group experienced any significant reductions in anxiety. The researchers concluded that their data failed to support the efficacy of St. John's wort for social phobia.[16]

A Combination of St. John's Wort and Valerian Appears to Be Useful for Comorbid Anxiety and Depression

In an open-label trial published in the journal *Phytomedicine*, researchers based in Germany compared the treatment of patients with comorbid depression and anxiety with St. John's wort combined with valerian extract, another anxiolytic herbal medicine used to treat insomnia and restlessness, or St. John's wort alone. The cohort consisted of 2,462 patients with mild-to-moderate depression; they were treated by 521 physicians. According to these researchers, large numbers of these patients were also dealing with anxiety. In fact, "the incidence of depressive disorders with comorbid generalized anxiety disorder is rated as being particularly high." The physicians treated these patients with either 500 mg valerian extract and 600 mg St. John's wort or 1,000 mg valerian and 600 mg St. John's wort. The physicians evaluated these patients before treatment and then three weeks and six weeks after treatment began, and the patients rated their levels of improvement on a scale ranging from "very markedly improved" to "deterioration." The physicians rated the efficacy of both combinations of treatment as very good or good in 87.2 percent of patients and poor in 1.6 percent; 83.2 percent of the patients reported a marked or very marked improvement. In 96.8 percent of the patients, tolerability was rated good or very good. The researchers concluded "that the combination of the two preparation as the basic therapy for mild to moderate depression comorbid with anxiety is effective."[17]

References and Further Readings

Akhondzadeh, S., H. R. Naghavi, M. Vazirian et al. "Passionflower in the Treatment of Generalized Anxiety: A Pilot Double-Blind Randomized Controlled Trial with Oxazepam." *Journal of Clinical Pharmacy and Therapeutics* 26 (2001): 363–7.

Dantas, Liliane-Poconé, Artur de Oliveira-Ribeiro, Liane-Maciel de Almeida-Souza, and Francisco-Carlos Groppo. "Effect of *Passiflora Incarnata* and Midazolam for Control of Anxiety in Patients Undergoing Dental Extraction." *Medicina Oral Patologia Oral y Cirugia Bucal* 22, no. 1 (January 1, 2017): e95–e101.

Farshbaf-Khalili, Azizeh, Mahin Kamalifard, and Maahsa Namadian. "Comparison of the Effect of Lavender and Bitter Orange on Anxiety in Postmenopausal Women: A Triple-Blind, Randomized, Controlled Clinical Trial." *Complementary Therapies in Clinical Practice* 31 (2018): 132–8.

Heidari-Fard, Solmaz, Sedighe Amir Ali-Akbari, Abulhasan Rafiei et al. "Investigating the Effect of Chamomile Essential oil on Reducing Anxiety in Nulliparous Women During the First Stage of Childbirth." *International Journal of Biology, Pharmacy and Allied Sciences* 6, no. 5 (2017): 828–42.

Kim, Myoungsuk, Eun Sook Nam, Yongmi Lee, and Hyun-Ju Kang. "Effects of Lavender on Anxiety, Depression, and Physiological Parameters." *Asian Nursing Research* 15 (2021): 279–90.

Kobak, Kenneth A., Leslie V. H. Taylor, Gemma Warner, and Rise Futterer. "St. John's Wort versus Placebo in Social Phobia." *Journal of Clinical Psychopharmacology* 25, no. 1 (February 2005): 51–8.

Lopresti, Adrian L., Peter D. Drummond Antonio M. Inarejos-García, and Marin Prodanov. "Affron, a Standardized Extract from Saffron (*Crocus sativus* L.) for the Treatment of Youth Anxiety and Depressive Symptoms: A Randomised, Double-Blind, Placebo-Controlled Study." *Journal of Affective Disorders* 232 (2018): 349–57.

Malsch, U. and M. Kiser. "Efficacy of Kava-Kava in the Treatment of Non-Psychotic Anxiety Following Pretreatment with Benzodiazepines." *Psychopharmacology* 157 (2001): 277–83.

Mao, Jun J., Sharon X. Xie, John R. Keefe et al. "Long-Term Chamomile (*Matricaria chamomilla* L.) Treatment for Generalized Anxiety Disorder: A Randomized Clinical Trial." *Phytomedicine* 23, no. 14 (December 15, 2016): 1735–42.

Mazidi, Mohsen, Maryam Shemshian, Seyed Hadi Mousavi et al. "A Double-Blind, Randomized and Placebo-Controlled Trial of Saffron (*Crocus sativus* L.) in the Treatment of Anxiety and Depression." *Journal of Complementary and Integrative Medicine* 13, no. 2 (June 1, 2016): 195–9.

Moazen-Zadeh, Ehsan, Seyed Hesameddin Abbasi, Hamideh Safi-Aghdam et al. "Effects of Saffron on Cognition, Anxiety, and Depression in Patients Undergoing Coronary Artery Bypasss Grafting: A Randomized Double-Blind Placebo-Controlled Trial." *Journal of Alternative and Complementary Medicine* 24, no. 4 (2018): 361–8.

Müller, Diethard, T. Pfeil, and V. von den Driesch. "Treating Depression Comorbid with Anxiety—Results of an Open, Practice-Oriented Study with St. John's Wort WS 5572 and Valerian Extract in High Doses." *Phytomedicine* No. 10 Supplement 4 (2003): 25–30.

Rafit, Forough, Farzaneh Ameri, Hamid Haghani, and Ali Ghobadi. "The Effect of Aromatherapy Massage with Lavender and Chamomile Oil on Anxiety and Sleep Quality of Patients with Burns." *Burns* 46 (2020): 164–71.

Sarris, Jerome and David J. Kavanagh. "Kava and St. John's Wort: Current Evidence for Use in Mood and Anxiety Disorders." *Journal of Alternative and Complementary Medicine* 15, no. 8 (2009): 827–36.

Sarris, Jerome, Gerard J. Byrne, Chand A. Bousman et al. "Kava for Generalised Anxiety Disorder: A 16-Week Double-Blind, Randomised, Placebo-Controlled Study." *Australian & New Zealand Journal of Psychiatry* 53, no. 3 (March 2020): 288–97.

Hydroxyzine

Introduction

Hydroxyzine is an antihistamine that competes with histamine for receptor sites, blocking the effects of histamine, a substance released by the body during an allergic reaction. While most antihistamines are available over the counter, hydroxyzine is sold only by prescription. It was approved decades ago by the Food and Drug Administration for three primary uses in adults and children—relief of the symptoms associated with anxiety, sedation before surgery, and the itchiness caused by skin conditions, such as atopic dermatitis. Other off-label uses of hydroxyzine include nausea and vomiting. Hydroxyzine is sold as hydroxyzine hydrocholoride (HCL) or hydroxyzine pamoate. Hydroxyzine pamoate is also sold under the brand name Vistaril.

In addition to being an antihistamine, hydroxyzine is a serotonin antagonist. It works like a selective serotonin reuptake inhibitor (SSRI); it stops serotonin from being reabsorbed into the brain's nerves or neurons, thus making more serotonin available in the brain. Serotonin plays a key role in lowering anxiety and balancing mood.

While some types of anti-anxiety medications take weeks to begin working, people taking hydroxyzine tend to see results quickly. Instead of weeks, relief may be felt in a few hours.

Regulation, Administration, and Costs

Like all prescription medications, hydroxyzine is regulated by the Food and Drug Administration. For anxiety, hydroxyzine HCL is sold in 10 mg, 25 mg, or 50 mg tablets and 10 mg/5 ml syrup; hydroxyzine pamoate is sold as 25 mg, 50 mg, or 100 mg capsules. Normally, hydroxyzine is taken three or four times per day (25 to 50 mg per dose) with or without food. The maximum daily dose for adults is usually 100 mg; health providers decide the proper dose for children. People with more sensitive stomachs may prefer to take it with food. Obviously, children on this medication will tend to be prescribed lower doses than most adults. Hydroxyzine is an inexpensive medicine, averaging about ten dollars per month; it should be covered by most health insurance.

Side Effects and Risks

Common side effects of hydroxyzine include blurred vision, confusion, dizziness, drowsiness, fatigue, irritability, dry mouth, headache, sexual problems, urinary retention, and constipation primarily in older adults. More serious side effects and risks include allergic reactions such as difficulty breathing, hives, and swelling of the lips, tongue, or face, confusion especially in older adults, increased heart rate, abnormal or irregular heartbeat, low blood pressure, and/or hallucinations. It is recommended that people taking hydroxyzine avoid alcohol, which may decrease the benefits of this medication and increase the risk of side effects. The symptoms of an overdose include many of the previously noted side effects and risks as well as decreased coordination, slowed reflexes, seizures, and coma. People who may have overdosed should seek emergency medical care. Hydroxyzine may also interact with a wide variety of other medications. To help reduce the chances of such an interaction, be sure to share a list of all medications and supplements with healthcare providers. Hydroxyzine should not be taken during the first trimester of pregnancy, and it should not be used during labor when it may harm the newborn. Because it may pass into breast milk and cause serious harm to a baby, nursing moms should not use this medicine or bottle feed their babies. Certain other people also should probably avoid this medication. These include the elderly, people with dementia or heart rhythm, liver, or kidney problems, and people who have low blood pressure or are dealing with convulsions and seizures.

Research Findings

Hydroxyzine Appears to Reduce the Anxiety Levels of People Dealing with Generalized Anxiety Disorder

In a multicenter, double-blind, placebo-controlled trial published in the journal *Human Psychopharmacology*, researchers from Belgium and France evaluated the ability of hydroxyzine to ease the symptoms of generalized anxiety disorder.

The trial was conducted in three geographic areas—north Paris, south France, and Dijon. The initial cohort consisted of 124 outpatients who had been dealing with generalized anxiety disorder for at least six months. For four weeks, sixty patients took 50 mg per day of hydroxyzine and sixty-four took a placebo. Patients were assessed four times—at baseline, after one week of treatment, after four weeks of treatment, and one week after stopping the therapy. Several scales were used to assess levels of anxiety including the Hamilton Anxiety Rating Scale. The final analyses included 110 patients—56 in the hydroxyzine group and 56 in the placebo group. The researchers learned that hydroxyzine is significantly more effective than placebo for the short-term control of GAD. Treatment-related adverse events were reported by fifty-two patients in the hydroxyzine group and twenty-two in the placebo group. These included sleepiness, dry mouth, weight gain, insomnia, and nervousness. Only three patients withdrew from the trial because of adverse events. The researchers concluded that their findings "confirmed the short-term anxiolytic efficacy of hydroxyzine under general practice conditions which are likely to be applicable to the majority of patients who present with generalized anxiety."[1]

In a sixty-two center, double-blind trial published in the journal *Psychopharmacology*, researchers from the UK and France compared the ability of hydroxyzine and buspirone to reduce levels of GAD. The cohort consisted of 244 patients with GAD; 70 percent of the patients were female, and the mean age for the cohort was forty-one years. For four weeks, they were treated with 50 mg hydroxyzine per day ($n = 81$) or 20 mg buspirone per day ($n = 82$) or a placebo ($n = 81$). Assessments with the Hamilton Anxiety Scale were conducted before, during, and after completion of the trial. Thirty-one patients did not complete the trial—ten in each of the interventions groups and eleven in the placebo group. A notable 39.5 percent of the hydroxyzine group reported one or more side effects; the most common side effect in the hydroxyzine group was somnolence (drowsiness), with about 10 percent rereporting this problem. The researchers found that during treatment 42 percent of the patients taking hydroxyzine and 36 percent on buspirone halved their Hamilton Anxiety Scale scores. Those on the placebo had a less impressive 29 percent. So, more patients improved on hydroxyzine than buspirone, and both treatments had better improvement than the placebo. The researchers concluded that hydroxyzine is likely to be proven an effective treatment for GAD, and it offers a "safer alternative to the benzodiazepines."[2]

In an eighteen-week, randomized, placebo-controlled, multicenter, parallel, double-blind trial published in the *Journal of Clinical Psychiatry*, researchers from France compared the use of 50 mg per day of hydroxyzine to 6 mg per day of bromazepam, a benzodiazepine, for the treatment of GAD. The cohort consisted of 334 patients with GAD, and, under the supervision of psychiatrists, 89 French general practitioners conducted the trial. For twelve weeks, 105 patients took hydroxyzine, 116 took bromazepam, a frequently used medication that is not currently available in the United States, and 113 took a placebo. The demographic characteristics of the groups were similar. Thus, the hydroxyzine group had a mean age of 43.6 years; the bromazepam group had a mean age of 44.9, and the placebo group had a mean age of 41.5 years. Each of the groups had about twice as many women as men. Before, during, and after the administration of the three interventions, patients visited the clinics multiple times. They also took a placebo for two weeks before and four weeks after the medications. The Hamilton Rating Scale was the primary tool used to assess the usefulness of the interventions. Fifty-six patients did not complete the trial—seventeen each in the medication groups and twenty-two in the placebo group. In the hydroxyzine group, drowsiness was the most frequent treatment-related adverse event. The researchers learned that hydroxyzine was an effective medication for the relief of GAD, and the results were statistically significant. "Its efficacy appeared progressively over time and was maintained up to day 84."[3]

Hydroxyzine Did Not Appear to Lower the Anxiety Levels of Patients Suffering from Pain

In a randomized, double-blind, controlled group trial published in the *American Journal of Emergency Medicine*, researchers based in France examined the ability of hydroxyzine to lower the anxiety levels of prehospital patients dealing with severe traumatic acute pain. The initial cohort consisted of 140 adult patients; they were divided into two groups with similar demographic characteristics. Seventy patients were treated with morphine and hydroxyzine, and seventy were treated with morphine and a placebo. The treatments were all administered in mobile intensive care units. (These units, which provide advanced life support services, are used throughout France.) Levels of anxiety were measured with the Face Anxiety Scale. Patients in the placebo group had more adverse events than those in the treatment group. For example, they had more than three times the rate of nausea as those in the hydroxyzine group. But, the adverse events were all mild to moderate. One person in the hydroxyzine group could not be included in the analyses. Although the researchers had hypothesized that the addition of hydroxyzine would reduce levels of anxiety more than a placebo, their findings failed to support this belief. The "addition of hydroxyzine to morphine in the prehospital setting did not reduce pain or anxiety in patients with severe pain."[4]

Hydroxyzine May Not Reduce Preoperative Anxiety

In a randomized, double-blind, controlled trial published in the journal *BioMed Research International*, researchers from Spain investigated the use of hydroxyzine to control preoperative anxiety in 127 boys and 41 girls between the ages of 2 and 16 years; they had a mean age of 7.4 years. A total of 165 major surgery interventions were analyzed. The children were initially divided into four groups. The first group took 2 mg/kg hydroxyzine in juice at least thirty minutes before surgery, and the children in the second group had only juice. The breakout of the Covid-19 pandemic forced the early ending of the study and prevented the completion of the remaining two groups, which added the presence of clowns to the protocols of the first two groups. Though the types of surgeries varied, they were all outpatient procedures. Anxiety levels were determined using a modified Yale scale specifically designed to measure preoperative anxiety. The researchers learned that hydroxyzine alone did not reduce levels of presurgical anxiety. However, the hydroxyzine as well as the presence of the parents and clowns appeared to be the most effective way to reduce the increasing levels of preoperative anxiety.[5]

In a double-blind, randomized, prospective controlled trial published in the *South African Medical Journal*, researchers from Johannesburg, South Africa, compared the administration of hydroxyzine and a placebo to anxious patients who are about to have gynecological surgery under general anesthesia. The cohort consisted of sixty female patients between the ages of twenty and sixty years. They were evenly placed in one of two groups; at baseline, there were no significant demographic differences between the groups. The women in one group received, depending upon their weight, either 50 or 100 mg hydroxyzine plus thiamine (vitamin B1) and the women in the other group received only thiamine. The average time interval between administration of the premedication and induction of anesthesia was 72.2 minutes. Anxiety levels were assessed with a visual analog scale the night before surgery, just before premedication, and at induction of anesthesia. The grading of the patients' anxiety levels was consistently higher than the patients own grading. In fact, throughout the preoperative period, seven patients in the hydroxyzine group and eight in the placebo group denied any anxiety. The researchers found that the preadministration of hydroxyzine did not lower anxiety levels in the women. Anxiety levels in both groups were not reduced by either hydroxyzine or thiamine. The researchers concluded that "hydroxyzine offers no significant advantage over a placebo in providing anxiolysis in the pre-operative period."[6]

Lorazepam and Midozolam Appear to Be Better Choices Than Hydroxyzine as a Surgical Premedicant

In a double-blind, placebo-controlled trial published in the journal *Anesthesia & Analgesia*, researchers based in Phoenix, Arizona, tested the efficacy and safety of hydroxyzine and lorazepam (Xanex) as a presurgery treatment. Before a surgical procedure, ninety patients were given either up to 100 mg of hydroxyzine or up to 4 mg lorazepam or 1 ml of normal saline; each group had thirty patients. One hour later, the patients given either medication were significantly more sedated that the patients given saline. Anxiety scores were low, and there was no significant difference between the two treated groups. Although not statistically significant, as further assessments were made, the patients in the lorazepam group were consistently more sedated than those in the hydroxyzine group, and they had less recall of the presurgical events. So, the patients on lorazepam were more satisfied with their overall experience. That is why the researchers recommended the use of lorazepam rather than hydroxyzine as a presurgery medicant. "The advantages of a longer duration of sedative effect, a greater effect on recall, and higher patient acceptance favor the use of lorazepam over hydroxyzine for surgical premedication."[7]

In a trial published in the *Journal of Anaesthesiology Clinical Pharmacology*, researchers from India wanted to learn if the benzodiazepine midazolam was superior to hydroxyzine and triclofos, a sedative, as a premedicant in children. The cohort consisted of sixty children, between the ages of two and eight years, who were scheduled for elective lower abdominal surgery. The children were evenly divided into three groups that were demographically similar; sixty minutes before surgery, after preparation by the anesthesiologist, parents gave their children 0.5 mg/kg midazolam or 0.5 mg/kg hydroxyzine or 75 mg/ kg triclofos. After administration, children and their parents relaxed in an undisturbed area. Assessments were conducted on the acceptability of drugs, level of sedation, and anxiety during separation and mask application. While 95 percent of the children in the other two groups remained sleepy and calm, only 65 percent in the hydroxyzine group had a similar response. And, though none of the children in the midazolam group and 5 percent of those in the triclofos group were combative or crying when the mask was placed on the face,

20 percent of those in the hydroxyzine group were combative and crying during mask application. Only one child in the hydroxyzine group complained of a dry mouth. The researcher concluded that "hydroxyzine did not prove to be as good a premedicant."[8]

Hydroxyzine May Reduce Anxiety Levels of Pediatric Dental Patients

In a retrospective study of the dental records and questionnaires published in the journal *European Archives of Paediatric Dentistry*, researchers based in of France evaluated the use of hydroxyzine to ease the anxiety of children prior to a single session of dental treatment. The children had an average age of 6.8 years; there were slightly more males than females. The average hydroxyzine dose was 1.63 mg/kg, and the medication compliance reached 85.9 percent. During an initial appointment, patients were instructed to take 1 to 2 mg/kg of hydroxyzine ninety minutes before their next scheduled appointment when their dental procedure would be performed. Of the more than 2,000 children who had treatment during the period studied, 210 (9.2 percent) were given a prescription for hydroxyzine. The dental procedures performed included restorations of permanent or deciduous teeth (first teeth or "baby teeth"), endodontic treatment of deciduous teeth, and extraction of permanent or deciduous teeth. Levels of anxiety were measured with the Venham's Clinical Anxiety Rating Scale. The final analyses included 184 children. In most cases, a notable 78.3 percent, the procedures were a success, and no adverse effects were observed. There were no overdoses or inappropriate uses of the hydroxyzine. The researchers learned that the children who were more anxious were more likely to have a therapeutic failure. The anxiety scores of the children with failed procedures were three times greater than the anxiety levels of the children who had successful procedures. The younger children were more difficult to treat than the older children. The researchers concluded that "conscious sedation with hydroxyzine following the maximum dosage recommendation for monotherapy is a good alternative for anxiety management during dental treatment."[9]

There Is Preliminary Evidence That Hydroxyzine May Be Useful for the Acute Exacerbation of Panic Disorder

In a case report published in the journal *Primary Care Companion for CNS Disorders*, researchers from Virginia described a 25-year-old man with a history of panic disorder. He arrived at an emergency department in Virginia complaining of chest pain, tachycardia, palpitations, hyperventilation, shortness of breath, sweating, nausea, and vomiting. In addition, he reported a sense of doom and the constant fear of having a panic attack; during the previous week, he had panic attacks three or four times per day. It was quickly determined that he did not have a myocardial infarction, and the blood tests were inconclusive. About a year ago, the man was placed on 40 mg per day of paroxetine (Paxil); after six months, that medicine was discontinued, and he began taking 75 mg per day of venlafaxine. Single and employed, he smoked a half pack of cigarettes each day but had no history of alcohol or drug abuse. Upon admission to the hospital's acute psychiatry unit, the man was placed on 25 mg hydroxyzine three times per day. The man promptly improved and had no panic attacks during his three-day hospital stay and at a one-month follow-up. The researchers commented that "an acute exacerbation of panic disorder was effectively managed by hydroxyzine in a healthy adult."[10]

There May Be an Association Between Hydroxyzine and the Long-Term Neurodevelopment of Young Children

In a population-based retrospective observational study published in the journal *Frontiers in Psychiatry*, researchers from Canada and Austria investigated the safety of the use of hydroxyzine in children under the age of five years. The researchers used 1997 to 2018 data on British Columbian children who were prescribed medications that act on the central nervous system. Focusing on psychotropic drug prescriptions in children five years of age or younger, the researchers soon learned that a liquid form of hydroxyzine was the most common medicine used on these young children. Most of the prescriptions were for hydroxyzine HCL 10 mg/5 ml oral solution. For each identified child, hydroxyzine prescription patterns were followed from birth through five years. Longitudinal patterns were noted for patients receiving one (short-term user), two to four (intermediate user), or more than four prescriptions (long-term user). After tracking the frequency of specific psychological and neuropsychiatric disorders, the researchers learned that a total of 24,371 children had been prescribed hydroxyzine; of these, 49.6 percent were prescribed before the age of two years. The vast majority, 70.7 percent, were given this prescription only once. Slightly less than 1,500 were given the medicine more than four times, and the remaining children received this prescription between two and four times.

The most frequent hydroxyzine users had an average of nine prescriptions, corresponding to a maximum exposure of 8.5 grams. The researchers determined that up to the age of ten, the more the children were exposed to hydroxyzine, the greater the incidence of tics, anxiety, and disturbances of conduct. The researchers concluded that they "found an association between the prevalence of mental disorders and the frequency of hydroxyzine prescription in preschool-age children." There is a need for the safety of hydroxyzine to be "reassessed," and "it should be provided for a limited duration only."[11]

References and Further Readings

Aleo, Esther, Amanda López Picado, Belén Joyanes Abancens et al. "Evaluation of the Effect of Hydroxyzine on Preoperative Anxiety and Anesthetic Adequacy in Children: Double Blind Randomized Clinical Trial." *BioMed Research International* (November 11, 2021): 7394042.

Boon, J. H. and D. Hopkins. "Hydroxyzine Premedication—Does It Provide Better Anxiolysis Than a Placebo?" *SAMJ* 86, no. 6 (June 1996): 661–4.

Chaudhary, Sujata, Reena Jindal, Gautam Girota et al. "Is Midzolam Superior to Triclofos and Hydroxyzine as Premedicant in Children?" *Journal of Anaesthiology Clinical Pharmacology* 30, no. 1 (January 2014): 53–8.

Darcis, T., M. Ferreri, J. Natens et al. "A Multicentre Double-Blind Placebo-Controlled Study Investigating the Anxiolytic Efficacy of Hydroxyzine in Patients with Generalized Anxiety." *Human Psychopharmacology* 10 (1995): 181–7.

Gober, Hans J., Kathy H. Li, Kevin Yan et al. "Hydroxyzine Use in Preschool Children and Its Effect on Neurodevelopment: A Population-Based Longitudinal Study." *Frontiers in Psychiatry* 12 (January 2022): Article 721875.

Houze-Cerfon, Charles-Henri, Frédéric Balen, Vanessa Houze-Cerfon et al. "Hydroxyzine Study." *American Journal of Emergency Medicine* 50 (December 2021): 753–7: 40.

Iskander, Joseph W., Benjamin Griffeth, and Christian Rubio-Cespedes. "Successful Treatment with Hydroxyzine of Acute Exacerbation of Panic Disorder in a Healthy Male: A Case Report." *Primary Care Companion for CNS Disorders* 13, no. 3 (2011): PCC.10l01126.

Lader, Malxolm and Jean-Claude Scotto. "A Multicentre Double-Blind Comparison of Hydroxyzine, Buspirone and Placebo in Patients with Generalized Anxiety Disorder." *Psychopharmacology* 139 (1998): 402–6.

Llorca, Pierre-Michel, Christian Spadone, Oliver Sol et al. "Efficacy and Safety of Hydroxyzine in the Treatment of Generalized Anxiety Disorder: A 3-Month Double-Blind Study." *Journal of Clinical Psychiatry* 63, no. 11 (2002): 1020–7.

Pouliquen, A., E. Boyer, J-L Sixou et al. "Oral Sedation in Dentistry: Evaluation of Professional Practice of Oral Hydroxyzine in the University Hospital of Rennes, France." *European Archives of Paediatric Dentistry* 22, no. 5 (October 2021): 801–11.

Wallace, George and Leonard J. Mindlin. "A Controlled Double-Blind Comparison of. Intramuscular Lorazepam and Hydroxyzine as Surgical Premedicants." *Anesthesia & Analgesia* 63 (1984): 571–6.

Hypnosis

Introduction

Also known as hypnotherapy, hypnosis is a trance-like mental state in which people experience heightened levels of attention, concentration, and suggestibility. Though hypnosis is frequently portrayed on big and small screens as "sleep-like," it is a state of hyperawareness and intense focusing. People are so engaged that they block out other distractions; they remain aware and do not lose control. Hypnosis has repeatedly been shown to have therapeutic properties for a host of different medical problems, including pain, irritable bowel syndrome and other gastrointestinal disorders, attention deficit hyperactivity disorder, asthma, dementia, nausea and vomiting from chemotherapy, and anxiety.

Though it is not completely clear how hypnosis works, it is known that it begins by quieting the conscious mind and taps into those parts of the brain where thoughts, beliefs, memory, and behaviors originate. In this state, the mind is more amenable to gentle guidance from the hypnotherapist.

While hypnotic-like trances have been used for thousands of years, they may be directly traced to a late eighteenth-century physician named Franz Mesmer. In the late nineteenth century Jean-Martin Charcot used it to treat women with "hysteria." His work is thought to have influenced Sigmund Freud.

Only a relatively small percentage of people—between 10 and 15 percent—are very responsive to hypnosis. People who are easily drawn into the world of fantasies are more susceptible, as are children. It may be challenging or impossible to hypnotize about 10 percent of adults.

Regulation, Administration, and Costs

There are no national regulations for hypnosis, and regulations vary from state to state; many states have no regulations. When searching for a therapist, try to locate a professional with good credentials and experience, especially in treating anxiety. There are many locations for hypnosis training; obviously, some are better than others. Search for a medical provider or psychotherapist with hypnosis training. Check to see if the potential candidate has been certified by the American Society of Clinical Hypnosis. Their program is open to health professionals with at least a master's degree; it requires forty hours of approved workshop training, twenty hours of individual training, and two years of practice in clinical hypnosis.

During a hypnosis session, which will probably be held in an office or online, the therapist will guide the patient/client through four stages. During the first stage, induction, the patient/client breathes deeply and relaxes muscles; during the second stage, deepener, the levels of relaxation deepen. The third stage, suggestions, is devoted to conveying a message that promotes improvements in the problem being addressed. During the last stage, emergence, the therapist guides the patients/client back, thus ending the session. There is no typical length to a hypnosis session, and the number of sessions required varies according to the problem addressed. While mild anxiety symptoms may be treated in a few session, more serious problems probably require many more sessions. Costs vary according to a therapist's training, background, and location. So, a physician conducting a session will cost more than a social worker or nurse, and a private therapist in a large city will be more expensive than one held in a suburban community-based therapist. A less trained therapist may cost less than $100, while a physician may well cost considerably more. Insurers may or may not cover hypnosis. If cost is an important concern, check with your provider before scheduling an appointment.

Side Effects and Risks

When conducted by a training professional, hypnosis is considered a very safe treatment. However, there are reports of memory loss, which is usually limited or temporary, and false and distorted memories. Other side effects include dizziness, headache, nausea, drowsiness, anxiety, distress, or sleep problems. Hypnosis may not be safe for people with profound mental illness.

Research Findings

Hypnosis May Be Useful for the Anxiety
Associated with a Dental Extraction

In a randomly controlled trial published in the journal *Patient Education and Counseling*, researchers from Germany wanted to learn if hypnosis would alleviate the anxiety experienced by some patients during a dental extraction. The cohort consisted of 102 patients who were about to have a dental extraction; fifty-one patients were assigned to receive the usual dental extraction procedure and fifty-one received the usual procedure and hypnosis. At baseline, the groups were demographically similar, as was their pre-procedure level of anxiety. Seventy patients reported having no past use of hypnosis. Ninety percent of the patients had positive attitudes toward hypnosis, and only seven had negatives attitudes toward the practice. Prior to and during treatment, the patients in the intervention group listened to standardized hypnotic suggestions from a portable CD player. The hypnotic suggestions consisted of a series of calming instructions. After the extraction, the patients in the intervention group were "dehypnotized," and the patients in both groups were asked to rate their before and after extraction levels of anxiety on a visual analogue scale. Though the post-extraction levels of anxiety were similar, the patients listening to hypnosis had significantly lower levels of anxiety during the procedure. And, more than 75 percent of the patients in the intervention group considered their hypnosis to be pleasant, and 80 percent of them believed that it enabled them to have "fear reduction" during the extraction. The researchers concluded that "hypnosis is beneficial as an adjunct intervention to reduce anxiety in dental patients undergoing tooth extraction."[1]

In a randomized controlled trial published in the journal *European Archives of Paediatric Dentistry*, researchers from India compared the ability of hypnosis and progressive muscle relaxation to reduce the anxiety and pain associated in dental extractions in children ages eight to twelve years. The cohort, which consisted of sixty children (thirty-six males and twenty-four females) undergoing a single primary molar extraction, were placed in one of three groups of twenty—hypnosis, progressive muscle relaxation, and control. All of the children had more than mild preoperative anxiety. Each of the children undergoing hypnosis was administered a hypnosis designed specifically for children undergoing extractions. Levels of anxiety were measured before and after extractions on all the children with the Visual Anxiety Facial scale. The researchers learned that the two interventions had similar significant lowering effects on anxiety. At the same time, the children in the control group had significant increases in anxiety. The researchers observed that "hypnosis was successful in resolving anxiety and the low anxiety state continued to be maintained till the end of the procedure with a long, calming effect."[2]

Hypnosis May Help Manage Anxiety in Cognitively Impaired Older Adults

In a single center, randomized, controlled pilot trial published in the journal *Alzheimer's Research & Therapy*, researchers from a university geriatric day hospital in France examined the ability of hypnosis to reduce the anxiety of cognitively impaired adults over the age of seventy years who were undergoing scheduled lumbar punctures. The cohort consisted of fifty outpatients, with a mean age of 77.2 years; 54 percent were women. They were assigned to receive hypnosis by a nurse or psychologist hypnotherapist or placed in the usual care/ control group. At baseline, both groups had similar demographic characteristics. During the hypnosis, the therapist spoke in a calm voice and delivered a series of suggestions, which triggered progressively stronger responses from the patient. When the patient reached "a state of modified consciousness," the procedure began. As the procedure progressed, the therapist guided the patient into a deeper "trance" state. After the spinal needle was removed, the therapist guided the patient out of hypnotized state. Levels of anxiety were noted by both the provider and patient. The researchers determine that the patients in the intervention group had significantly lower levels of anxiety than the patients in the control group. None of the patients had any immediate complications. The researchers concluded that "hypnosis appeared as a safe and well-accepted method in this context."[3]

Hypnosis May Help Burn Patients with Anxiety

In a randomized, blinded, placebo-controlled trial published in the journal *Burns*, researchers from Iran evaluated the ability of hypnosis to ease pain-related anxiety, a type of "anticipatory anxiety." The cohort consisted of sixty men with burns; they were all between the ages of eighteen and fifty years, with a mean age of 30.5 years. Having passed the emergency phase, the patients were in the acute phase of treatment; they had second- or third-degree burns, most often from fire. Ninety percent had previously been hospitalized for burns. Thirty were placed in the hypnotherapy group and thirty in the control group. Pain anxiety was measured with the Burn Specific Pain Anxiety Scale. The patients in the intervention group had four hypnosis sessions, which were held every other day; the patients in the control group had four neutral hypnosis sessions held every other day. Assessments were conducted at baseline and after the second, third, and fourth sessions. The researchers determine that the patients in the hypnosis group had significantly less pain anxiety than those in the control group. And, they concluded that hypnosis is an effective anxiety reducing tool in men with burns.[4]

In a prospective, randomized trial also published in *Burns*, researchers from Belgium compared the use of hypnosis and a stress reduction strategy for controlling dressing change anxiety and pain in severely burned patients. The cohort consisted of twenty-six patients, between the ages of eighteen and sixty five years, with a total burned surface area of 10 to 29 percent; they all required a hospital stay of at least fourteen days and ventilation assistance not more than five days. Eleven patients were placed in the hypnosis group and fifteen in the stress reduction group. Anxiety levels were measured on days one, three, five, seven, eight, ten, twelve, and fourteen. During wound care on days eight and ten, one psychologist administered both type of interventions. While asking the patients to focus on a pleasant life experience, the hypnotic state was induced using eye fixation, muscle relaxation, and permissive and indirect suggestions. When the patients had a vivid recollection of this experience, the hypnotic state was considered to be reached. At that point, patients assessed their anxiety with a visual analogue scale. During the first seven days, the levels of anxiety were similar in both groups. After the interventions began, before and during wound care, the patients in the hypnosis group had significantly lower levels of anxiety. "Hypnosis gives the patient the opportunity to escape the vicious circle of anxiety and pain." Still, the psychologist observed that the pain associated with dressing changes made it difficult for patients to maintain a hypnotic state.[5]

Hypnosis Appears to Ease the Anxiety That Cancer Patients May Experience

In a systematic review and meta-analysis published in the journal *Worldviews on Evidence-Based Nursing*, researchers from Taiwan examined studies on the use of hypnosis in adults and children to reduce the anxiety seen in cancer patients. They located twenty studies that met their criteria; thirteen were randomized controlled trials, and seven were single-group studies with pre- and post-test designs. There were a total of 878 participants, with 428 receiving hypnosis; eleven studies focused on adults and nine on children and adolescents between the ages of five and twenty years. Hypnosis was delivered by therapists in ten studies, by therapists and self-hypnosis in seven studies, and by self-hypnosis in only three studies. In the ten studies with information on hypnosis duration, the sessions ranged from fifteen to sixty minutes. Anxiety levels were measured in all of the studies but with varying tools. The researchers learned that some studies reported greater reductions in anxiety than others; these were studies that originated in Europe, had procedure-related stressors, were conducted on children or with mixed gender patients, and those with patients who had hematologic malignancies. Though the duration of hypnosis did not appear to have an effect on anxiety reduction, live therapists tended to be more effective in enabling patients to reach a deeper trance than audiotape-delivered hypnosis. The researchers noted that "hypnosis can alleviate anxiety for patients with cancer, particularly children or adolescents."[6]

Hypnosis for Hot Flashes in Postmenopausal Women Lowers Levels of Anxiety

In a single-masked, randomized, controlled trial published in the *Journal of Clinical Psychology in Medical Settings*, researchers from Waco, Texas, evaluated how the use of hypnosis to treat postmenopausal women with hot flashes impacts anxiety levels. The cohort consisted of 187 postmenopausal women with a minimum of seven hot flashes per day or fifty per week. The mean age of the group was 54.6 years and 138 were white, thirty-one were African-American, and eighteen were Native American, Asian, or Hispanic. The majority had attended college and were married. Ninety-three participants were placed in the hypnosis group and ninety-four in the control group. The participants completed five weekly forty-five-minute sessions of either hypnosis or a structured attention program. In addition, those in the hypnosis group were asked to practice daily self-hypnosis. Seven weeks after the sessions ended, a follow-up visit was held. Anxiety assessments were conducted with the State-Trait Anxiety Inventory, the Hospital Anxiety and Depression Scale–Anxiety subscale, and a visual analogue scale. While the subjects in the hypnosis group consistently had greater reductions in anxiety than the subjects in the structured attention program, the differences were not as pronounced as the researchers had anticipated. The anxiety reductions in the hypnosis group continued for weeks after the sessions ended. The researchers concluded that their "data provide initial support for the use of hypnosis to reduce symptoms of anxiety among postmenopausal women."[7]

Hypnosis Appears to Be Useful in Anxiety in Patients with Chronic Obstructive Pulmonary Disease (COPD)

In a randomized, sham-controlled, crossover trial published in the *International Journal of Chronic Obstructive Pulmonary Disease*, researchers from France and

Japan investigated the use of hypnosis to relieve anxiety and dyspnea in people with chronic obstructive pulmonary disease. The cohort consisted of twenty-one patients with COPD; there were thirteen men and eight women. Each of the patients had a clinical diagnosis of COPD and dyspnea, an intense feeling of the tightening of the chest; at admission, they had a mean age of 66.2 years. During the first of two individual fifteen-minute sessions, the patients received either hypnosis or sham hypnosis; in the second session, which was held twenty-four hours later, they had the alternative treatment. The sessions were administered in an identical manner by professionals in psychology, pulmonology, and/or palliative care, who were trained in hypnotherapy. Nineteen patients completed the trial. Two minutes after each session began and when the sessions ended, anxiety scores were measured with a shortened version of the State-Trait Anxiety Inventory questionnaire. The researchers learned that while the sham sessions induced a nonsignificant reduction in anxiety, the hypnosis sessions produced a significant reduction. And, they noted that they hoped that their findings "will be a seminal step towards the development of a long-duration hypnosis complementary protocol for the management (and self-management) of chronic anxiety in COPD patients."[8]

Hypnosis Does Not Appear to Be Effective for Preventing Anxiety During a Coronary Angiography

In a prospective, randomized trial published in the journal *BMC Complementary Medicine and Therapies*, researchers from France wanted to determine if hypnosis would help the anxiety experienced by patients undergoing coronary angiography, a procedure used to diagnose coronary artery disease. The cohort consisted of 169 patients who had a planned coronary angiography. Eighty-five were placed in the hypnosis group and eighty-four in the control group. At baseline, the patients in the two groups had almost the identical levels of anxiety. Before their procedures, the patients in the hypnosis group participated in a fifteen-minute hypnosis session. The sessions were conducted by four emergency physicians, a pediatric nurse, and a nurse anesthetist; they were all trained in hypnosis. The patients in the control group had a conversational interview with one of the same hypnotherapists. State and trait anxiety were measured the day before the procedure; state anxiety was measured immediately before the procedure. Again, the anxiety levels of the patients in both groups were almost identical. Interestingly, "most patients in the hypnosis group . . . thought hypnosis was effective on them compared to the control group."[9]

Hypnosis May Be Useful for Relief of Anxiety for Patients with Severe Chronic Diseases

In a nonrandomized clinical trial published in the journal *Annals of Palliative Medicine,* researchers from Italy evaluated the ability of two years of clinical and self-hypnosis to help relieve anxiety and pain in people with severe chronic diseases. The cohort consisted of fifty patients: there were fourteen men and thirty-six women. Twenty-five patients chose to be placed in the hypnosis group and twenty-five chose to serve as controls. At baseline, the two groups had similar demographic characteristics. A slight majority of the patients had rheumatic medical problems. That was followed by neurologic and oncologic diagnoses. All of the patients attended a two-hour hypnosis workshop; after the program, anxiety levels were measured with the Hamilton Anxiety Rating Scale. Then, for two years, the patients in the hypnosis group participated in weekly anxiety and pain workshops that included hypnosis and the teaching of self-hypnosis. The patients in the control group had conventional pharmacological therapy. Though the anxiety scores for the two groups were similar at baseline, after one year, the patients in the hypnosis group had significantly lower anxiety scores than those in the control group. By the end of the second year, thirteen subjects had either died or were no longer able to participate. Still, those in the hypnosis group continued to have significant decreases in anxiety. The researchers concluded that they observed "a significant statistical decrease in reported pain and anxiety among patients with advanced diseases receiving clinical hypnosis as an adjuvant therapy."[10]

Hypnosis Did Not Appear to Reduce Anxiety in Patients in the Intensive Care Unit

In a prospective, single-center, randomized trial published in the *European Journal of Anaesthesiology,* researchers from Belgium wanted to learn if hypnosis and virtual reality would relieve the anxiety and pain of cardiac surgery patients in intensive care units. The cohort consisted of 100 patients; there were 76 men and 24 workmen with a mean age of 66 years. The patients were placed in one of four groups—hypnosis, virtual reality, hypnosis and virtual reality, and control. Hypnosis consisted of a twenty-minute prerecorded session which was created and recorded by experts in clinical and experimental hypnosis; virtual reality consisted of a twenty-minute virtual reality session which was viewed on head-mounted display goggles. Anxiety assessments were conducted before and after each session. The researchers were unable to collect data from thirty patients. The researchers determined that there were no significant anxiety differences among the four groups, and no intervention was useful for anxiety. The available treatments were all equally ineffective. The researchers concluded that the interventions "did not show any differences in effectiveness, either between the techniques themselves or between the techniques and no treatment."[11]

References and Further Readings

Abensur Vuillaume, Laura, Charles Gentilhomme, Sandrine Weber et al. "Effectiveness of Hypnosis for the Prevention of Anxiety During Coronary Angiography (HYPCOR Study): A Prospective Randomized Study." *BMC Complementary Medicine and Therapies* 22, no. 1 (November 29, 2022): 315.

Anlió, Hernán, Bertrand Herer, Agathe Delignières et al. "Hypnosis for the Management of Anxiety and Dyspnea in COPD: A Randomized, Sham-Controlled Crossover Trial." *International Journal of Chronic Obstructive Pulmonary Disease* 15 (2020): 2609–20.

Brugnoli, Maria Paola, Giancarlo Pescue, Emaniela Pasin et al. "The Role of Clinical Hypnosis and Self-Hypnosis to Relief Pain and Anxiety in Severe Chronic Diseases in Palliative Care: A Two-Year Long-Term Follow-up of Treatment in a Nonrandomized Clinical Trial." *Annals of Palliative Medicine* 7, no. 1 (January 2018): 17–31.

Chen, Pei-Ying, Ying-Mei Liu, and Mei-Ling Chen. "The Effect of Hypnosis on Anxiety in Patients with Cancer: A Meta-Analysis." *Worldviews on Evidence-Based Nursing* 14, no. 3 (June 2017): 223–36.

Courtois-Amiot, Pauline, Anaïs Cloppet-Fontaine, Aurore Poissonnet et al. "Hypnosis for Pain and Anxiety Management in Cognitively *Impair14, no. 3 June 2017 ed* Older Adults Undergoing Scheduled Lumbar Punctures: A Randomized Controlled Pilot Study." *Alzheimer's Research & Therapy* 14 (2022): 120.

Frenay, Marie-Christine, Marie-Elisabeth Faymonville, Sabine Devlieger et al. "Psychological Approaches During Dressing Changes of Burned Patients: A Prospective Randomised Study Comparing Hypnosis Against Stress Reducing Strategy." *Burns* 27 (2001): 793–9.

Glaesmer, Heide, Hendrik Geupel, and Rainer Haak. "A Controlled Trial on the Effect of Hypnosis on Dental Anxiety in Tooth Removal Patients." *Patient Education and Counseling* 98, no. 9 (September 2015): 1112–15.

Jafarizadeh, Hossein, Mojgan Lotfi, Fardin Ajoudani et al. "Hypnosis for Reduction of Background Pain and Pan Anxiety in Men with Burns: A Blinded, Randomised, Placebo-Controlled Study." *Burns* 44 (2018): 108–17.

Roberts, R. Lynae, Joshua R. Rhodes, and Gary R. Elkins. "Effect of Hypnosis on Anxiety: Results from a Randomized Controlled Trial with Women in Postmenopause." *Journal of Clinical Psychology in Medical Settings* 28 (2022): 868–81.

Rousseaux, Floriane, Nadia Dardenne, Paul B. Massion et al. "Virtual Reality and Hypnosis for Anxiety and Pain Management in Intensive Care Units." *European Journal of Anaesthesiology* 39 (2022): 58–66.

Sabherwal, P., N. Kaira, R. Tyagi et al. "Hypnosis and Progressive Muscle Relaxation for Anxiolysis and Pain Control During Extraction Procedure in 8–12-Year-Old Children: A Randomized Controlled Trial." *European Archives of Paediatric Dentistry* 22 (2021): 823–32.

Magnesium

Introduction

Magnesium is a mineral that is found in abundance in the human body. It is contained in many foods, present in several medicines, and sold as a dietary supplement. In the human body, magnesium plays a role in a host of different functions, such as protein synthesis, muscle and nerve functioning, blood glucose control, and blood pressure regulation. In addition, it is involved in the transport of calcium and potassium across cell membranes, which is important to nerve impulse conduction, muscle contractions, and maintaining normal heart rhythm. And, some contend it may play a role in managing anxiety.

How is this accomplished? In the brain, magnesium blocks the activity of stimulating neurotransmitters and binds to calming receptors, triggering feelings of relaxation. Further, magnesium helps to regulate the release of stress hormones like cortisol, calming the body's nervous system.

On average, an adult body contains about 25 grams of magnesium; more than half is in the bones and the remainder is in the soft tissues. Since less than 1 percent is found in the blood serum, measuring blood serum levels of magnesium yields little usable information. Yet, even though there is little correlation between the amount of magnesium in the body and blood serum levels, the most commonly used method for assessing the body's magnesium status is the concentration of serum magnesium. Other methods include measuring magnesium concentrations in erythrocytes (blood cells that contain hemoglobin), salvia, or urine, or measuring ionized magnesium concentrations in blood, plasma, or serum. Still another alternative is a magnesium tolerance or a test in which urinary magnesium is measured after a parenteral (injectable) infusion of a dose of magnesium.

Regulation, Administration, and Costs

Since the US Food and Drug Administration does not regulate supplements, magnesium supplements are not regulated. Magnesium supplements are sold alone or as an ingredient in multivitamin supplements or combined with other dietary supplements, such as calcium. Forms of magnesium that are more readily absorbed by the body include magnesium aspartate, magnesium citrate, magnesium lactate, and magnesium chloride. Magnesium oxide and magnesium sulfate tend not to be absorbed as well. High doses of zinc may interfere with the absorption of magnesium. Magnesium is found in some laxative products as well as in some medications for heartburn and upset stomach.

The Recommended Dietary Allowance for magnesium varies according to age and sex. From birth to six months, the recommendation is 30 mg; from seven to twelve months, it is 75 mg. From one to three years, it is 80 mg, and from four to eight years, it is 130 mg. From nine to thirteen years, it is 240 mg. Between the ages of fourteen and eighteen years, males should take in 410 mg and females 360 mg. Pregnant females should take in 400 mg, and lactating females should take in 360 mg. Between the ages of nineteen and thirty years, males should take in 400 mg, and females and lactating females should take in 310 mg. Pregnant females should take in 350 mg. Males between the ages of thirty-one and fifty years should take in 420 mg, and females and lactating females should take in 320 mg. Pregnant females should take in 360 mg. And, finally, males fifty-one years and older should take in 420 mg and females 320 mg.

Magnesium is available in many different plant and animal foods and beverages. Foods that are high in fiber tend to have very good amounts of magnesium. Other good sources are green leafy vegetables, legumes, nuts, seeds, and fortified foods such as breakfast cereals. Some foods with abundant supplies of magnesium include pumpkin seeds, chia seeds, almonds, spinach, cashews, peanuts, soymilk, black beans, and edamame.

Prices for magnesium supplements vary widely. Many are inexpensive, but they may be moderately priced or even expensive. It may be a good idea to ask a knowledgeable healthcare provider for suggestions.

Side Effects and Risks

It is relatively easy to obtain sufficient amounts of magnesium from the diet. Just a few servings a day of foods rich in magnesium should be more than adequate. However, some groups are at risk for insufficient intake. These include people with gastrointestinal diseases, such as Crohn's disease and celiac disease, people with type 2 diabetes, people with alcohol dependence, and older adults. People in these groups should make an extra effort to ensure their intake is sufficient.

On the other hand, most people should not worry about taking in too much magnesium from food. In general, the kidneys will eliminate excess amounts in the urine. High doses from supplements or medications may cause unwanted side effects such as nausea, abdominal cramping, and diarrhea. Very large doses may result in magnesium toxicity, with symptoms such as nausea, vomiting, facial flushing, retention of urine, depression, lethargy, and hypotension. These may progress to muscle weakness, difficulty breathing, extreme hypotension, irregular heartbeat, and cardiac arrest. Because they may have problems excreting magnesium, people with impaired kidney function have an increased risk of magnesium toxicity. Several types of magnesium are more likely to cause diarrhea. These include magnesium carbonate, magnesium chloride, magnesium gluconate, and magnesium oxide. And magnesium supplements may interact with several medications such as antibiotics, bisphosphonates, diuretics, and proton pump inhibitors. For example, magnesium may decrease the absorption of oral bisphosphonates, such as alendronate, that are used to treat thinning bones and may make certain antibiotics insoluble. Taking diuretics with magnesium may increase the loss of magnesium in urine, and taking magnesium and prescription proton pump inhibitors may result in hypomagnesemia, an electrolyte disturbance caused by low serum magnesium levels. Before combining magnesium with these medications, it is best to check with a medical provider.

Research Findings

Short-Term Magnesium Supplementation May Help Open-Heart Surgery Patients with Anxiety, Depression, and Sleep Quality

In a single-blinded trial published in the journal *Magnesium Research*, researchers from Iran evaluated the ability of magnesium supplementation to aid anxiety, depression, and sleep quality after open-heart surgery. The cohort consisted of sixty open-heart surgery patients; they were divided equally into the intervention group and the control group. At baseline, the two groups were similar in gender, marital status, and underlying disease. Except on the two days after surgery and a half dose on the third day, from the day of hospitalization to the day of discharge, patients in the intervention group were given 500 mg magnesium per day. The patients in the control group did not receive any magnesium supplementation. Anxiety levels were measured with the Hospital Anxiety and Depression Scale, which has seven questions that address anxiety.

By the end of the trial, the mean level of magnesium in the intervention group was significantly higher than the control group, and the levels of anxiety in the intervention group decreased and increased in the control group. And, no serious side effects were reported. The researchers concluded that "taking magnesium supplementation may thus be a valuable intervention for such patients undergoing major surgery."[1]

When Combined with Hawthorn and California Poppy, Magnesium May Be Useful for Mild to Moderate Generalized Anxiety Disorder

In a double-blind, randomized, placebo-controlled, outpatient, multicenter trial published in the journal *Current Medical Research and Opinion*, researchers from France evaluated the efficacy and safety of magnesium to treat mild to moderate generalized anxiety disorder. The cohort consisted of 264 patients, 81 percent female, with a mean age of 44.6 years, who were being treated by twenty-two nonpsychiatric physicians. The patients had suffered from anxiety for a mean of eighty-six months; their symptoms included fatigue, tension, pain or muscle pain, palpitations or tachycardia, irritability, difficulty in falling asleep or interrupted sleep, feelings of over-excitement or exhaustion. For three months, 130 patients took the combination supplement and 134 took placebos. At baseline, the two groups were comparable on the parameters being studied, especially their initial Hamilton Anxiety Scale scores. Thirty-one patients ended the trial early, primarily because they believed the supplement was ineffective (six in the intervention group and eight in the placebo group), or they experienced undesirable side effects (three in each group). While the subjects in both groups had reductions in their levels of anxiety, the improvement in the intervention group was greater. At the end of the trial, the participating physicians commented that the study drug benefits were greater than its risk for 90 percent in subjects taking the study drug and 80 percent of those taking the placebo medication. Fifteen patients in the intervention group and thirteen in the placebo group reported an adverse event. These included digestive symptoms, such as nausea and morning sluggishness. While the researchers acknowledged that the difference between the two groups was small, it still demonstrated that the medication was "an effective and safe alternative symptomatic treatment for mild-to-moderate anxiety states in clinical practice."[2]

Magnesium and Vitamin B6 May Mildly Improve Anxiety-Related Premenstrual Symptoms

In a randomized, double-blind, placebo-controlled, crossover trial published in the *Journal of Women's Health & Gender-based Medicine*, researchers from the UK compared the use of magnesium, vitamin B6, magnesium plus vitamin B6, and a placebo for the treatment of anxiety-related premenstrual symptoms in women with an average age of thirty-two years. Each woman was assigned to take one of these supplement regimes daily for an entire menstrual cycle. So, for five consecutive months, they took daily doses of one of the following five alternatives for an entire month—no study supplements, 200 mg magnesium, 50 mg vitamin B6, 200 mg magnesium and 50 mg vitamin B6, or a placebo. During this time, the women recorded their daily menstrual symptoms and provided monthly urine samples for magnesium analysis. While forty-four women began the trial, thirty-seven completed the final cycle. The researchers found that after one month of the combination of magnesium supplementation and vitamin B6, the women obtained a small amount of relief from anxiety-related premenstrual symptoms. Because the absorption of magnesium appeared to be "poor," the researchers wondered if better relief might be obtained from two or more months of this therapy. And, they concluded that "in view of the modest effect found, further studies are needed before making general recommendations for the treatment of premenstrual symptoms."[3]

Dietary Intake of Magnesium May or May Not Be Related to the Incidence of Anxiety

In a study published in the *British Journal of Nutrition*, researchers from Iran and Canada investigated the association between dietary intake of magnesium and psychological disorders, such as anxiety and depression, in a cross-sectional group of Iranian adults. The cohort consisted of 3,172 Iranian adults; there were 1,398 men and 1,774 women. The mean age of the men was 38.4 years and the women was 35.1 years. During two phases, detailed data were collected on dietary intake and psychological health. Anxiety levels were assessed with the Iranian validated version of the Hospital Anxiety and Depression Scale. The researchers determined that the higher intake of magnesium among women was associated with a lower odds of anxiety. At the same time, among women, a deficient magnesium intake was positively associated with anxiety. The researchers commented that "further prospective studies are needed to confirm our findings."[4]

In a cross-sectional trial published in the *International Journal of Human Sciences*, researchers from Turkey evaluated magnesium intake in university students and its association with anxiety, depression, and eating behaviors. The cohort consisted of 386 randomly selected university students who had not been diagnosed with any psychiatric disorder and were not using any magnesium-containing nutritional supplements; there were 191 males and 195 females with an average age of 22.2 years. Data were collected in face-to-face interviews; among the measures used was the Beck Anxiety Scale. The researchers learned that the intake of magnesium was below the recommended daily allowance level in 156 students and above that level in 230 students. While the anxiety scores were slightly higher in the students with inadequate levels of magnesium, the difference was minimal. In fact, 28.8 percent of the students who consumed inadequate amounts of magnesium and 27 percent of the students who consumed adequate amounts of magnesium had anxiety. The researchers noted that "when anxiety scores were compared according to magnesium intake levels, there was no difference between magnesium intake groups among the anxiety scores." So, there appeared to be no significant association between magnesium intake and anxiety.[5]

In a study published in the *Australian and New Zealand Journal of Psychiatry*, researchers from Australia and Norway evaluated the association between magnesium intake and anxiety and depression in a large sample of community dwelling men and women. The sample consisted of 5,708 subjects between the ages of forty-six and forty-nine or seventy to seventy-four who participated in the Hordaland Health Study in western Norway; there were 2,461 men and 3,247 women. Dietary intake was assessed with a self-administered food frequency questionnaire, originally developed at the University of Oslo. Symptoms of anxiety and depression were self-reported using the Hospital Anxiety and Depression Scale. While the researchers found a significant inverse relationship between magnesium intake and depressive symptoms, the inverse relationship between magnesium intake and anxiety symptoms was weaker and not significant.[6]

People with Primary Hyperhidrosis and Elevated Levels of Anxiety Appear to Have Low Magnesium Levels

In a cross-sectional, case-control trial published in the *Journal of Cosmetic Dermatology*, researchers from Turkey investigated the association between vitamin D, magnesium deficiency, and the risk of anxiety and depression in people with primary hyperhidrosis, or excessive sweating. The cohort consisted of forty-nine people with primary hyperhidrosis; there were twenty-nine females and twenty males with a mean age of 24.9 years. The control group had forty-seven healthy and gender-matched individuals; there were twenty-eight females and nineteen males with a mean age of 25.5 years. Levels of anxiety were measured with the Hospital Anxiety and Depression Scale. Magnesium levels were measured with blood samples. The researchers learned that the anxiety scores of the subjects with primary hyperhidrosis were 1.3 times higher than those in the control group. There was no correlation between the severity of the disease and the anxiety scores. And, the subjects with primary hyperhidrosis had significantly lower magnesium levels (and vitamin D levels) than those without this disorder. Further, the females had significantly lower levels of magnesium than the males. The researchers suggested "that a relationship may exist between the identified vitamin D and magnesium deficiency and the association between primary hyperhidrosis and anxiety."[7]

Magnesium Supplementation Does Not Appear to Relieve Postpartum Anxiety

In a triple-blind, randomized controlled clinical trial published in the journal *Women & Health*, researchers from Iran tested the effects of magnesium and zinc supplements on the symptoms of anxiety and depression in postpartum women. The cohort consisted of ninety women who had given birth within the previous forty-eight hours. The women were assigned to one of three groups, each with thirty-three subjects. The women in each of the groups had similar socio-demographic and obstetric characteristics. For eight weeks, the women in one group, with a mean age of 26.4 years, took one 32 mg magnesium sulfate tablet per day; the women in a second group, with a mean age of 29.4 years, took one 27 mg zinc sulfate tablet per day; and the women in the third group, with a mean age of 27.6 years, took a placebo. To determine serum values of magnesium and zinc, blood samples were taken at the beginning and end of the trial. At the beginning of the study, the serum levels of the three groups were similar. Both at the beginning and end of the trial, levels of anxiety were measured with the Spielberger State-Trait Anxiety Inventory and levels of depression were measured with the Edinburgh Postnatal Depression Scale. At baseline, no statistically significant differences were found between the groups in levels of anxiety or depression. Two subjects in the magnesium group and two in the zinc group failed to complete all the requirements of the study. By the end of the trial, there were still no significant differences between the groups in levels of anxiety or depression. Neither supplement appeared to have any impact on the development of postpartum and depressive symptoms in non-depressed women. The researchers recommended that future studies should focus on "different doses with longer follow-ups."[8]

There May Be an Association Between Pregnancy, Magnesium Levels, Restless Leg Syndrome, and Anxiety

In a case-control study published in the journal *Biological Trace Element Research*, researchers from Turkey examined the clinical and psychiatric causes of restless leg syndrome, a common medical problem during pregnancy. The researchers compared a number of different factors, including levels of serum calcium, magnesium, potassium, and sodium, in 134 healthy pregnant women and 119 pregnant women with restless leg syndrome, diagnosed during the second trimester. At baseline, no statistical differences were found between the groups in terms of age, gestational week, the last menstrual cycle, and body mass index (BMI). Measurements of anxiety, depression, and sleep quality were also calculated. The researchers determined that the women in the restless leg syndrome group had statistically significant lower levels of magnesium and higher levels of anxiety. In fact, there was a significant relationship between the level of anxiety severity and restless leg syndrome. In the restless leg syndrome group, 52.9 percent of the women had moderate anxiety and 16.8 percent had severe anxiety. This stands in contrast to the fact that none of the women in the control group had any symptoms of severe anxiety.[9]

Obsessive-Compulsive Disorder May Be Linked to Insufficient Levels of Several Trace Elements, Including Magnesium

In another study published in the journal *Biological Trace Element Research*, researchers from Bangladesh analyzed the relationship between magnesium, zinc, copper, manganese, iron, and calcium and obsessive-compulsive disorder. The cohort consisted of forty-eight subjects with OCD, forty-two males and six females with a mean age of 24.71 years, and forty-eight healthy controls, forty-two males and six females with a mean age of 21.33 years. They were matched for sex, age, and socioeconomic status. The subjects were evaluated with a semi-structured questionnaire. Ten milliliter blood samples were drawn from all of the subjects, and the Yale-Brown Obsessive Compulsive Scale was used to measure the severity of the illness of the subjects with OCD.

The researchers learned that the subjects with mild and moderate OCD had significantly lower levels of magnesium (and iron and zinc) than the control subjects. "This imbalance of the elemental homeostasis may play a role in the etiology of OCD."[10]

References and Further Readings

Anjom-Shoae, Javad, Omid Sadeghi, Ammar Hassanzadeh Keshteli et al. "The Association Between Dietary Intake of Magnesium and Psychiatric Disorders Among Iranian Adults: A Cross-Sectional Study." *British Journal of Nutrition* 120, no. 6 (September 2018): 693–702.

De Souza, M. C., A. F. Walker, P. A. Robinson, and K. Bolland. "A SYnergictic Effect of a Daily Supplement for 1 Month of 200 mg Magnesium Plus 50 mg Vitamin B6 for the Relief of Anxiety-Related Premenstrual Symptoms: A Randomized, Double-Blind, Crossover Study." *Journal of Women's Health & Gender-Based Medicine.*" 9 (November 2, 2000): 131–9.

Fard, F. E., M. Mirghafourvand, S. Mahammad-Alizadeh et al. "Effects of Zinc and Magnesium Supplements on Postpartum Depression and Anxiety: A Randomized Controlled Clinical Trial." *Women & Health* 57, no. 9 (2017): 1115–28.

Hanus, Michel, Jacqueline Lafon, and Marc Mathieu. "Double-Blind, Randomised, Placebo-Controlled Study to Evaluate the Efficacy and Safety of a Fixed Combination Containing Two Plant Extracts *Crataegus oxyacantha* and *Eschscholtzia californica* in Mild-to-Moderate Anxiety Disorders." *Current Medical Research and Opinion* 20, no. 1 (2004): 63–71.

Jacka, Felice N., Simon Overland, Robert Stewart et al. "Association Between Magnesium Intake and Depression and Anxiety in Community-Dwelling Adults: The Hordaland Health Study." *Australian and New Zealand Journal of Psychiatry* 43 (2009): 45–52.

Kircali Haznedar, Nagihan and Pelin Bilgiç. "Evaluation of Dietary Magnesium Intake and Its Association with Depression, Anxiety and Eating Behaviors." *International Journal of Human Sciences* 16, no. 1 (2019): 345–54.

Manav, Vildan, Cemre Büsra Türk, Asude Kara Polat et al. "Evaluation of the Serum Magnesium and Vitamin D Levels and the Risk of Anxiety in Primary Hyperhidrosis." *Journal of Cosmetic Dermatology* 21 (202): 373–9.

Saba, Sara, Fakhrudin Faizi, Mojtaba Sepandi, and Batool Nehrir. "Effect of Short-term Magnesium Supplementation on Anxiety, depression and Sleep Quality in Patients After Open-Heart Surgery." *Magnesium Research* 35, no. 2 (2022): 62–70.

Shohag, Hasanuzzaman, Ashik Ulllah, Shalahuddin Qusar et al. "Alteration of Serum Zinc, Copper, Manganese, Iron, Calcium, and Magnesium Concentrations and the Complexity of Interelement Relations in Patients with Obsessive-Compulsive Disorder." *Biological Trace Elements Research* 148 (2012): 275–80.

Yilirim, Engin and Hakan Apaydin. "Zinc and Magnesium Levels of Pregnant Women with Restless Leg Syndrome and Their Relationship with Anxiety: A Case-Control Study." *Biological Trace Element Research* 199 (20): 1674–85.

Melatonin

Introduction

Melatonin is a hormone that is naturally made in the pineal gland of the brain. With the assistance of the amino acid tryptophan, the pineal gland creates the neurotransmitter serotonin. Serotonin is then used to make melatonin. After it is produced, melatonin enters the bloodstream and cerebrospinal fluids and travels throughout the body.

Melatonin regulates circadian rhythms, the day and night wake/sleep cycles. During the day, the body produces less melatonin, which encourages wakefulness; at night, the body makes more melatonin, which signals the body to sleep. Most often, melatonin supplementation is used to help people fall asleep and stay asleep. But, people use melatonin for other conditions, such as chronic pain, jet lag, depression, dementia, and, of course, anxiety.

The body begins to make more melatonin about two hours before a person's usual bedtime. Levels peak around 3 to 4 am and then lower. Melatonin production is also affected by the seasons. When the days are shorter, more is made, and less is made when the days are longer. Certain conditions and medical problems are associated with lower levels of melatonin. These include aging, extreme pain, cancer, mood disorders, bipolar disorder, type 2 diabetes, and dementia. When melatonin levels are low, people are at increased risk for sleep problems, such as trouble falling asleep and sleep disturbances. It is not uncommon for sleep disorders to worsen anxiety, and anxiety may easily contribute to disrupted sleep and sleep disorders.

The vast majority of the studies on anxiety and melatonin focus on using melatonin to calm anxiety in patients before a surgical procedure. It is believed that melatonin increases levels of the neurotransmitter aminobutyric acid (GABA) in certain parts of the brain. Higher levels of GABA having a calming effects and reduce the symptoms of anxiety. This is beneficial for both the patient and the surgical team.

There are few, if any, studies on using melatonin for problems such as generalized anxiety disorder, obsessive-compulsive disorder, or social anxiety disorder. Since it encourages sleep and may only be used for a relatively short period of time, it is understandable why researchers would be reluctant to devote their limited research dollars to a product that has little potential widespread use for most anxiety problems.

Regulation, Administration, and Costs

The US Food and Drug Administration does not regulate supplements. As a result, there are no regulations regarding melatonin. There are two types of melatonin supplements: natural melatonin is made from the pineal gland of animals, and synthetic melatonin is manufactured. Some people caution against using the natural form which may be contaminated with a virus. While melatonin is mostly sold as pills, liquids, and gummies, it is also available as transdermal patches and rectal suppositories. A typical bedtime dose for adults generally ranges from 0.3 to 5 mg. But, recommendations go as high as 12 mg per day. It is probably better to start with a lower dose and increase the dose as needed. Childhood doses should be no more than 3 mg per day, and adolescent doses should be no more than 5 mg per day. Prices for melatonin vary from very inexpensive to moderate. Even the most costly brands are not expensive.

Side Effects and Risks

For most people, especially for the short-term use, melatonin appears to be safe. No one recommends taking this supplement for more than six months. But, melatonin has been associated with a number of different side effects including headaches, sleepiness, strange dreams or night sweats, dizziness, stomach cramps, dry mouth, irritability, agitation, and nausea. Though more serious side effects are rare, they include blurry vision or watery eyes, feeling faint or passing out, confusion, vertigo, unexplained bruising, and blood in the urine. And, after using melatonin, people are cautioned not to drive or use machinery for at least four to five hours.

However, there are many people who should probably avoid melatonin. These include women who are trying to become pregnant or already pregnant and women who are breastfeeding. There is insufficient evidence to know if it is safe during pregnancy and breastfeeding. Melatonin might increase bleeding in people with bleeding disorder and exacerbate the symptoms of depression. It may elevate blood pressure levels in people taking certain blood pressure medications and increase the risk of seizures in those with seizure disorders. Since melatonin may alter the immune functioning of the body, it should not be taken by those who have received a transplant and are on medication to suppress the immune system. As for children, melatonin is possibly safe for the short-term use in children. There is very limited evidence that melatonin may interfere with adolescent development.

Research Findings

Melatonin Appears as Useful as Midazolam for Preoperative Anxiety in People over the Age of Sixteen Years

In a trial published in the *Journal of Anaesthesiology Clinical Pharmacology*, researchers from India compared the administration of 0.4 mg/kg of oral melatonin, 0.2 mg/kg of oral midazolam, a benzodiazepine, or a placebo for preoperative anxiety, cognition, and psychomotor function. The cohort consisted of 120 patients between the ages of sixteen and fifty-five years; they were divided into three demographically similar groups of forty. Sixty to ninety minutes before their elective surgery began, they were given one of the three alternatives, which were similar in appearance. With a visual analog scale, assessments were conducted before and after surgery. There were four dropouts in the melatonin and another four in the placebo group; there were three dropouts in the midazolam group. These occurred primarily because the waiting time before surgery lasted longer than anticipated—more than ninety minutes. The researchers found no significant difference between melatonin and midazolam; they resulted in similar reductions in preoperative anxiety. Both interventions were statistically better at reducing anxiety than the placebo. Why would melatonin be a preferable choice? It "does not impair the general cognitive and psychomotor function."[1]

Melatonin May or May Not Be Useful for Children with Presurgical Anxiety

In a randomized, double-blind, placebo-controlled trial published in the *European Journal of Anaesthesiology*, researchers from Saudi Arabia and Iowa City, Iowa, compared the use of melatonin and midazolam before minor elective surgery in children. They divided 105 children between the ages of two and five into seven groups, each with fifteen children. At baseline, all of the children had similar demographic characteristics. Then, the children were assigned to take one of the following premedications—melatonin 0.1, 0.25, or 0.5 mg/kg and 15 mg/kg acetaminophen, midazolam 0.1, 0.25, or 0.5 mg/kg and 15 mg/kg acetaminophen, or acetaminophen 15 mg/kg. Assessments were conducted before and after administration of the study drug or placebo, on separation from parents, and introduction of the anesthesia mask. Two weeks after the surgery, the parents completed the Post Hospitalization Behaviour Questionnaire, which included six categories of questions on anxiety. The researchers learned that there was no difference in anxiety between the groups when the children were in the preoperative holding area. However, upon separation from the parents and the introduction of the mask, the children taking the 0.25 or 0.5 mg/kg doses of melatonin or midazolam had less anxiety than the children in the control group. The researchers commented that their findings "indicated that melatonin may be an attractive alternative to midazolam."[2]

Melatonin May or May Not Be Useful to Reduce Anxiety Before Dental Surgery

In a randomized, double-blind, prospective, clinical trial published in the *Journal of Oral and Maxillofacial Surgery*, researchers from Turkey examined the anxiolytic effects of oral melatonin and oral midazolam in patients undergoing surgery for an impacted third molar. The cohort consisted of ninety patients who had similar demographic characteristics. The patients were then placed in one of three groups. After anxiety and other assessments were conducted, thirty patients received 0.4 mg/kg oral melatonin, thirty took 0.2 mg/kg oral midazolam, and the remaining thirty were given a multivitamin. One hour later and immediately before surgery, the researchers evaluated the patients with the same tests. All of the surgeries were performed by the same surgical team. The researchers learned that the post-medication reduction in anxiety was lowest in the midazolam group. However, the differences between midazolam and melatonin were not statistically significant. The researchers commented that "patients and surgeons reported high satisfaction with the surgical process when a premedication dose of melatonin was administered, and patient recovery was rapid."[3]

In a randomized, prospective trial published in the *Journal of Cellular & Molecular Anesthesia*, researchers from India compared the use of low-dose oral melatonin and oral midazolam for elective surgical anxiety in children. The cohort consisted of seventy children between the ages of two and ten years; they were divided into two groups. About ninety minutes before surgery, thirty-five children, with a mean age of 6.171 years, were given 0.2 mg/kg oral melatonin (maximum 5 mg); the other thirty-five children, with a mean age of 5.286, were given 0.5 mg/kg oral midazolam (maximum 20 mg). Levels of anxiety were measured before administration of the drug and ninety minutes later. While the levels of anxiety between the two groups were initially not statistically different, the second assessment determined that the children in the melatonin group had statistically significant higher levels of anxiety. So, the midazolam reduced anxiety significantly better than melatonin. The researchers concluded that "low-dose melatonin (0.2mg/kg) is not an adequate premedicant for children to alleviate preoperative anxiety compared to midazolam."[4]

Melatonin Seems to Be as Useful as Alprazolam for Presurgical Anxiety in Adults

In a trial published in the journal *Anesthesia Essays and Researches*, researchers from India compared the use of melatonin and alprazolam (Xanax), a benzodiazepine, for anxiety in adults who are about to undergo surgical procedures under general anesthesia. A total of ninety adults were randomly placed in one of three groups—3 mg melatonin (two tablets), 0.25 mg oral alprazolam (two tablets), or two tablets of a multivitamin (placebo). At baseline, the three groups had similar demographic profiles. Each intervention was administered 120 minutes before the induction of anesthesia. The researchers learned that while the patients in both intervention groups had significant reductions in levels of anxiety, the reduction in anxiety was greater in the melatonin group than that of the alprazolam group. Still, the researchers cautioned that more studies are needed "with different doses of melatonin and a larger sample size to find out an optimal and safe dose of melatonin as well as to prove its efficacy over benzodiazepine."[5]

Elderly May Not Obtain the Same Presurgical Anxiety-Reducing Benefits from Melatonin

In a randomized, prospective, double-blind trial published in the journal *Anesthesia & Analgesia*, researchers from Italy investigated the use of melatonin to reduce presurgical anxiety in people over the age of sixty-five years. The researchers enrolled 150 patients; seventy-five were placed in the melatonin group and given 10 mg oral melatonin before their surgeries, and seventy-five were placed in the placebo group. They were scheduled to have abdominal, thoracic, endocrinologic, vascular, or skin surgery. At the preoperative evaluation, each patient was administered the Mini Mental Status Examination. On the day of the surgery, information was collected on demographic statistics, and levels of anxiety and depression were measured both before and after surgery. Researchers coordinated an additional assessment seven days later. The analyses were performed on sixty-seven patients in the melatonin group and seventy-one in the placebo group. The researchers learned that neither the melatonin nor the placebo reduced the levels of anxiety in these patients. When compared to the placebo, melatonin "does not significantly reduce anxiety in elderly patients undergoing elective surgery."[6]

Melatonin May Help with the Anxiety and Pain Associated with Tourniquet in Intravenous Regional Anesthesia

In a randomized, double-blind, prospective clinical trial published in the journal *Advanced Biomedical Research*, researchers from Iran evaluated the ability of melatonin to help with the anxiety and pain associated with elective hand surgery using a tourniquet and intravenous regional anesthesia. The cohort consisted of fifty patients who had surgery for such problems as carpal tunnel syndrome, trigger finger, tendon release, and tendon repair. Twenty-five patients received 6 mg of oral melatonin ninety minutes before their surgeries and twenty-five, who served as controls, received placebos. At baseline, both groups were similar in terms of age and gender. Several anxiety and pain assessments were conducted. The researchers learned that the patients in the control group had significantly higher levels of anxiety (and pain). The researchers concluded that "the use of this drug at different doses and in different surgeries can reduce the pain and anxiety of patients during and after surgery."[7]

Melatonin Did Not Consistently Help with Anxiety from Wisdom Teeth Extraction

In a randomized, single-center, prospective, placebo-controlled trial published in the *Singapore Medical Journal*, researchers from Singapore tested the ability of melatonin to ease the anxiety that people experience when they have their wisdom teeth removed. The cohort consisted of seventy-six patients between the ages of twenty-one and sixty-five years who were scheduled for elective extraction of all four wisdom teeth under general anesthesia. Ninety minutes before the procedure the patients received either 6 mg melatonin or an identical in appearance placebo. Visual analog scale scores measure 60 and 30 minutes after the premedication was administered and again 30, 60, 90, 120 minutes and 4 hours after surgery. The final analyses included thirty-six patients in the melatonin group and thirty-seven in the placebo group. The researchers learned that melatonin appeared to have a gender-specific effect on anxiety. When compared to patients receiving placebos, female patients had faster reductions in anxiety than male patients. "A positive analgesic and anxiolytic effect of *melatonin was demonstrated in female patients but not male patients.*" However, more studies are needed before a definitive determination may be made.[8]

Melatonin May Reduce Anxiety in Patients Having Cataract Surgery Under Topical Anesthesia

In a trial published in the journal *Anesthesia & Analgesia*, researchers from Saudi Arabia examined the ability of melatonin to improve anxiety and other aspects of cataract surgery conducted under topical anesthesia. The researchers randomly assigned forty patients over the age of sixty years to one of two groups of twenty patients. At baseline, each of the groups had similar demographic characteristics. Ninety minutes before the surgery the patients received either 10 mg melatonin or a placebo. Upon arrival in the operating room, patients were asked about their levels of anxiety; levels of anxiety were assessed again at the end of the surgery. The researchers learned that after premedication, the anxiety levels decreased significantly in the melatonin group, and the scores were significantly lower than the placebo group. One patient in the melatonin group complained of dizziness, and another patient in the control group had nausea. The researchers concluded "that oral melatonin premedication for patients undergoing cataract surgery under local anesthesia provided anxiolytic effects."[9]

In randomized, placebo-controlled, double-blind clinical trial published in the *Indian Journal of Ophthalmology*, researchers from Iran also evaluated the use of melatonin before the same type of surgery. Sixty patients were assigned to receive either 3 mg sublingual melatonin or a placebo sixty minutes before their surgeries; the twelve male and eighteen female patients in the melatonin group had a mean age of 63.5 years, and the seventeen male and thirteen female patients in the placebo group had a mean age of 70.38 years. At baseline, there were no significant differences between the demographic characteristics of the two groups. During their preoperative visits, patient verbal anxiety scores ranged from 0 to 10. Anxiety scores for each patient were recorded before premedication, sixty minutes after premedication, on arrival at the operating room, during the operation, and before discharge from the recovery room. The researchers found that after melatonin, premedication anxiety scores significantly decreased in the melatonin group but increased in the placebo group. Throughout the surgery and recovery, the patients who were treated with melatonin continued to have significantly less anxiety than those in the placebo group. The researchers concluded that "melatonin is a valuable premedicant for patients undergoing cataract surgery under topical anesthesia."[10]

Melatonin Supplement Labelling May Be Alarmingly Incorrect

In a study published in the *Journal of Clinical Sleep Medicine*, researchers from Ontario, Canada, analyzed thirty melatonin supplements from sixteen different brands for amounts of melatonin and serotonin. They included liquid, capsule, and tablet formulations that were purchased in local stores. The researchers determined that the melatonin content varied between samples and lots. They found no observed pattern between individual brands, type of supplement, or labeled value. The most dramatic misrepresentation was a chewable tablet that had a 478 percent higher amount of melatonin than was indicated on the label. In contrast to the label claim of 1.5 mg melatonin, it had 9 mg, though that was even variable between lots. One supplement had 83 percent less melatonin than the amount on the label. The capsule products had the most variability; the products with the lowest levels of variability had the simplest mix of ingredients, generally tablets or sublingual tablets. The researchers noted that they were surprised to find that lot to lot variability was also high. It ranged from 0.37 percent to 466 percent. Serotonin was found in eight of the thirty samples tested. Serotonin content ranged from a low of 1.21 mg/mL to as high as 74.27 mg/mL. When two lots were available, serotonin was found in both. And, serotonin lot to lot variability was high, ranging from 1.25 percent to 133 percent. The researchers concluded that "melatonin content did not meet label within a 10 percent margin of the label claim in more than 71 percent of supplements and an additional 26 percent were found to contain serotonin. It is important that clinicians and patients have confidence in the quality of supplements."[11]

In a research letter published in *JAMA: Journal of the American Medical Association*, researchers from Somerville, Massachusetts and the University of Mississippi compared the amounts of melatonin listed in the labels of twenty-five bottles of melatonin gummies to the actual amounts contained in the gummies. One product contained no detectable melatonin. Instead, it had 31.3 mg of cannabidiol (CBD), a phytocannabinoid derived from cannabis which children should never be using. In the products that contained melatonin, the actual quantity of melatonin ranged from 74 to 347 percent of the labeled quantity. Only three products or 12 percent contained a quantity of melatonin that was within 10 percent of the declared amount. Five products indicated that they had CBD in quantities ranging from 10.6 to 31.3 mg. The actual quantity of CBD ranged from 104 to 118 percent of the labeled amount. The researchers noted that children who consume these gummies could be exposed to between 40 and 130 times higher quantities of melatonin. As for the CBD, the FDA has not approved it for any use in healthy children. The researchers advised clinicians to tell parents that the pediatric use of melatonin gummies "may result in ingestion of unpredictable quantities of melatonin and CBD."[12]

Many Studies Have Reported Adverse Events Associated with Melatonin

In a comprehensive systematic review of studies on oral melatonin published in the journal *Complementary Therapies in Medicine*, researchers from Australia examined the adverse events that have been associated with this supplement. They identified fifty controlled studies of oral melatonin supplementation in humans that included statistical analyses of adverse events. Of these articles, twenty-six did not mention any significant adverse events between the intervention and control, and twenty-four reported at least one statistically significant adverse event. All of the studies involved some method of control, and sample sizes ranged from 6 to 392, with a total of 3,803 and an average of 76 participants. Study participants were most often healthy; these were followed by people having surgical procedures. Study participants often had neurological or mental health conditions, sleep disorders, or a combination of both. Other frequent medical problems included endocrine abnormalities, cardiovascular conditions, asthma, fibromyalgia, and cancer. Melatonin doses generally ranged from 2 mg to 10 mg, but variations ranged from 0.3 mg to 1,600 mg. While typically taken at bedtime, in these studies, melatonin was also administered before a procedure or outcome measure test, or at multiple time-points throughout the day. Study durations ranged from one-day single administration to 3.5 years of daily dosing. The researchers learned that the most frequently reported adverse events were reductions in psychomotor and neurocognitive function or fatigue and excessive sleepiness. To avoid these problems, the researchers advised taking melatonin at bedtime, not before activities requiring alertness. In addition, the researchers observed that melatonin may impact endocrine parameters, especially reproductive factors and glucose metabolism, including alterations to sex hormones in both men and women, suppression of ovulation and sperm count, and reductions in insulin activity. But, other studies appear to dispute these findings. The researchers noted that "adverse events are generally minor, short-lived, easily managed and likely avoidable if dosing is applied in accordance with the circadian rhythm of endogenous melatonin." Still, they underscored the need for more research, especially since melatonin is increasingly being used for a greater number of medical problems.[13]

References and Further Readings

Abbasivash, Rahman, Sohrab Salimi, Behzad Ahsan et al. "The Effect of Melatonin on Anxiety and Pain of Tourniquet in Intravenous Regional Anesthesia." *Advanced Biomedical Research* 8 (November 27, 2019): 67.

Capuzzo, Maurizia, Barbara Zanardi, Elisa Schiffino et al. "Melatonin Does Not Reduce Anxiety More than Placebo in the Elderly Undergoing Surgery." *Anesthesia & Analgesia* 103, no. 1 (July 2006): 121–3.

Cohen, Peter A., Bharathi Avula, Yan-Hong Wang et al. "Quantity of Melatonin and CBD in Melatonin Gummies in the US." *JAMA: Journal of the American Medical Association* 329, no. 16 (2023): 1401–2.

Erland, Lauren A. E. and Praveen K. Saxena. "Melatonin Natural Health Products and Supplements: Presence of Serotonin and Significant Variability of Melatonin Content." *Journal of Clinical Sleep Medicine* 13, no. 2 (2017): 275–81.

Foley, Hope M. and Amie E. Steel. "Adverse Events Associated with Oral Administration of Melatonin: A Critical Systematic Review of Clinical Evidence." *Contemporary Therapies in Medicine* 42 (2019): 65–81.

Gooty, Sunanda, Davi Sai R. Priyanka, Ravikanth Pula et al. "A Comparative Study of Effect of Oral Melatonin versus Oral Midazolam as Premedicant in Children Undergoing Surgery Under General Anesthesia." *Journal of Cellular & Molecular Anesthesia* 7, no. 3 (2022): 160–7.

Ismail, Salah A. and Hany A. Mowafi. "Melatonin Provides Anxiolysis, Enhances Analgesia, Decreases Intraocular Pressure, and Promotes Better Operation Conditions During Cataract Surgery Under Topical Anesthesia." *Anesthesia & Analgesia* 108, no. 4 (April 2009): 1146–51.

Khare, Arvind, Beena Thada, Neena Jain et al. "Comparison of Effects of Oral Melatonin with Oral Alprazolam Use as a Premedicant in Adult Patients Undergoing Various Surgical Procedures Under General Anesthesia: A Prospective Randomized Placebo-Controlled Study." *Anesthesia Essays and Researches* 12, no. 3 (July–September 2018): 657–62.

Khezri, Marzieh and Hamid Merate. "The Effects of Melatonin on Anxiety and Pain Scores of Patients, Intraocular Pressure, and Operating Conditions During Cataract Surgery Under Topical Anesthesia." *Indian Journal of Ophthalmology* 61, no. 7 (2013): 319–24.

Patel, Tushar and Madhuri S. Kurdi. "A Comparative Study Between Oral Melatonin and Oral Midazolam on Preoperative Anxiety, Cognitive, and Psychomotor Functions." *Journal of Anaesthesiology Clinical Pharmacology* 31, no. 1 (January–March 2015): 37–43.

Samarkandi, A., M. Niaguib, W. Riad et al. "Melatonin vs. Midazolam Premedication in Children: A Double-Blind, Placebo-Controlled Study." *European Journal of Anaesthesiology* 22, no. 3 (March 2005): 189–96.

Seet, Edwin, Chen Mei Liaw, Sylvia Tay, and Chang Su. "Melatonin Premedication versus Placebo in Wisdom Teeth Extraction: A Randomised Controlled Trial." *Singapore Medical Journal* 56, no. 12 (2015): 666–71.

Torun, Aysun Caglar and Ezgi Yüceer. "Should Melatonin Be Used as an Alternative Sedative and Anxiolytic Agent in Mandibular Third Molar Surgery." *Journal of Oral and Maxillofacial Surgery* 77 (2019): 1790–5.

Mindfulness Meditation

Introduction

Tracing back thousands of years to the practices of the Eastern traditions, meditation focuses on mind and body integration. It is designed to calm the mind and improve overall well-being. One type of meditation, known as mindfulness, mindfulness meditation, or mindfulness-base stress reduction (MBSR), involves focusing intensely, without interpretation or judgment, on the sensations and feelings of the immediate meditative moment. It teaches people how to decelerate their negative thoughts. Mindfulness involves breathing methods, guided imagery, and practices that relax the body and mind and help reduce stress. As a result, it has the potential to be quite useful for anxiety disorders and other problems, including stress, pain, depression, insomnia, and high blood pressure.

Though a microbiologist by training, Jon Kabat-Zinn, PhD, was one of the first people to introduce mindfulness to the West. Having learned about mindfulness as a graduate student, Kabat-Zinn became an advocate for the practice, and in 1979, he created MBSR and founded the Stress Reduction Clinic, now known as the Center for Mindfulness, at the UMASS Memorial Health, UMASS Memorial Medical Center, in Worcester, Massachusetts. There, he and his associates taught mindfulness to patients in coursework that has been replicated a countless number of times; they also conducted extensive scientific research on the usefulness of mindfulness for many different problems. Kabat-Zinn was a key leader in transforming mindfulness from an Eastern religious practice into an integral component of mainstream secular society.

In the United States, the various types of meditation have grown dramatically in popularity. According to a 2017 survey published by the National Center for Health Statistics (NCHS), a division of the Centers for Disease Control and Prevention, the percentage of adults who practice some form of mantra-based meditation, mindfulness meditation, or spiritual meditation in the previous twelve months tripled between 2012 and 2017, from 4.1 percent to 14.2 percent. Among children aged four to seventeen years, the percentage increased from

0.6 percent in 2012 to 5.4 percent in 2017.[1] A few years earlier, in 2012, another NCHS survey found that meditation was primarily used for general wellness, improving energy and aiding memory or concentration. Almost one-third, a notable 29.2 percent, used meditation to relieve anxiety, while 21.6 percent used it for stress and 17.8 percent used it for depression. In fact, mental health problems were the most important reason for using meditation.[2]

Regulation, Administration, and Costs

While there are academic programs in which people may study how to teach mindfulness, there do not appear to be any federal or state regulations on the teaching or practicing of mindfulness. It is not uncommon for mindfulness classes to be held at workplaces, community centers, hospitals, clinics, or places of worship, and mindfulness classes may also be combined with other activities. Thus, a stress reduction class may incorporate mindfulness into its program. Or, mindfulness may be combined with cognitive behavioral therapy. (See entry on cognitive behavioral therapy.) A typical mindfulness teacher-led meditation class may consist of about eight weekly sessions that usually last at least thirty to sixty minutes.

Though techniques vary, mindfulness meditation tends to involve deep breathing and an acute awareness of body and mind. Most mindfulness meditation sessions begin by sitting in the comfortable position on a chair or with legs crossed on a meditation cushion on the floor, with the head, neck, and back straight but not stiff. Hands should drop to the top of the legs. When sitting in a chair, feet should touch the floor. While breathing through the nose, people focus their attention on moving their breath into and out of the body. Expect physical sensations or thoughts to interrupt the breathing, and it is normal for the mind to wander. There is no need to block or eliminate these thoughts. But, when the time is right, gently redirect attention to the breathing. Of course, this same practice may be followed while walking, whether outside or in a quiet inside pacing area, or even while doing laps in a pool or lying on a flat surface, such as a bed.

When meditating by oneself, it is useful to begin with short mindfulness sessions of five or ten minutes. Setting a timer may help. Eventually, the sessions may increase to at least forty-five minutes. People who have the time and inclination may meditate in the morning and at night. It is not uncommon for people who practice alone at home to do so under the guidance of a free online app.

Costs vary. Those who are concerned about the costs associated with mindfulness meditation should practice at home or consider classes led by volunteers in a community setting. Such classes are probably free or very inexpensive. For sessions led by trained paid teachers, students should expect to pay a minimum of $15 to $25 per class. There are mindfulness meditation coaches that work directly with students in person and online. These sessions may easily start at $60 or more for thirty minutes. While the beginning salary of a mindfulness coach tends to be modest, those who rise to the top of the field may make a six-figure income. Sessions with those coaches tend to be very expensive and beyond the reach of most people. While it is possible for mindfulness to be covered by insurance, especially for those sessions held in a medical setting, do not assume that it is. It is best to check.

Side Effects and Risks

Though mindfulness is generally believed to be safe and effective, there are reports of side effects and risks. Because people practicing mindfulness are encouraged to directly face their current concerns and existing habits, they may experience uncomfortable reactions, thoughts, emotions, and sensations. On occasion, this has the potential to result in a worsening of a person's mental health status, including symptoms of anxiety and depression. And, in very rare instances, mindfulness practiced extensively or too many hours per day may trigger psychosis and mania. People with severe symptoms, such as untreated trauma, active suicidal ideation, or substance abuse, should probably not participate in mindfulness meditation.

Research Findings

Mindfulness May Help College and University Students Obtain Relief from Anxiety

In a pilot trial published in the *Journal of American College Health*, researchers from Minnesota investigated the use of guided mindfulness meditation on anxiety and stress in pre-healthcare college students. The cohort consisted of thirty-three students, twenty-two females and eleven males, between the ages of nineteen and twenty-two years. After preliminary testing, over an eight-week period the students were told to devote five to twelve minutes per day to guided meditation. Large numbers of students failed to come close to that goal. On average, the students completed 252.26 minutes or 55.8 percent of their total 452.25 mindfulness training. Since there were variations in the amount of time the students spent on mindfulness, the researchers subdivided the cohort into four quartiles. The students in Group 4 spent the most training time and those in Group 1 the least. Groups 2 and 3 were in-between. The researchers learned that the students in Group 4 had the most improvement in anxiety and stress, while the students in Group 1 had no significant improvement. Still, the students generally believed that they were helped by the intervention; a notable 71.1 percent found the intervention to be "very beneficial, somewhat beneficial, or beneficial." The researchers concluded that "actionable ideas for college students considering meditation as a tool to reduce stress and anxiety include dedicating 5 to 10 minutes per day to self-care in the form of meditation."[3]

In a randomized, controlled trial published in the journal *Healthcare*, researchers from Indonesia evaluated the ability of mindfulness breathing meditation to reduce anxiety, stress, and depression among Indonesian university students. The cohort consisted of 122 students from sixteen universities; 61 students (41 women) were placed in the intervention group and 61 (51 women) served as controls. Though the subjects in the intervention group tended to be a few years older than the subjects in the control group, both groups otherwise had similar demographics. Before the intervention began, researchers measured the levels of anxiety, stress, and depression among the subjects. For four weeks, every day, the subjects in the intervention meditated fifteen minutes. During the first two weeks, the intervention was carried out with guidance on Zoom meetings. At the end of the trial, the students completed an anxiety, depression, and stress questionnaire. The researchers learned that at baseline, there were no significant differences between the groups in anxiety, depression, and stress. By the end of the trial, the intervention group had significantly less anxiety and stress and less, but not significantly less, depression. The researchers concluded that "the use of mindfulness breathing meditation could be applied to all university students and so forth to develop psychosocial status and mindful attentiveness to one's needs."[4]

Mindfulness May Help Nursing Students Deal with Anxiety and Stress

In a randomized, quasi-experimental trial published in the journal *Nurse Education in Practice*, researchers from Spain evaluated the use of an intensive online mindfulness program to aid in the anxiety and stress associated with a challenging clinical nursing simulation. The cohort consisted of forty-two undergraduate nursing students, between the ages of eighteen and forty-two years; twenty-one were placed in the intervention group and twenty-one in the control group. Eighty-one percent were women. The students in the intervention group took part in a ten-day, at home, intensive online mindfulness program. All of the students then participated in small group forty to fifty-minute prebriefing sessions, which was followed by the actual ten to twelve-minute clinical simulation observed by other students. The sessions ended with a fifteen to twenty-minute debriefing. It is important to note that 95.23 percent of the subjects had previously participated in a clinical simulation, but only 33.33 percent had prior work experience in health care. The researchers conducted a number of different physiological and psychological measures to assess levels of anxiety and stress. During the prebriefing, though both groups demonstrated levels of anxiety and stress, the levels were significantly lower in the intervention group. The levels decreased during the debriefing phase. The researchers observed that the "intensive and online mindfulness intervention for nursing students prior to simulation can alleviate anxiety and psychophysiological stress caused by clinical simulation, one of the most popular and evidently useful teaching strategies today."[5]

Mindfulness May Be Useful for Anxiety in Women Diagnosed with Breast Cancer

In a systematic review published in the journal *Current Oncology*, researchers from Austria examined the ability of mindfulness to reduce the levels of anxiety and depression and improve the quality of life in women diagnosed with breast cancer. The researchers located only six studies, published since 2018 in English or German, that addressed this issue. In every study, the sample sizes were under 100, and the duration of the trials was relatively brief, ranging from four to eight weeks. Most of the studies had a low risk of bias. Still, the researchers determined that four of the studies found improvement in anxiety scores after the mindfulness intervention. But, in two of these studies, the benefits were limited to the early and intermediate follow-up periods, and did not last into the later stage of their follow-up research. The researchers concluded that "all these data support the trend that MBSR training can have a positive influence on anxiety scores up to 12 months after completion of the intervention." Though, as a group, these studies failed to determine definitively if the benefits continued longer than one year, mindfulness may still be employed as an adjunct therapy "to improve the psychological care of breast cancer patients."[6]

Mindfulness May Be Useful for Up to Six Months of Cancer-Related Anxiety

In a systematic review and meta-analysis published in *JAMA Network Open*, researchers from Canada studied the use of mindfulness for the anxiety associated with cancer. The researchers included twenty-eight randomized controlled trials with 3,053 adults who participated in mindfulness therapy or were placed in some type of control group. The trials, which were all published in English, were conducted in thirteen countries from four continents; breast cancer was the most common diagnosis. The median duration of the intervention was eight weeks. Because of the nature of the interventions and the fact that subjects reported their own levels of anxiety, blinding was not possible. As a result, all of trials were considered at high risk for bias. The researchers learned that mindfulness interventions for adults with cancer were associated with reductions in the severity of anxiety for short-term anxiety, defined as one month or under, and medium-term anxiety, defined as six months or under. This did not prove to be true for long-term anxiety, defined as more than six and less than twelve months. The authors commented "that mindfulness-based interventions should be considered an effective treatment option for reducing short-term and medium-term anxiety among adults with cancer."[7]

Mindfulness May Help People with Social Anxiety Disorder

In a systematic review and meta-analysis published in the journal *Psychiatry Research*, researchers from China evaluated the use of mindfulness for social anxiety disorder. The researchers located 11 randomized controlled two or three-armed trials with 729 patients and five single-arm trials with 132 patients that met their criteria. Sample sizes ranged from nine to fifty-eight subjects, with a mean of twenty-seven, and the age range of the subjects was eighteen to fifty-nine years, with a median of thirty-nine years. Interventions lasted between eight and twelve weeks. The risk of bias for all of the studies was generally low. The researchers found that mindfulness was significantly superior to no treatment and equivalent to certain active treatments such as aerobic exercise. Yet, it was significantly less effective than evidence-based treatment (EBT), such as cognitive behavior therapy (CBT), a finding they had not anticipated. On the contrary, the researchers had expected that it would be equivalent in usefulness to EBT in alleviating social anxiety disorder symptoms. Still, because 40 to 50 percent of patients tend not to respond to CBT, the researchers commented that mindfulness "may be an effective and safe alternative therapy to CBT," with longer durations of mindfulness more effective than those that continue for shorter periods of time.[8]

Mindfulness May Be as Useful as Escitalopram for Reducing Anxiety

In a randomized, clinical trial published in *JAMA Psychiatry*, researchers from several locations in the United States but based in Washington, DC compared the efficacy of mindfulness meditation and escitalopram (Lexapro) for treating anxiety disorders. The initial cohort consisted of 276 adults with a diagnosed anxiety disorder from three academic medical centers in the United States; 59 percent white, 20 percent Asian, 15 percent African-American, and 75 percent female. One hundred and thirty-six subjects participated in a mindfulness program and 140 were placed on escitalopram. The mindfulness program included eight 2.5-hour weekly classes, and forty-five minutes of daily practice at home. A day-long retreat weekend class was held during the fifth or sixth week. Escitalopram was initiated at 10 mg per day orally; if well tolerated, it was increased to 20 mg per day on the second week. The subjects in both groups received baseline assessments and periodic and follow-up evaluations. One hundred and two subjects in the mindfulness group and 106 in the escitalopram group completed the trial. While frequent adverse events occurred in the subjects of both groups, no serious adverse events were reported. The most common adverse event in the mindfulness group was, ironically, increased anxiety; the most common adverse events in the escitalopram group were insomnia or sleep disturbance, nausea, fatigue, and headache. At the twelve-week follow-up, 49 percent of the mindfulness group and 78 percent of the escitalopram group were still continuing their treatment. By the twenty-four-week follow-up, those percentages were 28 percent and 52 percent, respectively. The researchers learned that the subjects in both groups experienced similar reductions in anxiety; there were no significant differences in outcomes. And, the reductions in anxiety continued during the follow-up periods. The researchers concluded that "MBSR was shown to be a well-tolerated treatment option with comparable effectiveness to a first-line medication for patients with anxiety disorders."[9]

Mindfulness May Have a Limited Effect on Anxiety in Children and Adolescents

In a systematic review and meta-analysis published in the journal *Child Care and Family Psychology Review*, researchers from Australia and the UK examined the ability of mindfulness to help children and adolescents with anxiety. The researchers identified twenty randomized controlled trials with 1,582 subjects, eighteen years or younger, that met their criteria. Seven of the studies were conducted in the United States, four in Spain, three in Iran, two in Australia, and one each in Hong Kong, Chile, France, and Canada. Sample sizes ranged from 14 to 364; subjects ranged in age from 4 to 18 years; mean ages in the studies varied from 5.1 to 16.8 years. Twelve of the studies were conducted in schools; the remainder were in clinics. Total mindfulness training times ranged from 270 to 2,160 minutes; 793 subjects were trained in mindfulness and 789 served as controls. Intervention duration times ranged from four to twenty-four weeks. The researchers learned that the mindfulness programs showed a significant yet small overall mean effect on anxiety. However, this reduction was substantially reduced to a small and nonsignificant mean effect when the three trials from Iran were excluded. Although school-based programs were more effective than those conducted in clinics, the difference between the two was not statistically significant. The researchers concluded that "across Western youth populations, the most likely outcome is that MBIs [mindfulness-based interventions] have no beneficial effect in anxiety symptoms reduction."[10]

It Is Not Clear If Mindfulness Helps People Undergoing Hemodialysis Cope with Their Anxiety and Depression

In a randomized, controlled trial published in the *Clinical Journal of the American Society of Nephrology*, researchers from Canada and Hungary noted that up to 50 percent of people undergoing hemodialysis suffer from anxiety and/or depression. As a result, they wanted to learn if these patients would benefit from a brief mindfulness intervention. The initial cohort consisted of forty-one patients on maintenance hemodialysis in Montreal, Canada. All of these patients were diagnosed with anxiety and/or depression. They had a mean age of sixty-five years, and 24 percent were female, 49 percent white, and 49 percent were married. On average, they had ten or more medical problems, including kidney failure, with the most common comorbidities being hypertension, diabetes, dyslipidemia, coronary artery disease, arrhythmias, and peripheral vascular disease. Forty-six percent were on psychiatric medications. Twenty-one were assigned to receive eight weeks of ten to fifteen-minute individually administered chairside mindfulness meditation interventions. These were conducted three times per week, during hemodialysis treatments. Patients were encouraged to practice mindfulness at home. The patients in the control group received their usual treatment; patients in both groups were given psychoeducational material on anxiety and depression. Fifteen patients completed the intervention; of the fifteen, the mean number of sessions completed was twenty out of twenty-four. Symptoms of anxiety and depression were measured with the Patient Health Questionnaire and the General Anxiety Disorder-7. The researchers determined that the patients "appreciated the mindfulness meditation intervention." Still, their findings were not statistically significant. "Although meditation seemed associated with self-reported subjective benefits, we did not detect statistically significant effects on depression and anxiety symptom scores with our small sample."[11]

References and Further Readings

Burgstahler, Matthew S. and Mary C. Stenson. "Effects of Guided Mindfulness Meditation on Anxiety and Stress in a Pre-Healthcare College Student Population: A Pilot Study." *Journal of American College Health* 68, no. 6 (August–September, 2020): 666–72.

Cramer, Holger, Helen Hall, Matthew Leach et al. "Prevalence, Patterns, and Predictors of Meditation Use Among US Adults: A Nationally Representative Survey." *Scientific Reports* 6 (2016): 36760.

Hoge, Elizabeth A., Eric Bui, Mihriye Mete et al. "Mindfulness-Based Stress Reduction vs Escitalopram for the Treatment of Adults with Anxiety Disorders: A Randomized Clinical Trial." *JAMA Psychiatry* 80, no. 1 (January 2023): 13–21.

Komariah, Maria, Kusman Ibrahim, Tuti Pahria et al. Effect of Mindfulness Breathing Meditation on Depression, Anxiety, and Stress: A Randomized Controlled Trial Among University Students." *Healthcare* 11 (2023): 26.

Ladenbauer, Severin and Josef Singer. "Can Mindfulness-Based Stress Reduction Influence the Quality of Life, Anxiety, and Depression of Women Diagnosed with Breast Cancer?—A Review." *Current Oncology* 29 (2022): 7779–93.

Liu, Xiaoyu, Pengcheng Yi, Lijun Ma et al. "Mindfulness-Based Interventions for Social Anxiety Disorder: A Systematic Review and Meta-Analysis." *Psychiatry Research* 300 (2021): 113935.

Oberoi, Sapna, Jiayu Yang, Roberta L. Woodgate et al. "Association of Mindfulness-Based Interventions with Anxiety Severity. In Adults with Cancer." *JAMA Network Open* (August 2020): e2012598.

Odgers, Katarzyna, Nicole Dargue, Cathy Creswell et al. "The Limited Effect of Mindfulness-Based Interventions on Anxiety in Children and Adolescents: A Meta-Analysis." *Clinical Child and Family Psychology Review* 23 (2020): 407–26.

Thomas, Zoë, Marta Novak, Susanna Gabriela et al. "Brief Mindfulness Meditation for Depression and Anxiety Symptoms in Patients Undergoing Hemodialysis." *Clinical Journal of the American Society of Nephrology* 12, no. 12 (December 7, 2017): 2008–15.

Torné-Ruiz, Alba, Mercedes Reguant, and Judith Roca. "Mindfulness For Stress and Anxiety Management in Nursing Students in a Clinical Simulation: A Quasi-Experimental Study." *Nurse Education in Practice* 66 (2023): 103533.

Mirtazapine

Introduction

Mirtazapine is an atypical antidepressant that is used primarily for the treatment of major depressive disorder. Because it has sedative and anxiolytic properties, mirtazapine is often used off-label for panic disorder, post-traumatic stress disorder, obsessive-compulsive disorder, generalized anxiety disorder, and social anxiety disorder. Although it is not completely understood how mirtazapine works, it is believed to support neurotransmitter activity between nerve cells in the brain by increasing the levels of serotonin and norepinephrine.

First synthesized in 1989, in 1994, mirtazapine was approved for use for major depressive disorder in the Netherlands. Two years later, in 1996, the US Food and Drug Administration approved its use for moderate and severe depression in adults. It was probably around that time that mirtazapine was first prescribed off-label for the symptoms of the various types of anxiety. Mirtazapine is not approved for use in children, and it is unclear whether people under the age of eighteen may safely take this medication.

Initial improvements from mirtazapine may be seen after a week or two. But, the full effects may not be apparent for six to eight weeks.

Regulation, Administration, and Costs

Like all prescription medications, mirtazapine is regulated by the FDA. It is sold as a generic drug and with the brand names Remeron and Remeron SolTab. The recommended starting dose is 15 mg per day. Because it has sedative properties, mirtazapine is taken at bedtime with or without food. It is available as an immediate release oral tablet and an orally disintegrating/dissolving tablet. Orally disintegrating/dissolving tablets must remain in their original packaging. When patients do not respond to the 15 mg dose, they may be increased to a maximum of 45 mg per day.

Mirtazapine is a moderately priced drug, averaging about $30 to $45 per month. It should be covered, at least in part, by health insurance.

Side Effects and Risks

A number of different side effects and risks have been associated with mirtazapine. The following side effects and risks occur in more than 10 percent of the people who take this medication: drowsiness, increase in appetite and weight gain, xerostmia (dry mouth), increase in serum cholesterol, constipation, sedation, thrombocytopenia (low platelet count in blood resulting in increased risk for bleeding), angle closure glaucoma, low white count and subsequent increased risk for infection, bone marrow suppression, neutropenia, and hypertriglyceridemia. The consumption of alcohol may increase the risk of these side effects.

Mirtazapine should never be combined with a monoamine oxidase inhibitor (MAO). Patients should stop taking a MAO at least fourteen days before beginning mirtazapine. Combining both drugs increases the risk of taking in too much serotonin and developing serotonin syndrome. Similar problems may occur when mirtazapine is combined with linezolid and intravenous methylene blue. The symptoms of serotonin syndrome include agitation, restlessness, insomnia, confusion, as well as hypertension (high blood pressure), rapid heart rate, dilated pupils, loss of muscle coordination, and muscle rigidity.

Taking mirtazapine with other sedative drugs may result in dangerous levels of sleepiness. In addition, mirtazapine may interact with the supplements St. John's Wort and tryptophan, as well as seizure and migraine medications. Other medications that should not be combined with mirtazapine include diazepam, tramadol, cimetidine, ketoconazole, and medications for mood disorders, such as lithium, and antipsychotics.

While it is dangerous to combine mirtazapine with many other medications, overdosing on mirtazapine rarely results in fatalities. For example, even when seven to twenty-two times the maximum dose of mirtazapine was taken, there were no significant adverse cardiac events. The most common overdose reactions were tachycardia, confusion, memory problems, drowsiness, mild hypertension, and mild CNS depression. Other signs and symptoms of overdose include disorientation and impaired memory.

Mirtazapine has been known to cause severe allergic reactions. Symptoms of an allergic reaction include trouble breathing, swelling of the face, tongue, eyes, or mouth, severe rash with skin swelling, a painful reddening of the skin with blisters, and itchy welts.

Mirtazapine should never be suddenly discontinued; patients should always slowly and gradually taper off this medication. The sudden stoppage may trigger the discontinuation syndrome, with symptoms such as depression, panic attacks, tinnitus, restlessness, vertigo, decreased appetite, insomnia, nausea, vomiting, diarrhea, and hypomania or mania.

As with some other medications, on occasion, mirtazapine worsens levels of anxiety and/depression, and it has been known to cause suicidal ideation. Patients taking mirtazapine need to be closely monitored for mood changes.

Animal studies have shown adverse reactions to the fetus when the mom has taken mirtazapine during the pregnancy. However, many believe that mirtazapine appears to be safe for pregnant women to take. Discuss the individual situation with a medical provider. It is known that mirtazapine is passed to babies during breastfeeding, and children should not take mirtazapine. Since the kidney function of seniors may be slowed, seniors may take longer to remove the drug from their bodies. So, the side effects in seniors may be more noticeable and continue for longer periods of time.

Like certain other antidepressants, there is a FDA Black Box warning for mirtazapine. In short-term studies, antidepressants were found to increase the risk of suicidality in children, adolescents, and young adults under the age of twenty-four years. The risk is highest during the first few months of treatment.

Research Findings

Mirtazapine Appears to Be Useful for Panic Disorder

In an open-label, three-month trial published in the journal *International Clinical Psychopharmacology*, researchers from Italy evaluated the efficacy and tolerability of mirtazapine for panic disorder. The cohort consisted of twenty-seven female and eighteen male patients, mean age of 36.4 years, with panic disorder, with or without agoraphobia. Eleven of the patients had a comorbid diagnosis of major depression. Patients were frequently assessed with structured psychiatric interviews, and their symptoms were rated with psychometric scales. After a diagnosis of panic disorder was established, each participant was placed on an initial daily dose of 15 mg of mirtazapine and then raised to a fixed dose of 30 mg per day for the remainder of the trial. The most common reported adverse events were drowsiness in eight patients and weight gain in seven patients. Because of adverse events, three subjects withdrew from the trial. The researchers learned that mirtazapine appeared to be effective in controlling the symptoms of panic disorder. A statistically significant improvement was seen in the first two weeks of treatment and continued until the end of the study. The researchers concluded that mirtazapine "is well tolerated for the treatment of panic disorder when administered at a starting dose of 15 mg/day and increased to 30 mg/day after a few days of treatment."[1]

In a double-blind, randomized, flexible-dose, eight-week trial published in the *Brazilian Journal of Medical and Biological Research*, researchers from Brazil compared the effects of mirtazapine and fluoxetine (Prozac) on the symptoms of panic disorder. The cohort consisted of twenty-seven patients who had a minimum of three panic attacks two weeks before the enrollment. During the first two weeks of the trial, the patients were assigned to daily doses of 15 mg mirtazapine ($n = 14$) or 10 mg fluoxetine ($n = 13$). The patients taking mirtazapine had a mean age of 36.1 years, and those taking fluoxetine had a mean age of 36.4 years. Women comprised 86.7 percent of the mirtazapine group and 66.7 percent of the fluoxetine group. In both groups, the median duration of the illness was thirty-six months. At the beginning of the third week, the doses were raised to 30 mg mirtazapine and 20 mg fluoxetine. But, half of the patients did not require the full doses. After baseline assessments, patients, who kept panic attack diaries, were evaluated at the end of weeks 1, 2, 4, 6, and 8. Doses could be decreased if adverse effects were noticed. Twenty-two patients completed the entire trial. The adverse effects most often reported by the mirtazapine group were drowsiness and weight gain. During the trial, none of the patients had even a single panic attack. So, both drugs were considered to be effective for panic attacks. The researchers concluded that "mirtazapine is an antipanic agent with an effectiveness comparable to that of fluoxetine."[2]

Mirtazapine May or May Not Help with Social Anxiety Disorder

In a randomized, double-blind trial published in *International Clinical Psychopharmacology*, researchers from the Netherlands tested the use of mirtazapine for social anxiety disorder, also known as social phobia. The cohort consisted of sixty subjects with social anxiety disorder; there were thirty-four women and twenty-six men with a mean age of 38.6 years. At baseline, the two groups had similar demographic characteristics and levels of social anxiety, and they only had social anxiety disorder and not have any other axis 1 or 2 disorders. For twelve weeks, thirty subjects were assigned to take 30 to 45 mg per day of mirtazapine and thirty were assigned to take a placebo. Two subjects from the mirtazapine group and one from the placebo group did not complete the study. By the end of the trial, though the subjects in the mirtazapine group had gained more weight, the subjects in both groups experienced similar reductions in social anxiety. The researchers commented that this was the first study of its kind which "failed to find the superior efficacy of mirtazapine as compared with placebo."[3]

In an eight-week, open-label trial published in the *Journal of Anxiety Disorders*, researchers from Boston, Massachusetts, studied the use of mirtazapine for children and adolescents with social anxiety. The initial cohort consisted of eighteen children and adolescents between the ages of eight and seventeen years. Although the starting dose was 15 mg per day at bedtime for all of the subjects, the doses were adjusted for each individual patient. The mean final daily dose was 28.75 mg. Eight patients achieved the maximum 45 mg dose. The patients were seen and evaluated weekly. Measures used included the Clinical Global Impressions Scale-Social Phobia and the Liebowitz Social Anxiety Scale for Children and Adolescents. The most frequently reported adverse events were sleepiness, especially in the morning, and irritability. Another adverse effect was an average weight gain of 3.27 kg or 7.21 pounds. Still, seven patients did not report any adverse events. The researchers determine that 56 percent of the subjects had their social anxiety symptoms "much" to "very much improved." All the patients exceeded the cutoff score for social anxiety at baseline; 39 percent had a remission of their social anxiety symptoms and 22 percent had a remission of all their anxiety symptoms. Significant improvements were seen during the first two weeks of treatment. Yet, eleven patients, a notably large 61 percent, did not complete the entire study; four of these patients discontinued because of adverse events. "The others discontinued due to study burden (22 percent), insufficient response (6 percent), or to pursue herbal treatment (6 percent)." The researchers concluded that "larger controlled trials are needed to further evaluate efficacy and safety."[4]

When Added to Sertraline, Mirtazapine Makes Sertraline a Better Treatment for the Symptoms of Post-Traumatic Stress Disorder

In a trial published in the journal *Depression and Anxiety*, researchers from New York City investigated the ability of mirtazapine and sertraline (Zoloft), a selective serotonin reuptake inhibitor (SSRI), to treat the symptoms of post-traumatic stress disorder. The initial cohort consisted of thirty-eight adults with PTSD; they were recruited at an academic medical center and a private mental health clinic with mostly Spanish-speaking patients. The sample was about two-thirds female, and a single team of researchers conducted the trial at both settings. The subjects were randomized to receive twenty-four weeks of double-blind treatment with sertraline plus mirtazapine or sertraline and a placebo. At baseline, the subjects in both groups had moderate to severe PTSD. The subjects received periodic assessments by a single psychiatrist. Mirtazapine doses were initiated at 30 mg per day and could be increased to 45 mg per day or reduced to 15 mg per day. Both treatments were well tolerated, and there were no serious adverse events. Two subjects were excluded from the final analyses. The researchers determined that sertraline plus mirtazapine was a more clinically effective treatment for PTSD than sertraline alone, and the subjects in the combined group had a significantly greater rate of remission. Both treatments were well tolerated, with significantly increased appetite but not weight gain. The researchers commented that their "findings suggest that the combination of mirtazapine plus a SSRI warrants further study as a PTSD treatment."[5]

In a twenty-four-week trial published in the journal *Psychiatry and Clinical Neuroscience,* which was a continuation of an earlier eight-week study, researchers from Korea tested the use of mirtazapine alone for treating PTSD. The cohort was quite small, only twelve patients; they were all diagnosed with chronic PTSD. They had a mean age of 34.3 years, and nine were male. The causes of the PTSD were road traffic accidents in nine subjects, violence in two subjects, and rape in one subject. The average daily dose of mirtazapine was 27.2 mg, and the average maximum daily dose was 35.7 mg. The researchers used several measurement tools, such as the Impact of Event Scale-Revised and the Short PTSD Rating Interview, to evaluate the effectiveness of the medication. The researchers found that the symptoms of PTSD were significantly reduced during the course of the trial. And, the therapeutic effects of mirtazapine on PTSD were maintained or increased from eight to twenty-four weeks. At week eight, three patients had their score levels reduced by 50 percent; by week twenty-four, eight had their score levels reduced by 50 percent. The researchers noted that "long-term treatment with mirtazapine can be helpful in maintaining the short-term effects and relieving some symptoms of PTSD." And, they concluded that "further and better-designed studies are required to confirm the long-term efficacy of mirtazapine on PTSD."[6]

Mirtazapine May Help People with Preoperative Psychological Stress, Including Anxiety

In a trial published in the journal *Acta Anaesthesiologica Taiwanica*, researchers from Taiwan examined the ability of mirtazapine to help preoperative patients who are psychologically distressed with symptoms such as anxiety. The cohort consisted of seventy-nine patients who were about to have major abdominal surgery. They were placed in two groups. The fifty patients who chose the interventional treatment group took 30 mg of orodispersible mirtazapine (mirtazapine that disintegrates in the mouth) each night from preoperative day 0 to postoperative day 3. The twenty-nine patients in the other group took only the usual medications. Patients in both groups were evaluated both before and after the operation with measures, such as the Hospital Anxiety and Depression Scale (HADS) and Athens Insomnia Scale (AIS), that asked about anxiety, depression, and insomnia. The researchers learned that mirtazapine reduced the HADS scores of the patients in two days. "Mirtazapine can decrease HADS and AIS day indexes in the postoperative period and improve patients' quality of life immediately after the operation."[7]

Mirtazapine May Help Ease Anxiety in Children and Adolescents with Autism Spectrum Disorder

In a ten-week, double-blind, placebo-controlled, pilot trial published in the journal *Neuropsychopharmacology*, researchers from several locations in the United States but based in Boston, Massachusetts, investigated the use of mirtazapine for anxiety in children and adolescents with autism spectrum disorder (ASD). The initial cohort consisted of thirty children and adolescents with ASD, 80 percent male, between the ages of five to seventeen years. All of the children, who had clinically significant levels of anxiety, were randomized to take 7.5 to 45 mg per day of mirtazapine ($n = 20$) or a placebo ($n = 10$). Subjects were evaluated in-person at weeks 2, 4, and 6 and by telephone at weeks 1, 3, 5, and 8. A final in-person visit was conducted at week ten. One of the subjects assigned to mirtazapine withdrew at four weeks because of symptoms of irritability and aggression. The remaining twenty-nine subjects completed the entire trial. At the end of the trial, nine (47 percent) of the mirtazapine subjects and two (20 percent) of the placebo subjects were rated "very much improved" or "much improved." Mirtazapine was found to be safe and well tolerated; there were no serious adverse events or suicidalities reported. The most common adverse events were sedation and drowsiness, which were reported by 60 percent of the subjects in each group. Fifty percent of those on mirtazapine, and 20 percent of those on the placebo had an increase in appetite. The researchers concluded that mirtazapine "may have potential efficacy for treating anxiety in youth with ASD."[8]

People with Obsessive-Compulsive Disorder Who Fail to Respond to Sertraline Monotherapy May Respond Well to Mirtazapine/Sertraline Combination Therapy

In a twelve-week trial published in the journal *International Clinical Psychopharmacology*, researchers from Iran assessed the efficacy of adding mirtazapine to sertraline (Zoloft), a SSRI, treatment for obsessive-compulsive disorder. The cohort consisted of sixty-one patients who suffered from OCD but failed to benefit from at least twelve weeks of sertraline monotherapy. The subjects were randomly assigned to have either mirtazapine or a placebo added to their current sertraline treatment. The subjects began with 7.5 mg of mirtazapine per day; when appropriate, doses were then increased weekly by 7.5 mg increments. Though the doses ranged from 15 to 45 mg per day, the mean daily dose of mirtazapine was 39.56 mg per day. Twenty-two patients in the mirtazapine group and twenty-three in the placebo group completed the trial. OCD symptoms were measured using the Yale-Brown Obsessive Compulsive Scale (Y-BOCS). The researchers learned that mirtazapine decreased the symptoms of OCD significantly more than the placebo. The average Y-BOCS score decreased by approximately ten points in the placebo group, but the average decrease in the mirtazapine group was significantly more. For some subjects, the benefits were quite notable. Nine patients (40.90 percent) in the mirtazapine group and one patient (4.34 percent) in the placebo group had at least a 35 percent decrease in their Y-BOCS scores. The researchers observed that their findings showed that "serotonin enhancers other than SSRIs can also help in alleviating OCD symptoms." At the same time, the researchers acknowledged that they had a limited number of subjects from a single center, and the trial was relatively brief.[9]

It May Be Safe for Pregnant Women to Take Mirtazapine

In a register-based nationwide cohort study published in the journal *Arta Psychiatrica Scandinavica*, researchers from Denmark examined the relationship between mirtazapine exposure during pregnancy and the risk of specific adverse pregnancy outcomes. The researchers determined that there were 1,650,649 pregnancies registered in Denmark from 1997 to 2016. Of these pregnancies, 1945 were exposed to mirtazapine. There were live births in 1,192,539 of these pregnancies, with 897 exposed to mirtazapine. Among the mirtazapine-exposed children, thirty-one (3.5 percent) were diagnosed with a major congenital malformation compared to 152 (4.3 percent) among the unexposed children. Spontaneous abortions occurred in 237 (12.5 percent) of the pregnancies exposed to mirtazapine and 931 (12.3 percent) of the unexposed pregnancies. There were five stillbirths (0.3 percent) among the exposed and twenty-eight (0.4 percent) among the unexposed. Neonatal death occurred in three infants (0.3 percent) among the exposed and twenty cases (0.6 percent) among the unexposed. The researchers noted that they "found no association between mirtazapine exposure in pregnancy and increased risk of major congenital malformations, spontaneous abortion, stillbirth, or neonatal death."[10]

References and Further Readings

Chou, Wei-Han, Feng-Sheng Lin, Chih-Peng Lin et al. "Mirtazapine, in Orodispersible Form, for Patients with Preoperative Psychological Distress: A Pilot Study." *Acta Anaesthesiologica Taiwanica* 54 (2016): 16–23.

Kim, Won, Chi-Un Pae, Jeong-Ho Chae et al. "The Effectiveness of Mirtazapine in the Treatment of Post-Traumatic Stress Disorder: A 24-Week Continuation Therapy." *Psychiatry and Clinical Neurosciences* 59, no 6 (December 2005): 743–7.

McDougle, Christopher J., Robyn P. Thom, Caitlin T. Ravichandran et al. "A Randomized Double-Blind, Placebo-Controlled Pilot Trial of Mirtazapine for Anxiety in Children and Adolescents with Autism Spectrum Disorder." *Neuropsychopharmacology* 47 (2022): 1263–70.

Mowla, Arash and Haniyeh Baniasadipour. "Is Mirtazapine Augmentation Effective for Patients with Obsessive-Compulsive Disorder Who Failed to Respond to Sertraline Monotherapy? A Placebo-Controlled, Double-Blind, Clinical Trial." *International Clinical Psychopharmacology* 38 (2023): 4–8.

Mrakotsky, Christine, Bruce Masek, Joseph Biederman et al. "Prospective Open-Label Pilot Trial of Mirtazapine in Children and Adolescents with Social Phobia." *Journal of Anxiety Disorders* 22 (2008): 88–97.

Ostenfeld, Anne, Tonny Studsgaard Petersen, Lars Henning Pedersen et al. "Mirtazapine Exposure in Pregnancy and Fetal Safety: A Nationwide Cohort Study." *Acta Psychiatrica Scandinavica* 145, no. 6 (2022): 557–67.

Ribeiro, L., J. V. Busnello, M. Kauer-Sant'Anna et al. "Mirtazapine versus Fluoxetine in the Treatment of Panic Disorder." *Brazilian Journal of Medical and Biological Research* 34, no. 10 (October 2019): 1303–7.

Sarchiapone, M., M. Amore, S. De Risio et al. "Mirtazapine in the Treatment of Panic Disorder: An Open-Label Trial." *International Clinical Psychopharmacology* 18, no. 1 (2003): 35–8.

Schneier, Franklin R., Raphael Campeas, Jaime Carcamo et al. "Combined Mirtazapine and SSRI Treatment of PTSD: A Placebo-Controlled Trial." *Depression and Anxiety* 32 (2005): 570–9.

Schutters, Sara I. J., Harold J. G. M. Van Megan, Jantien Frederieke Van Veen et al. "Mirtazapine in Generalized Social Anxiety Disorder: A Randomized, Double-Blind, Placebo Controlled Study." *International Clinical Psychopharmacology* 25 (2010): 302–4.

Music Therapy

Introduction

Music therapy is the use of musical interventions to accomplish a wide variety of therapeutic goals, including the promotion of wellness, easing of stress, alleviation of pain, enhancement of memory, and, of course, the reduction in the levels of anxiety. Although the informal use of music for healing may be traced to ancient times, today music therapy is an established health profession which treats the physical, emotional, and cognitive needs of people of all ages. While the music therapist may be a well-trained musician, it is not necessary for clients to have any musical background. In fact, music therapists tailor the music therapy program for anyone from a trained professional musician to someone who never sang or played an instrument.

The modern practice of music therapy began to evolve after the First and Second World Wars when community musicians visited hospitals to perform for veterans. It soon became apparent that the music helped the veterans improve both emotionally and physically. Over time, academic programs were designed and expanded. Currently, there are over 9,000 board-certified music therapists in the United States.

Regulation, Administration, and Costs

Regulation of the music therapy profession varies from state to state. The majority of states appear to have no regulations. Normally, a professional music therapist earns an undergraduate, master's, or doctoral degree in a music therapy from a program approved by the American Music Therapy Association. In addition to academic coursework in musical and clinical foundations, music therapy principles, and psychology, a bachelor's degree requires 1,200 hours of clinical training, including a supervised internship. After completing an undergraduate degree, in order to earn the credential MT-BC (Music Therapist-Board

Certified), music therapists take the national board certification examination, which is administered by the Certification Board for Music Therapists (CBMT). This certification provides an objective national standard for the profession. Graduate degrees delve more deeply into advanced clinical practices and devote time to conducting research. People considering music therapy for their anxiety should locate a therapist who has experience treating people with anxiety disorders. And potential clients should be aware that not everyone who works as a music therapist has obtained this training or certification, especially in states where there is little or no regulation. If certification is an important determinant, be sure to ask the prospective therapist before scheduling an appointment.

Music therapy is offered in both individual and group formats; group sessions tend to be more structured than individual sessions. Therapists may be employed in many settings, such as medical and mental health inpatient and outpatient hospital environments, rehabilitation programs, nursing homes and long-term care facilities, adult day care programs, community clinics and mental health agencies and centers, physical therapy programs, private practices, and educational and correctional facilities. There are even independent music therapy companies. Music therapists may work alone or in conjunction with other therapeutic specialists.

During the first music therapy session, the music therapist assesses the needs of the client(s) and develops a treatment plan which includes a variety of music-based activities, such as listening to music, singing or humming along to music, song discussion, improvisation, dancing, responding to music, songwriting, recording music, and playing musical games. Although the focus tends to be more on engaging with music and less on the technical aspects of music, music therapists may even provide instruction on how to play an instrument. Sometimes, the therapist may ask what feelings the music creates. Often, music therapy, which offers an accepting, participatory environment, works when other types of therapy, which rely almost exclusively on verbal communication, have been less effective. It is important for clients to feel some type of connection with their therapist. If this fails to occur during the first or second session, it is probably a good idea to find a new therapist.

Individual music therapy is more expensive than group therapy, and music therapy will cost more in a large, expensive city than a less costly locale. Sessions, which usually take between thirty and sixty minutes, but may be shorter or longer, tend to range between $50 to $125 or more. Insurance may or may not cover this form of therapy. It is best to check with the provider.

Side Effects and Risks

While music therapy tends to be a very positive, life-affirming treatment for anxiety, in some instances, it has the potential to trigger unwanted, negative, and painful past memories. The "wrong" music or uncomfortable lyrics may increase anxiety, adding to distress. Further, music therapy may not be useful for people who dislike and reject all types of music. And, ironically, people already suffering from an anxiety disorder may find the volume, acoustics, and the type of instrument overstimulating and anxiety-provoking.

Research Findings

Music May or May Not Be Useful for Preoperative, Intraoperative, or Postoperative Anxiety

In a randomized, controlled trial published in the *Journal of Clinical Oncology*, researchers from Cleveland, Ohio, and Danville, Pennsylvania, investigated the use of live and prerecorded music therapy for several issues, including anxiety levels in women undergoing ambulatory surgery for breast cancer. The cohort consisted of 201 female patients with potential or known breast cancer at two hospitals in Ohio. The women had a mean age of fifty-nine years and 74.6 percent were white. The most common surgeries were biopsy, lumpectomy, and re-excision. The women were assigned to receive either patient-selected live music preoperatively with therapist-selected recorded music intraoperatively (n = 68) or patient-selected recorded music preoperatively with therapist-selected recorded music intraoperatively (n = 68), or the usual preoperative care with noise-blocking earmuffs intraoperatively (n = 65). Several anxiety assessments, such as the Global Anxiety-Visual Analog Scale, were conducted. The researchers determined that both treatment groups had significantly greater reductions in preoperative anxiety. The average reduction of anxiety in the live treatment group was 42.5 percent and 41.3 percent in the recorded treatment group. The researchers concluded that their findings "support the use of music therapy facilitation in the surgical arena."[1]

In a randomized, controlled trial published in the *International Archives of Otorhinolaryngology*, researchers from India tested the efficacy of music therapy on anxiety and pain in patients undergoing nasal septal surgery, a procedure used to correct a deviated nasal septum. The cohort consisted of fifty-nine patients.

Twenty-nine patients had both conventional medicine and music therapy; the music was delivered through headphones and "played at a comfortable level." There were two sessions per day each lasting thirty minutes; the sessions were held just before the surgery and for two postoperative days. Thirty patients were treated only with conventional medicine. At baseline, the patients in both groups were demographically similar. Pre- and postoperative anxiety was assessed using the Generalized Anxiety Disorder-7 scale. The researchers found that when compared to the patients in the conventional treatment group, the patients in the music therapy group had statistically significant reductions in anxiety. The researchers commented that "listening to music may have a wide range of therapeutic effects in patients by relieving anxiety, stimulating sedation, relaxing and reducing emotional and stress response to unpleasant stimuli by distraction."[2]

In a single-blind trial published in the journal *Anesthesia Progress*, researchers from Japan investigated the use of music on preoperative anxiety in an outpatient operating room for patients about to undergo dental surgery under intravenous sedation (IVS). All of the patients indicated that they were afraid or very afraid of their upcoming procedure. Sixty adult patients with dental anxiety were divided into two groups. The patients in the music group listened to music via wireless earphones in the operating waiting room for at least ten minutes until immediately before sedation; the patients in the control group wore earphones but did not listen to this music. The anxiety levels of the patients were objectively measured using heart rate variability (HRV) analysis; the subjective levels of anxiety were measured with a visual analog scale (VAS). The researchers observed that the HRV and VAS values of the music listening group were similar to those of the no music group; there were no significant differences between the two groups. And, they concluded "that music intervention failed to reduce preoperative anxiety in patients with dental fear in the outpatient OR [operating room]."[3]

In a multicenter, prospective, randomized, controlled trial published in the journal *Complementary Therapies in Medicine*, researchers from Turkey examined the use of music therapy for anxiety in patients during a carotid endarterectomy procedure conducted under regional (not general) anesthetic. The initial cohort consisted of seventy patients; there were thirty-five patients in the music therapy group and thirty-five in the control. Patients in both groups had similar demographic characteristics. The patients in the music group selected one of four types of music—Turkish folk music, Turkish classical music, Turkish popular music, or Turkish art music. The patients in the control group listened to operating room noise. While only half of the patients heard music, all of the patients wore headphones. The four vascular surgeons who performed the procedures were blinded to the study groups. Using the State-Trait Anxiety Inventory (STAI), preoperative and postoperative levels of anxiety were assessed by the same two trained research assistants. Intraoperative anxiety was also measured. Sixty-four patients were included in the analyses. Unexpectedly, the researchers learned that listening to music during the procedure was associated with significantly higher levels of anxiety than the regular noise from the operating room. The researchers concluded that "a well-controlled operating room environment, continuous sensible discussion between the operating room team and providing rational answers or positive feedback to the patient may be more advantageous than listening to music."[4]

Music Therapy May Slightly Improve the Anxiety Levels of Breast Cancer Patients Undergoing Chemotherapy

In a randomized trial published in the *Journal of Cellular Physiology*, researchers from Rome, Italy, and Philadelphia, Pennsylvania, compared the use of music therapy and virtual reality for patients undergoing chemotherapy. The cohort consisted of ninety-four patients undergoing their second infusion of chemotherapy. Thirty were placed in the music therapy group, thirty in the virtual reality group, and thirty-four in the control group. Both the music therapy and the virtual reality interventions continued for twenty minutes. Anxiety levels were measured before and after the treatments. Two patients from the virtual reality group were too ill to complete the trial. The researchers learned that the patients in all three groups had high levels of anxiety before the chemotherapy. Although all three groups had lower levels of anxiety after the chemotherapy, the reductions were significant only in the two intervention groups. However, it should be noted that the difference in the music therapy group "barely reached the level of significance." The researchers concluded that virtual reality therapy was more useful than music therapy in relieving the anxiety of these patients.[5]

While Appearing to Be Effective for Anxiety, the Relief That Music Therapy Provides May Be Relatively Brief

In a meta-analysis published in the journal *Psychiatry Research*, researchers from China examined the overall effectiveness of music therapy for anxiety. They reviewed thirty-two randomized controlled trials with 1,924 subjects; the trials were published in English from 2003 to 2021. The smallest trial included only 13 subjects, while the largest had 184. Music therapy ranged in duration from one to twenty-four sessions, with an average of 7.5 sessions. Eight studies with 368 subjects mentioned follow-up; in those studies, follow-up ranged from one to sixteen weeks, with an average of 7.75 weeks. While the researchers learned that music therapy significantly reduced anxiety at intervention, the relief was not sustained. At follow-up, music therapy did not significantly decrease the anxiety scores of the subjects. The researchers noted that future research "should focus on pragmatic approaches to integrate MT [music therapy] within existing health services."[6]

Music Therapy Seems to Reduce Anxiety in Critically Ill Patients

In a systematic review and meta-analysis published in the journal *Minerva Anestesiologica*, researchers from Milan, Italy, examined the ability of music therapy to reduce the anxiety and stress experienced by critically ill patients. The researchers located ten randomized controlled clinical trials and one quasi-randomized trial, with a total of 959 patients, that met their criteria. Study sizes ranged from 17 to 373 patients, with a median size of 60 patients. While none of the studies mentioned any adverse events, all of the studies reported a significant reduction in the levels of anxiety at the end of the music intervention. The majority of the studies used a single intervention. Because the studies lacked blinding, which was impossible given that the intervention was music therapy, they all had some degree of inherent bias. The benefits of music therapy were observed "even when music therapy was provided in a short, single intervention." The researchers concluded that "since music therapy is an easy intervention to implement, we suggest to consider it among the non-pharmacological strategies for anxiety and stress management in critically ill patients."[7]

Music Therapy May Reduce the Anxiety and Stress of Women During Cesarean Delivery

In a single-center, randomized, controlled trial published in the journal *BMC Pregnancy and Childbirth*, researchers from Germany evaluated the effectiveness of music therapy for anxiety and stress levels of women having a caesarean delivery. From March 2015 to August 2017, the researchers recruited 304 pregnant women with an indication for cesarean and no serious comorbidities. The women had a mean age of 33.6 years and a mean gestation age of 268.5 days. The researchers used several tools to measure anxiety and stress levels, such as the State-Trait Anxiety Inventory. Levels of anxiety were measured a week or two before the surgery, at admission, during skin suture, and two hours later. For the 154 women in the music group, slow-tempo continuous music began when they entered the operating room. There were 150 women in the control group; they received the usual care. Using both subjective and objective measures, the researchers found that music therapy reduced anxiety and stress. And, 96 percent of the women in the music group indicated that they would want to hear music again if they had another caesarean. The researchers concluded "that music during caesarean has an anxiety and stress soothing effect on the wake patient."[8]

Music Therapy May Benefit People Having a Colonoscopy

In a randomized, controlled trial published in the journal *Complementary Therapies in Clinical Practice*, researchers from Turkey investigated the effect of music therapy on anxiety, pain, and patient comfort in people undergoing a colonoscopy. The cohort consisted of 112 patients having a first-time colonoscopy in the endoscopy unit of a hospital in west Turkey. During the procedure, fifty-six patients listened to thirty minutes of music therapy and fifty-six patients received usual care. The researchers collected data before, during, and after the colonoscopy with an information form, an observation form, a visual analog scale, and the Spielberger State-Trait Anxiety Inventory. The researchers determined that the music therapy reduced anxiety and pain and enhanced comfort. And, they concluded that "since music therapy is an inexpensive, simple, noninvasive, and nonpharmacological method without any side effects, it might be useful as an adjunct to analgesics and sedatives for patients undergoing colonoscopy."[9]

Music Therapy Appears to Reduce Anxiety and Depression in Mothers of Preterm Infants

In a prospective, randomized, controlled trial published in the journal *BMC Psychology*, researchers from Brazil tested the ability of music therapy to lower the anxiety and depression experienced by mothers of preterm infants. The cohort consisted of twenty-one mothers of preterm infants who were admitted to the neonatal intensive care unit of a tertiary hospital between August 2015 and September 2017. Ten mothers were placed in the music therapy group and eleven in the control group. The women, who were between the ages of eighteen and forty years, were evaluated for anxiety, depression, and heart rate variability (HRV), medical problems that have the potential to deteriorate under such stressful circumstances. Conducted by music therapists, the women had individual weekly music therapy sessions, lasting for thirty to forty-five minutes. The sessions continued as long as the infants were hospitalized; the mothers attended an average of seven sessions. Among the measures used to assess the women was a Brazilian Portuguese version of the Beck Anxiety Inventory. The researchers found that the women in the music therapy group demonstrated statistically significant improvements in both anxiety and depression. The researchers noted that more studies are needed with larger sample sizes. Still, the researchers concluded that music therapy was "a reliable and low-cost therapy" that is easily able to be added to overall care.[10]

Music Therapy May Be Similarly Beneficial for the Parents of Premature Infants

In a mixed-methods pilot trial published in the *International Journal of Environmental Research and Public Health*, researchers from Switzerland and Austria evaluated the ability of creative music therapy to alleviate the anxiety, stress, and depressive symptoms of parents of premature infants. The initial cohort consisted of sixteen parent couples ($n = 32$) with premature infants being treated in a hospital in Zurich, Switzerland. Ten couples were randomly allocated to the music therapy group and six to the control group. A minimum of twenty minutes of music therapy was offered two to three times per week in the morning, after feeding time, with a trained and experienced music therapist; the infants and parents had at least eight sessions. If a parent could not be present, the sessions were still conducted with the infant. All of the couples completed questionnaires that asked about their levels of anxiety and depression and degrees of parental attachment at two weeks postpartum, at approximate neonatal intensive care unit hospitalization halftime, and two weeks after the infant was discharged. In addition, semi-structured interviews were conducted with the parents. Because several infants were transferred to other hospitals, by the final analysis, there were only seven couples in the music therapy group and three in the control group. When compared to the control group, the parents in the music therapy group had significant reductions in anxiety from the first and second evaluation, and there was a trend toward a significant reduction in the second to third evaluation. The researchers concluded that there is a need "for a more extensive powered follow-up study."[11]

Music Therapy May Ease the Anxiety and Depression of Alzheimer's Patients

In a trial published in *The Journal of Alternative and Complementary Medicine*, researchers from Spain examined the use of music therapy to treat the anxiety and depression associated with Alzheimer's disease. The cohort consisted of twenty-five patients with mild Alzheimer's disease; they had a mean age of 78.38 years. There were twice as many males as females, and all of the subjects were taking similar medications. The music therapy protocol was applied by a music therapist to groups of twelve to thirteen for sixty minutes. In order to quantify levels of anxiety and depression, salivary cortisol levels were measured before and after therapy. The researchers learned that the levels of cortisol decreased after therapy; there appeared to be a linear relationship between anxiety and depression and levels of cortisol. "A short period of music therapy can be an alternative medicine to improve emotional variables in Alzheimer's patients."[12]

References and Further Readings

Çelebi, Dilruba, Emel Yilmaz, Semra Tutcu Sahin, and Hakan Baydur. "The Effect of Music Therapy During Colonoscopy on Pain, Anxiety and Patient Comfort: A Randomized Controlled Trial." *Complementary Therapies in Clinical Practice* 38 (2020): 101084.

Chirico, Andrea, Patrizia Maiorano, Paola Indovina et al. "Virtual Reality and Music Therapy as Distraction Interventions to Alleviate Anxiety and Improve Mood States in Breast Cancer Patients During Chemotherapy." *Journal of Cellular Physiology* 235, no. 6 (June 2020): 5353–62.

de la Rubia, Orti, José Enrique, Maria Pilar Garcia-Pardo, Carmen Cabañés Iranzo et al. "Does Music Therapy Improve Anxiety and Depression in Alzheimer's Patients?" *The Journal of Alternative and Complementary Medicine* 42, no.1 (2018): 33–6.

Gogoularadja, Avinash and Satvinder Singh Bakshi. "A Randomized Study on the Efficacy of Music Therapy on Pain and Anxiety in Nasal Septal Surgery." *International Archives of Otorhinolaryngology* 24, no. 2 (2020): e232–e236.

Hepp, Philip, Carsten Hagenbeck, Julius Gilles et al. "Effects of Music Intervention During Caesarean Delivery on Anxiety and Stress of the Mother of a Controlled, Randomized Study." *BMC Pregnancy and Childbirth* 18 (2018): 435.

Kavakli, Ali Sait, Nilgun Kavrut Oztruk, Hilal Yavuzel Adas et al. "The Effects of Music on Anxiety and Pain in Patients During Carotid Endarterectomy Under Regional Anesthesia: A Randomized Controlled Trial." *Complementary Therapies in Medicine* 44 (June 2019): 94–101.

Kehl, Selina M., Pearl La Marca-Ghaemmaghami, Marina Haller et al. "Creative Music Therapy with Premature Infants and Their Parents: A Mixed-Method Pilot Study on Parents' Anxiety, Stress and Depressive Symptoms and Parent-Infant Attachment." *International Journal of Environmental Research and Public Health* 18, no. 1 (2021): 265.

Lu, Guangli, Ruiying Jia, Dandan Liang et al. "Effects of Music Therapy on Anxiety: A Meta-Analysis of Randomized Controlled Trials." *Psychiatry Research* 304 (October 2021): 114137.

Palmer, Jaclyn Bradley, Deforia Lane, Diane Mayo et al. "Effects of Music Therapy on Anesthesia Requirements and Anxiety in Women Undergoing Ambulatory Breast Surgery for Cancer Diagnosis and Treatment: A Randomized. Controlled Trial." *Journal of Clinical Oncology* 33, no. 28 (October 1, 2015): 3162–8.

Ribeiro, Mayara K. A., Tereza R. M. Alcântara-Silva, Jordana C. M. Oliveira et al. "Music Therapy Intervention in Cardiac Autonomic Modulation, Anxiety, and Depression in Mothers of Preterms: Randomized Controlled Trial." *BMC Psychology* 6 (2018): 57.

Umbrello, Michele, Tiziana Sorrenti, Giovanni Mistraletti et al. "Music Therapy Reduces Stress and Anxiety in Critically Ill Patients: A Systematic Review of Randomized Clinical Trials." *Minerva Anestesiologica* 85, no. 8 (August 2019): 886–98.

Wakana, Keiichiro, Yukifumi Kimura, Yukie Nitta, and Toshiaki Fujisawa. "The Effect of Music on Preoperative Anxiety in an Operating Room: A Single-Blind Randomized Controlled Trial." *Anesthesia Progress* 69, no. 1 (2022): 24–30.

Probiotics

Introduction

Probiotics are living microorganisms, such as bacteria and yeasts, that are thought to promote health when consumed or applied to the body. Or, as the World Health Organization issued in 2001, probiotics are "live microorganisms which when administered in adequate amounts confer a beneficial health effect on the host."[1] Probiotics may be found in a wide variety of dietary supplements, yogurt and other fermented foods, and beauty products. While many people consider all bacteria to negatively impact the body, there are bacteria that support the body and its functioning. They may play a role in digesting food, killing disease-causing cells, or producing vitamins. In fact, many of the microorganisms in probiotic products are the same or similar to microorganism already in the body.

Probiotics are identified by their specific strain, which includes the genus, the species, the subspecies, when applicable, and the strain designation. The seven core genera of microbial organisms most often used in probiotic products are *Lactobacillus, Bifidobacterium, Saccharomyces, Streptococcus, Enterococcus, Escherichia, and Bacillus.*

When people consume probiotics, the probiotics travel to the intestines and join the other microorganisms already in the body. These microorganisms are called the gut microbiome. The microbiome is responsible for digesting food, breaking down toxins, supporting the immune system, and making the body's energy and vitamins and hormones.

In recent years, there has been a growing interest in the association between gastrointestinal and brain health. This has led to the concept of "gut-brain-axis" and research on whether certain agents, such as probiotics, may improve gut health and, in turn, contribute to the well-being of the brain. Increasingly, researchers have found evidence of associations between gut microbiota and both gastrointestinal and extra-gastrointestinal diseases. In fact, there is now fairly strong proof that dysbiosis (imbalances in the gut microbiome) and inflammation of the gut are directly linked to psychiatric illnesses, including anxiety and depression. Probiotics are able to restore normal microbial balance, which supports the prevention and treatment of anxiety.

Probiotics may be traced to ancient times. It is believed that the Roman naturalist Pliny the Elder used fermented milk to treat intestinal problems. Many centuries later, in the late 1800s, the scientist Ilya Mechnikov, who later won a Nobel Prize, noted that despite their extreme poverty and harsh weather conditions, the rural residents of Bulgaria lived longer than the residents of other wealthier European populations. The reason, according to Mechnikov, was their diet which was rich in yogurt and fermented milk products. And, so, Michnikov and his colleagues began drinking sour milk, which introduced probiotics, meaning "for life," into the modern world. Around the same time, Henri Tissier, who worked at the Pasteur Institute, isolated *Bifidobacterium* from the gut flora of breast-fed infants. Tissier maintained that these bacteria reduced diarrhea in babies.[2] Fast-forward, decades later, probiotics are now a multibillion dollar business that just keeps growing and expanding exponentially.

It should be noted that probiotics are not the same as prebiotics. Prebiotics are nondigestible food components that selectively stimulate the growth or activity of desirable microorganisms. Symbiotics are products that combine prebiotics and probiotics.

Regulation, Administration, and Costs

The type of probiotic regulation by the US Food and Drug Administration depends on its intended use—as a food ingredient, dietary supplement, or medication. Normally, in order to be an ingredient in a food product, the probiotic must be approved by the FDA as a food additive or as a generally recognized as safe (GRAS) item for consumption. Foods containing probiotics may not claim that they treat, cure, mitigate, or prevent a disease. When probiotics are sold as dietary supplements, they do not require FDA approval, but they may not make health claims. And, if a probiotic product is sold as a medication, it needs to meet stricter requirements, such as FDA-approved clinical trials proving that it is safe and effective for the intended use. Prescription probiotics may be prescribed for gastrointestinal problems or anxiety and other mental health issues (off-label).

Currently, labeling regulation require manufacturers to list the total weight of the microorganisms on the Supplement Fact labels. But this mass may consist of both live and dead microorganisms. For probiotics to support health, the microorganisms need to be alive. So, consumers should look for the number of CFUs (colony forming units or the number of viable cells) at the end of the product's shelf life, not at the time of manufacture. Many probiotic supplements have one to ten billion CFU per dose, but some contain much higher amounts. Higher CFUs do not necessarily mean the product is more effective.

Probiotics are found naturally in many foods, such as apple cider vinegar, some cheeses, some pickles, kafir, kimchi, sauerkraut, tempeh, kombucha, and miso. While the probiotics in fermented foods, such as yogurt, may be active when sold, they may not survive the transit through the stomach or be adequately digested in the intestine. As dietary supplements, probiotics are available in a wide variety of forms, such as tablets, capsules, powders, gummies, and liquids, and these may have different strains and doses. There is still too little definitive research on the benefits of probiotics, dosages, and the people who may most benefit from consuming probiotics, and there are no official government recommendations for the use of probiotics in healthy people.

Prices of probiotics vary. Thus, a food product containing probiotics may or may not cost more than a similar food product without probiotics. And, probiotic supplements range in price from somewhat inexpensive to very expensive. The actual cost of a prescription probiotic would depend on the individual product and the medical insurance coverage.

Side Effects and Risks

Normally, probiotics have only minimal side effects in healthy adults. These include bloating, flatulence or gas, diarrhea, and headaches. Generally, these stop within a few days or weeks. Rarely, probiotics may cause a skin rash or itching. But, people with weakened immune systems or a serious illness may have more side effects, such as bacterial or fungal infections. In fact, the American Gastroenterology Association recommends that people with Crohn's disease, ulcerative colitis, and *C. difficile* only use probiotics if they are part of a clinical trial.[3]

And, it is possible that probiotics may interact with other medications. However, at present, information on such interactions is very limited. Still, people who begin probiotics because they are taking an antibiotic should be sure to take the medication and supplement at least two hours apart. Some additional risks possibly associated with probiotics include becoming resistant to antibiotics, developing an infection, or being exposed to a harmful substance created by the probiotic.

Research Findings

Lactobacillus plantarum P8 May Alleviate Stress and Anxiety in Stressed Adults While Improving Memory and Cognition

In a twelve-week randomized, double-blind, and placebo-controlled trial published in the journal *Clinical Nutrition*, researchers from Malaysia investigated the effects of the probiotic *Lactobacillus plantarum* P8 on psychological, memory, and cognitive parameters in 103 moderately stressed adults; stress levels were determined from scores on Cohen's Perceived Stress Scale. Fifty-two subjects were placed on the probiotic, and fifty-one took the placebo. As part of the overall evaluation, all of the subjects were assessed with the Depression, Anxiety, and Stress Scale (DASS-42) questionnaire. While the placebo only reduced anxiety from moderate at week zero to mild at week twelve, the probiotic lowered anxiety levels from moderate at week zero to normal at week twelve. The researchers concluded that the probiotic "reduced some stress and anxiety symptoms . . . followed by enhanced memory and cognitive abilities."[4]

Regulating the Intestinal Microbiota with Probiotics Appears to Improve Anxiety, but Not as Well as Some Other Interventions

In a systematic review published in the journal *General Psychiatry*, researchers from China searched for evidence supporting the use of probiotics or non-probiotics to improve intestinal microbiota and anxiety. The researchers located twenty-one studies, with 1,503 subjects, that met their criteria, including ten studies with patients who had IBS, six studies with healthy controls, and other studies with patients with chronic illnesses, such as rheumatoid arthritis, obesity, and type 2 diabetes. In fourteen studies, probiotics were used to regulate intestinal microbiota and six studies used an alternative, such as making dramatic dietary adjustments, including the low FODMAP diet. In seven studies, the probiotic product contained only one kind of probiotic; two studies used a product with two kinds of probiotics; and, the other five studies used at least three kinds of probiotics. The overall quality of the studies was high. The researchers learned that more than half of the twenty-one studies found that regulating intestinal flora effectively improved anxiety symptoms. Of the fourteen studies that used probiotics as the intervention, 36 percent improved anxiety, while six of the seven studies using non-probiotics also improved anxiety, and they were 86 percent effective. Clearly, the non-probiotic interventions were significantly better at improving anxiety than the probiotic interventions. The researchers concluded that "more relevant clinical intervention studies should be carried out with the unified anxiety assessment scales and statistical methods being used to clarify the relationship between intestinal flora adjustment and improvement of anxiety symptoms."[5]

Lactobacillus rhamnosus HN001 May Be Useful in the Prevention and Treatment of Postpartum Depression and Anxiety

In a randomized, double-blind, placebo-controlled trial published in the journal *EBioMedicine*, researchers from New Zealand evaluated the ability of the probiotic *Lactobacillus rhamnosus* HN001 to help prevent and treat postpartum depression and anxiety. The initial cohort consisted of 423 women from Auckland and Wellington, New Zealand, who were recruited at fourteen to sixteen weeks gestation. The women received either the probiotic supplement ($n = 212$) or a placebo ($n = 211$), which they took from enrollment until up to six months after birth, while they were breastfeeding. The women were interviewed at baseline and when the children were about six and twelve months, and they were asked to complete a questionnaire about their psychological well-being. The Edinburgh Postnatal Depression Scale evaluated maternal mood. One hundred and ninety-three women in the probiotic group and 187 women in the placebo group were included in the final analyses. The researchers learned that the prevalence of depression and anxiety in the women taking the probiotic was significantly lower than the women on the placebo. Still, the researchers cautioned that "not all probiotic strains have the same effect on health, and it is possible that the results found using HN001 are not generalizable to other probiotic strains."[6]

Multispecies Probiotics May Be Helpful for Anxiety in Adolescents

In a randomized, double-blind, placebo-controlled trial published in the *Journal of Affective Disorders*, researchers from Houston, Texas, tested the ability of multispecies probiotics to reduce anxiety in healthy young adults. The initial cohort consisted of eighty-six college students, 75.6 percent female, with an average age of 20.59 years. Twenty-four subjects were Hispanic, twenty-three African-American, twenty Caucasian, and fourteen Asian/Pacific Islander. The students were divided into five groups and given one of five different supplements to take: probiotics with high CFU and high species count, probiotics with high CFU and low species count, placebo supplement, probiotics with low CFU and high species count, and probiotics with low CFU and low species count. High CFU was defined as having between forty and fifty billion viable count of bacteria and low CFU count had between ten and twenty billion viable count of bacteria. High species count was defined as having between sixteen and twenty different bacteria, while the low species count probiotics had between ten and fifteen different bacteria. The subjects completed a survey at baseline and at twenty-eight days of treatment when the trial ended. The researchers learned that the probiotics improved panic anxiety, neurophysiological anxiety, negative affect, worry, and increased mood regulation. And, CFU levels were more important in calming anxiety than the species counts. Further, the subjects with higher levels of anxiety reported better improvements than those with normal levels of anxiety. The researchers concluded "that probiotics may have the therapeutic potential to treat anxiety, however, further research is necessary to make that determination."[7]

Probiotics May Help Anxiety in People with Multiple Sclerosis

In a trial published in the journal *Clinical Nutrition*, researchers from Iran investigated the use of probiotics in people with multiple sclerosis for various problems, including anxiety. The initial cohort consisted of sixty people with multiple sclerosis; for twelve weeks they were randomly assigned to one of two groups—a probiotic capsule group or a placebo group. The probiotic capsules contained *Lactobacillus acidophilus*, *Lactobacillus casei*, *Bifidobacterium bifidum*, and *Lactobacillus fermentum*. Each group had twenty-five females and five males. Among the assessments made was a depression, anxiety, and stress scale (DASS), administered at baseline and when the intervention ended. Fifty-four subjects, twenty-seven in each group, completed the trial, and the rate of compliance was high—more than 90 percent in each group. The researchers learned that compared to the placebo, the probiotic significantly improved DASS scores, thus lowering levels of anxiety.[8]

Intake of Probiotics Improved the Mental Health of Petrochemical Workers

In a six-week, randomized, double-blind, placebo-controlled trial published in the journal *Nutritional Neuroscience*, researchers from Iran examined the ability of probiotics to improve the mental health and anxiety levels of petrochemical workers. The initial cohort consisted of seventy-five male and female workers; they were divided into three groups. The mean age, height, weight, and BMI at baseline and six weeks were not significantly different between the groups. Twenty-five subjects were placed on 100 g per day of probiotic yogurt and one placebo, twenty-five subjects took one probiotic capsule per day plus 100 g per day of conventional yogurt, and twenty-five subjects took 100 g per day of conventional yogurt and one placebo tablet. Dietary and physical activity records were taken at weeks one, three, and five. Compliance rates were high; throughout the study, more than 90 percent of the yogurts and capsules were consumed. Seventy subjects completed the trial. Mental health parameters, including a general health questionnaire (GHQ) and DASS scores, were measured. After six weeks, there was a significant improvement of GHQ and DASS scores in the probiotic yogurt and the probiotic capsule groups. There was no significant improvement in the conventional yogurt group. The researchers concluded that "the consumption of probiotic yogurt or a multispecies probiotic capsule had beneficial effects on mental health parameters in petrochemical workers."[9]

Probiotics May or May Not Be Useful for the Anxiety Associated with Chronic Fatigue Syndrome

In a randomized, double-blind, placebo-controlled, pilot trial published in the journal *Gut Pathogens*, researchers from Canada examined the use of probiotics for the emotional problems, especially anxiety, associated with chronic fatigue syndrome (CFS). The researchers noted that past studies found that CFS patients have alterations in their intestinal microbial flora. The initial cohort consisted of thirty-nine CFS patients. For eight weeks, the subjects took either a total of twenty-four billion CFUs of *Lactobacillus casei* strain Shirota (LcS) or a placebo. Thirty-five subjects, twenty-seven females and eight males, completed the trial. Assessments were conducted before and after the intervention with the Beck Depression and Beck Anxiety Inventories. The researchers noted that there was a statistical difference in the anxiety scores between those taking the probiotic and those on the placebo; those taking the probiotic had significant improvements in anxiety. The researchers commented that the probiotic that they used may play a role "in mediating some of the emotional symptoms of CFS and other related conditions." But, it was a small study "and broad conclusions cannot be drawn at this time."[10]

More Studies May Be Needed to Determine If Probiotics Are Truly Useful for Anxiety

In a systematic review and meta-analysis published in the journal *Neuroscience & Biobehavioral Reviews*, researchers from Rhode Island reviewed the relationship between prebiotics and probiotics and depression and anxiety. They located thirty-four controlled, clinical trials that met their criteria; of these, twenty-nine were on probiotics. Slightly over one-fourth of the studies had an overall low risk of bias, and 41.2 percent had an overall high risk. The remainder had an unclear risk of bias. Among the studies reviewed, *Lactobacillus* received the most interest. Still, it did not appear to have an effect on anxiety, regardless of whether it was considered alone or in combination with prebiotics or other probiotics. Still, the researchers observed that the majority of the studies were underpowered to detect significant effects. And, they found "general support" for the belief that probiotics had some effect on depression and anxiety, "with small pooled effects in both cases." However, their findings are qualified because of "the relative rarity of trials with psychiatric samples and the prevalence of non-clinical samples in the literature."[11]

Probiotics Did Not Appear to Help Depression and Anxiety in People with Irritable Bowel Syndrome

In a systematic review and meta-analysis published in the *Journal of Clinical Medicine*, researchers from Germany examined the ability of probiotics to improve depression, anxiety, and quality of life in people with irritable bowel syndrome (IBS). The researchers located twenty-five randomized, double-blind, placebo-controlled trials with 4,717 subjects that met their criteria; of these, eleven, with a total of 1,977 subjects, were eligible for meta-analysis. The trials, which were published between 2005 and 2021, were conducted in Europe ($n = 19$), Asia ($n = 11$), United States ($n = 4$), and Africa ($n = 1$). The median age of the subjects was forty-two years, and 68 percent were female. The duration of interventions ranged from four to twenty-four weeks. Twenty trials used a single strain probiotic and fifteen used a multi strain. The overall risk of bias was low in nineteen studies, with some concerns in ten studies and a high risk in six studies. The researchers did not observe any differences in degrees of depression and anxiety and only a slight improvement in the quality of life between the intervention and placebo groups. So, in these subjects, probiotics did not have any notable effect on anxiety.[12]

References and Further Readings

Kouchaki, Ebrahim, Omid Reza Tamtaji et al. "Clinical and Metabolic Response to Probiotic Supplementation in Patients with Multiple Sclerosis: A Randomized, Double-Blind, Placebo-Controlled Trial." *Clinical Nutrition* 36 (2017): 1245–9.

Le Morvan de Sequeira, Charlotte, Marie Kaeber, Sila Elif Cekin et al. "The Effects of Probiotics on Quality of Life, Depression and Anxiety in Patients with Irritable Bowel Syndrome: A Systematic Review and Meta-Analysis." *Journal of Clinical Medicine* 10, no. 16 (August 8, 2021): 3497.

Lew, Lee-Ching, Yan-Yan Hor, Nur Asmaa et al. "Probiotic *Lactobacillus plantarum* P8 Alleviated Stress and Anxiety While Enhancing Memory and Cognition in Stressed Adults: A Randomised, Double-Blind, Placebo-Controlled Study." *Clinical Nutrition* 38 (2019): 2053–64.

Liu, Richard, Rachel F. L. Walsh, and Ana E. Sheehan. "Prebiotics and Probiotics for Depression and Anxiety: A Systematic Review and Meta-Analysis of Controlled Clinical Trials." *Neuroscience & Biobehavioral Reviews* 102 (July 2019): 13–23.

Mohammadi, A. A., S. Jazaueri, K. Khosravi-Darani et al. "The Effects of Probiotics on Mental Health and Hypothalamic-Pituitary-Adrenal Axis: A Randomized, Double-Blind, Placebo-Controlled Trial in Petrochemical Workers." *Nutritional Neuroscience* 19, no. 9 (November 2016): 387–95.

Rao, A. Venket, Alison C. Bested, Tracey M. Beaulne et al. "A Randomized, Double-Blind, Placebo-Controlled Pilot Study of a Probiotic in Emotional Symptoms Off Chronic Fatigue Syndrome." *Gut Pathogens* 1, no. 1(2009): 6.

Slykerman, R. F., F. Hood, K. Wickens et al. "Effects of *Lactobacillus rhamnosus* HN001 in Pregnancy on Postpartum Symptoms of Depression and Anxiety: A Randomised Double-Blind Placebo-Controlled Trial." *EBioMedicine* 24 (2017): 159–65.

Tran, Nhan, Masha Zhebrak, Christine Yacoub et al. "The Gut-Brain Relatioship: Investigating the Effect of Multispecies Probiotics on Anxiety in a Randomized Placebo-Controlled Trial of Healthy Young Adults." *Journal of Affective Disorders* 252 (2019): 271–7.

Yang, Beibei, Jinbao Wei, Peijun Ju, and Jinghong Chen. "Effects of Regulating Intestinal Microbiota on Anxiety Symptoms: A Systematic Review." *General Psychiatry* 32 (2019): e100056.

Psilocybin

Introduction

Though it may be made synthetically, psilocybin is a naturally occurring psychedelic substance that is found primarily in the so-called "magic mushrooms" of the *Psilocybe* genus. These mushrooms, which are grown in tropical and subtropical regions of the United States, South America, and Mexico, typically contain 0.2 to 0.4 percent psilocybin. Mushrooms with psilocybin are sold fresh or dried and have long, slender stems topped by caps with dark gills on the underside. Fresh mushrooms have white or off-white gray stems; the caps are dark brown around the edges and light brown or white in the center. Dried mushrooms tend to be rusty brown with off-white areas. Psilocybin mushrooms may be eaten, brewed as a tea, or added to other foods to cover their bitter flavor; dried mushrooms have higher amounts of psilocybin than fresh mushrooms.

When ingested psilocybin is transformed into a pharmacologically active ingredient known as psilocin, which affects several different serotonin receptors in the brain. Known to be dose-dependent, psilocybin alters perception, cognition, and emotions. Psilocybin acts as a catalyst for a therapeutic process. As such, it is believed to increase the intensity of psychotherapy and may trigger profound thoughts, and it is beleived to be especially useful for treatment-resistant anxiety and depression.

Hoping to induce hallucinations and altered states of consciousness, since prehistoric times, psilocybin has been used in different cultures and with indigenous people in some countries. Research on psilocybin and other psychedelic drugs dramatically escalated in the 1960s when they became popular for recreational purposes. It has been estimated that over 1,000 clinical papers involving about 40,000 subjects were published during that time period.[1] In the late 1950s, Swiss chemist Albert Hofmann and his colleagues identified and synthesized purified psilocybin from the mushroom *P. mexicana*. (Hofmann is better known for his research on and experimentation with lysergic acid diethylamide or LSD, which is similar in structure to psilocybin but far more potent; that is why Hofmann is often mentioned as the "father of LSD.")

However, the increased misuse of psychedelic drugs during the 1960s when they became popular for recreational purposes led to a widespread prohibition of production. Though this prohibition made research on psilocybin more difficult, some research projects, with promising results, continued.

Regulation, Administration, and Costs

Following the 1971 United Nations Convention on Psychotropic Substances, the US federal government passed laws classifying psilocybin as illegal. The US Drug Enforcement Administration (DEA) now lists psilocybin as a Schedule 1 drug and considers it a drug with a high potential for abuse. Further, as a Schedule 1 drug, the DEA maintains there is no safe way to administer psilocybin, and it has no legitimate medical purpose. There are many both inside and outside the scientific world who consider this classification to be too rigid.

So, it should not be surprising that several US cities have passed measures making the prosecution of citizens possessing psilocybin unlikely. Seattle, Washington, decriminalized magic mushrooms; Denver, Colorado, voters passed a ballot measure prohibiting the city from using money to prosecute people for magic mushrooms and related offenses. City councils in Oakland and Santa Cruz, California took similar steps. The list keeps growing. In 2020, Oregon passed a law decriminalizing magic mushrooms, and the state decided to build a framework for regulating their therapeutic use. (Decriminalizing is not the same as legalization. While psilocybin remains illegal, the actual prosecution of people for possession is deprioritized or discouraged.) For now, psilocybin remains illegal and strictly controlled at the national level in most countries. However, there are notable exceptions. At present, Jamaica does not have any regulations on the cultivation of psilocybin mushrooms. That is probably one of the reasons that Jamaica has become a popular destination for psychedelic retreats. Portugal has decriminalized all drugs. Some countries ban the mushrooms but not the spores, because the spores do not contain psilocybin. Canada classifies magic mushrooms as a Schedule 3 drug. Other countries just don't enforce their laws. Indigenous people in some South American countries had fought their governments to enable them to continue to use psychedelic plants. And, in the United States, certain research undertakings and trials have been permitted.

For the treatment of anxiety, psilocybin is normally used in very small doses, such as 0.5 g; these are known as microdoses. Why is this important? Very small doses reduce the risk of hallucinations. The effects of psilocybin usually take between twenty minutes and two hours to begin, and they last for about four to six hours.

Since psilocybin is illegal in the United States, it is a bit challenging to obtain an exact cost estimate. At the same time, in larger cities, such as New York City and Los Angeles, and the parts of the country where psilocybin prosecutions no longer occur, it is more readily available, and there may even be some degree of competitive pricing. That said, it is estimated that a gram sells for between $7 and $15, with an average of around $10. Seven grams costs between $55 and $75. Some dealers sell psilocybin coated in chocolate and in capsules and gummies.

Side Effects and Risks

Psilocybin has been associated with a wide number of side effects including headache, dizziness, nausea, vomiting, sleepiness, muscle weakness, lack of coordination, insomnia, impaired concentration, unusual body sensations, migraines, confusion, and overactive reflexes. Ironically, anxiety may also be a side effect.

When used in higher doses, psilocybin may cause visual and auditory hallucinations. It may also distort an individual's sense of time and reality, as well as perceptions of the world. People may feel separated from their bodies, a feeling known as disassociation. Though it is well known that people illegally experiment with psilocybin on their own, with friends, and in recreational settings all over the country, psilocybin may only be used with a higher degree of safety under the close monitoring of a highly trained medical professional.

Psilocybin is not considered to be addictive, and it does not cause compulsive use. Because psilocybin causes such an intense experience, people may actually limit their use. Of course, many people become psychologically addicted to psilocybin. While it is possible to overdose on psilocybin, it is believed that dying from an overdose is rare. Still, the symptoms of an overdose are anxiety, panic attacks, vomiting, diarrhea, agitation, paranoia, psychosis, seizures, and coma. An overdose typically lasts for six to eight hours, but some of the effects may be felt for days.

The experience of being on a psychedelic medication is not necessarily pleasurable. It may make people feel scared or emotionally intense, as well as overwhelmingly fearful. They may have confused reactions that may lead to dangerous behavior in unmonitored settings. At future times, it may trigger terrifying flashbacks. And, there is always the possibility of eating poisonous mushrooms, which may cause stomach pains, vomiting, diarrhea, muscle spasms, delirium, even death. People who may have eaten poisonous mushrooms should seek emergency medical care.

There are certain people who should not take psilocybin. These include people with a history or family history of psychosis. It may be dangerous for people with schizophrenia or bipolar disorder. Since psilocybin may temporarily raise blood pressure and heart rate, people with existing heart problems should avoid this drug.

Research Findings

Psilocybin Treatment May Be Useful for Anxiety in Patients with Advanced-Stage Cancer

In a double-blind, placebo-controlled pilot trial published in the journal *Archives of General Psychiatry*, researchers from California and New Mexico evaluated the safety and efficacy of using psilocybin to treat patients with advanced-stage cancer and anxiety. The cohort consisted of twelve adults who were treated in a clinical research unit of a large public sector academic medical center; they were diagnosed with acute stress disorder or generalized anxiety disorder or anxiety disorder from cancer, or adjustment disorder with anxiety. The subjects ranged in age from thirty-six to fifty-eight years; eleven of the subjects were women. Though all the subjects were in the advanced stage of their cancer, they had initially been diagnosed with breast cancer, colon cancer, ovarian cancer, peritoneal cancer, salivary gland cancer, or multiple myeloma. The duration of their primary cancers ranged from two months to eighteen years. All of the subjects completed the three months' assessment; eleven completed the four months' assessment, and six completed the six-month assessment. During the follow-up period, two subjects became too ill to continue participating, and two died. While four subjects had no prior history of the use of a hallucinogen, eight did have such an experience. Each subject had two treatment sessions spaced several weeks apart. During one session, they received 0.2 mg/kg active psilocybin and during the other session they received a placebo. After treatment, the subjects were monitored for six hours. Various measurements were taken from two weeks prior to the first treatment to up to six months after the second. Psychological measures included the Beck Depression Inventory, the Profile of Mood Status, and State-Trait Anxiety Inventory. The researchers found that at one and three months after treatment, psilocybin significantly reduced levels of anxiety, and there were no clinically significant adverse events. The researchers concluded that their findings "established the feasibility and safety of administering moderate doses of psilocybin to patients with advanced-stage cancer and anxiety."[2]

Psilocybin May Help People with Anxiety and Depression Triggered by Dealing with Their Life-Threatening Cancer

In a double-blind, placebo-controlled crossover trial published in the *Journal of Psychopharmacology*, researchers from New York City and Palo Alto, California, examined the use of psilocybin to treat anxiety and depression in people with life-threatening cancer. The cohort consisted of twenty-nine patients with life-threatening cancer, as well as cancer-related anxiety and depression; most of them were recruited from NYU Langone's Perlmutter Cancer Center, an academic medical facility. The mean age of the patients was fifty-three years, and 60 percent were female. Ninety-three percent were white. Nearly two-thirds of the patients had either stage 3 or stage 4 cancer. The types of cancers included breast or reproductive, gastrointestinal, hematologic, and others. Almost all of the patients met the criteria for adjustment disorder; the remainder had generalized anxiety disorder. Although 59 percent of the patients had been treated with an antianxiety medication or antidepressant in the past, when the trial began, no patient was on a psychotropic medication. The patients were randomly assigned to receive treatment with a single dose of 0.3 mg/kg of psilocybin or the vitamin supplement niacin (250 mg), both in conjunction with nine total pre- and post-treatment sessions of psychotherapy delivered by a dyadic therapy team. Seven weeks after their first treatment, the patients were randomly assigned to receive the alternate treatment. Multiple assessments were conducted during the approximately nine months that the trial was conducted. There were no serious medical or psychiatric adverse events from either the psilocybin or niacin. The researchers determined that psilocybin treatment resulted in "immediate, substantial, and sustained improvements in anxiety and depression." After 6.5 months, 60 to 80 percent of the patients had clinically significant reductions in anxiety or depression. The researchers concluded that "psilocybin administered in conjunction with appropriate psychotherapy could become a novel pharmacological-psychosocial treatment modality for cancer-related psychological and existential distress."[3]

In a continuation of the previous research study published in the *Journal of Psychopharmacology*, researchers from Palo Alto, New York City, New Haven, Connecticut, and Aurora and Denver, Colorado, located the sixteen patients who were still alive and found that fifteen of these patients agreed to participate in a follow-up study. Data were collected on an average of 3.2 (range of 2.3 to 4.5 years) and 4.5 (range of 3.5 to 5.5 years) years after the psilocybin administration. Between the first and second data collection, one patient died; so, the final analysis had fourteen patients. Seventy-one percent reported either a partial or complete remission of their cancers, and 29 percent were in the active stages of their disease. Ninety-three percent had cancer-related adjustment disorder with anxious and/or depressed features; 7 percent had generalized anxiety disorder. There was a higher proportion of reproductive cancers in this sample and no one had a digestive cancer. Seventy-one percent rated the psilocybin treatments the single or top-five most spiritually significant experience(s) of their lives. Eighty-six percent maintained that it increased life satisfaction or well-being. All of the subjects said they had moderate, strong, or extremely positive behavioral changes that they attributed to psilocybin. The researcher determined that the combination of psychotherapy and psilocybin was associated with large and significant reductions in anxiety and depression. And, they commented that their "findings have meaningful implications for the clinical management of cancer-related existential distress."[4]

Another trial on anxiety and depression in people dealing with life-threatening cancer was also published in the *Journal of Psychopharmacology*. In this two-session, randomized, double-blind, crossover trial, researchers from Baltimore, Maryland, compared the use of very low dose (1 or 3 mg/70kg) and very high dose (22 or 30 mg/70kg) psilocybin in fifty-one patients with potentially life-threatening diagnoses of cancer who were dealing with anxiety and/or depression. Sixty-five percent had recurrent or metastatic cancer; the types of cancer included breast, upper aerodigestive, gastrointestinal, genitourinary, hematologic, and other. Those who received the low dose during the first session received the high dose during the second session; conversely, those who received the high dose during the first session had the low dose at the second session. The sessions were approximately five weeks apart. The researchers conducted assessments and evaluations before, during, and after the sessions. While no serious adverse events occurred, during the sessions there were some transient problems. For example, 34 percent of the subjects in the high-dose session and 17 percent in the low-dose session had moderate increases in blood pressure, and 32 percent of the subjects in the high-dose session and 12 percent in the low-dose session had some form of psychological discomfort. The researchers determined that the high-dose psilocybin produced large decreases in levels of anxiety and depression, and these benefits were sustained in 80 percent of the subjects for six months. The researchers concluded that future research should be conducted on a larger and more diverse sample "to establish the generality and safety of psilocybin treatment of psychological distress associated with life-threatening cancer."[5]

Psilocybin Appears to Be Useful for the Symptoms of Obsessive-Compulsive Disorder

In a modified, double-blind trial published in the *Journal of Clinical Psychiatry*, researchers from Tucson, Arizona, and San Antonio, Texas, investigated the safety, tolerability, and efficacy of psilocybin in nine patients with obsessive-compulsive disorder. Five of the subjects were unable to work because of their OCD symptomatology. Patients were required to abstain from using antidepressants or nutritional or pharmaceutical supplements. The seven male and two female patients, who ranged in age from twenty-six to sixty-two years, had up to four treatments of psilocybin. The doses ranged from 20 mg/kg to 300 mg/kg; the higher doses were hallucinogenic. In total, the patients ingested twenty-nine doses. Testing days were separated by at least one week. Set in a controlled environment, each session was conducted in an outpatient clinic over an eight-hour period. The subjects then spent the night in a psychiatric or medical-surgical unit of the hospital, where they were closely observed. One subject experienced transient hypertension, but no other adverse events were noted. The Yale-Brown Obsessive Compulsive Scale and a visual analog scale were administered at baseline and at four, eight, and twenty-four hours after psilocybin ingestion. During one or more of the sessions, notable but variable decreases in OCD symptoms were seen in all of the subjects. Because of discomfort with hospitalization, after the first testing sessions, two subjects refused further participation. Still, psilocybin appeared to be safe and well tolerated. It also was associated with transient relief of OCD symptoms in subjects with treatment-resistant OCD that lasted for more than twenty-four hours. Interestingly, five of the subjects described their experiences as very psychologically and spiritually enriching, and four subjects on the high dose had positive transcendental feelings, such as the "exploration of other planets, visiting past-life reincarnations, and interacting with deities." The researchers concluded that their trial "confirms and extends anecdotal reports of acute reduction in OCD symptoms with exposure to psilocybin."[6]

In a case report published in the *Journal of Psychoactive Drugs*, physicians from Mexico described the case of Mr. J. C, a thirty-year-old, 90 kg, married man who was treated for OCD for over a year. His symptoms included obsessive thoughts, compulsions, checking behaviors, rumination, worry, and anxiety. Although he had been prescribed a wide variety of medications, they were only partially effective. When he began eating psilocybin containing mushrooms, he was taking fluoxetine, fluvoxamine, and risperidone. Under the watchful eye of a friend, he consumed 2 g of dried mushrooms in his home. For the first hour after ingestion, he felt only a sense of disassociation. But, his OCD symptoms completely disappeared for the entire hour and were significantly reduced for two weeks. Warned by his medical professionals about such consumption, the man nevertheless continued to eat 2 g of dried mushrooms every two weeks. His dissociation symptoms did not reoccur, and he did not have another adverse effect. Further, his OCD symptoms continued to be significantly reduced. According to the researchers, thanks to the mushrooms, the man was able "to perform most of his daily tasks and work without interruptions, meaningfully improving his well-being and quality of life."[7]

When Compared to Non-Microdosers, Adults Who Microdose Psychedelics Have Lower Levels of Anxiety and Depression

In a study published in the journal *Scientific Reports*, researchers from multiple locations but based in British Columbia, Canada, compared a sample of 4,050 adult microdosers to a sample of 4,653 adult non-microdosers. The data were collected between November 2019 and July 2020 from self-selected respondents recruited via media. Because of the application used, the study was only available to users of iPhones. In order to be included in the microdosing group, a subject had to be a current microdoser; the non-microdoser group included people who had never microdosed as well as those who microdosed in the past. The thousands of subjects who responded were from eighty-four countries. Eighty-five percent of the microdosers noted that they used psilocybin, usually in combination with non-psychedelic substances such as Lion's mane mushrooms, chocolate, and/or niacin. A far lower 11 percent indicated that they used LSD. Most of the people who responded, 5,413 or 62.2 percent, were from the United States. The next largest group was from Canada—1,104 people or 12.7 percent. Other countries with larger numbers of participants were, in descending order, Australia, Great Britain, Russia, the Netherlands, and Denmark. The majority of the microdosers microdosed one to four times per week. The most frequent reasons for microdosing were anxiety, depression, and symptoms of post-traumatic stress disorder. In their various analyses, the researchers consistently found that microdose users demonstrated lower levels of anxiety, depression, and stress. Females were more likely than males to report microdosing to improve mood and decrease anxiety. The researchers concluded that their "examination of a large international sample of adults highlights the prominence of therapeutic and wellness motivations for microdosing drugs and identified lower levels of anxiety and depression among microdosers relative to controls."[8]

Psilocybin May Be Safer Than Many People Realize

In a study published in the *Journal of Psychopharmacology*, researchers from London and Australia examined the twelve-month prevalence of adverse reactions to psilocybin/magic mushrooms that require emergency medical treatment. They used data from the 2017 Global Drug Survey, a large anonymous online survey of patterns of drug use conducted between November 2016 and January 2017. The researchers learned that 9,233 people noted that they used magic mushrooms. Of these, nineteen (0.2 percent) sought emergency treatment. Seeking emergency care was far more likely to occur among younger people. In fact, "young age" was the only predictor of needing emergency treatment; neither first-time use nor the frequency of use in the past year were predictors. The most commonly cited symptoms were psychological including, ironically, anxiety/panic attacks, paranoia/suspiciousness, and seeing and hearing things. Though less frequent, there were physical reactions such as passing out/unconsciousness, difficulty breathing, and seizures. Eight of the respondents were admitted to the hospitals, and all except for one indicated that they returned to normal within twenty-four hours. The majority of those who required emergency medical care noted that they used the mushrooms as well as other substances during the same session, with 37 percent reporting the use of cannabis and 32 percent using alcohol. The researchers concluded that "psilocybin mushrooms are a relatively safe drug, with serious incidents rare and short-lasting."[9]

But, There Are Reports of Dangerous Behaviors and Fatalities Following Psilocybin Ingestion

In a case report published in the *Journal of Forensic Sciences*, physicians and researchers from France noted that there are instances of dangerous behavior and death from indirect causes under the influence of magic mushrooms, such as psilocybin. They described the case of an eighteen-year-old male who was at home with three friends. The male and two of his friends consumed psilocybin, and the third friend consumed cannabis. During the evening the male isolated himself in the bathroom before emerging naked. Soon, he was acting unusually aggressive and excited. Suddenly, he had an urge to jump from the balcony. When the friend who consumed cannabis tried to stop him, the male managed to jump, with a fatal result. The deceased male, who had no known medical or psychiatric history, had been consuming hallucinogenic mushrooms to overcome his shyness. In his room, the police found several growing mushroom plants and cannabis. The cause of death was determined to be "multiple trauma secondary to an accidental high fall under the influence of psilocybin mushrooms." No other psychoactive substances were detected in his body. "The victim's inexplicable behavior leading to a fatal fall can be linked toxicologically to the sole influence of the psychedelic mushrooms."[10]

References and Further Readings

Agin-Liebes, G. I., T. Malone, M. M. Yalch et al. "Long-Term Follow-up of Psilocybin-Assisted Psychotherapy for Psychiatric and Existential Distress in Patients with Life-Threatening Cancer." *Journal of Psychopharmacology* 34, no. 2 (February 2020): 155–66.

Griffiths, Roland R., Matthew W. Johnson, Michael A. Carducci et al. "Psilocybin Produces Substantial and Sustained Decreases in Depression and Anxiety in Patients with Life-Threatening Cancer: A Randomized Double-Blind Trial." *Journal of Psychopharmacology* 30, no. 12 (2016): 1181–97.

Grob, Charles S., Alicia L. Danforth, Gurpreet S. Chopra et al. "Pilot Study of Psilocybin Treatment for Anxiety in Patients with Advanced-Stage Cancer." *Archives of General Psychiatry* 68, no. 1 (January 2011): 71–8.

Honyiglo, Emma, Angélique Franchi, Nathalie Cartiser et al. "Unpredictable Behavior Under the Influence of 'Magic Mushrooms': A Case Report and Review of the Literature." *Journal of Forensic Sciences* 64, no. 4 (2018): 1266–70.

Johnson, Matthew W. and Roland R. Griffiths. "Potential Therapeutic Effects of Psilocybin." *Neurotherapeutics* 14 (2017): 734–40.

Kopra, E. I., J.A. Ferris, A. R. Winstock et al. "Adverse Experiences Resulting in Emergency Medical Treatment Seeking Following the Use of Magic Mushrooms." *Journal of Psychopharmacology* 36, no. 8 (2022): 965–73.

Lugo-Radillo, Agustin and Jorge Luis Cortes-Lopez. "Long-Term Amelioration of OCD Symptoms in a Patient with Chronic Consumption of Psilocybin-Containing Mushrooms." *Journal of Psychoactive Drugs* 53, no. 2 (2021): 146–8.

Moreno, Francisco A., Christopher B. Wiegand, E. Keolani Taitano, and Pedro L. Delgado. "Safety, Tolerability, and Efficacy of Psilocybin in Nine Patients with Obsessive-Compulsive Disorder." *Journal of Clinical Psychiatry* 67 (2006):1735–40.

Rootman, Joseph M. Pamela Kryskow, Kalin Harvey et al. "Adults Who Microdose Psychedelics Report Health Related Motivations and Lower Levels of Anxiety and Depression Compared to Non-Microdosers." *Scientific Reports* 11 (2021): 22479.

Ross, Stephen, Anthony Bossis, Jeffrey Guss et al. "Rapid and Sustained Symptoms Reduction Following Psilocybin Treatment for Anxiety and Depression in Patients with Life-Threatening Cancer: A Randomized Controlled Trial." *Journal of Psychopharmacology* 30, no. 12 (2016): 1165–80.

Reflexology

Introduction

Also known as zone therapy, reflexology is the application of pressure to specific areas of the feet and sometimes the hands (rarely ears); these areas are believed to correspond to specific muscle groups or organs of the body. The nerve endings of the feet and hands are thought to be directly connected to the rest of the body. Thus, in foot reflexology, pinching the top of the toes is thought to help sinus problems, and applying pressure to the heel is useful for low back and sciatic nerve pain. Pressing on particular areas of the feet or hands promotes health benefits, such as the relaxation of tension and anxiety, improvement in circulation, and support of normal functioning. For example with foot reflexology for anxiety, begin by pressing on the big toe. Then, slowly slide down the side of the foot pressing gently until the heel. Repeat the process going back up to the big toe. With hand reflexology for anxiety, press just below the crease of the wrist on the outer hand. Place pressure on the little dent.

According to reflexology, the foot is divided into five zones that run from toe to heel. The big toe is zone #1 and the pinky toe is zone #5. At the same time, the human body is divided into ten zones that run from head to foot. Zone #1 aligns with the left and right center of the body, and zone #5 aligns with the left and right side of the body. Placing pressure on a zone in the foot may relieve pain in that zone of the body. A similar system exists for hands.

There are several theories behind reflexology. One suggests that reflexology stimulates the central nervous system, which relaxes the body and improves breathing, blood flow, the immune response, and other areas. Another theory contends that reflexology changes the way the brain perceives pain. Placing pressure on extremities makes the brain less inclined to perceive pain as deeply; it reduces the way the brain registers pain. And, a third theory suggests that when the vital energy or *qi* (pronounced chee) that flows throughout the body is blocked by stress, aches, pain, and illness follow. By supporting vital energy, reflexology enables it to continue to flow throughout the body, lessening the chances of pain and ill health. It is important to add that Western medicine practitioners do not necessarily accept these beliefs or the theories behind them, although those who practice a more integrative form of medicine may adhere to some aspects. And, reflexology should never be used as a substitute for regular medical care.

Reflexology is believed to have truly ancient roots. It was first recorded on the Egyptian tomb of Ankhamor in 2,330 BC along with other medical procedures. In the United States, the modern practice of reflexology was primarily developed by two doctors, William H. Fitzgerald, who wrote in 1917 about ten vertical zones that extend the length of the body, and Joe Shelby Riley, who developed a map of horizontal zones going across the body and a detailed map of reflex points on the feet and hands. Eunice Ingham, a physiotherapist who worked with Riley, designed the foot maps and reflexology charts that are still in use today.[1]

Regulation, Administration, and Costs

The American Commission for Accreditation of Reflexology Education and Training (ACARET) sets the standards for reflexology education, and it credentials those involved with educating students of reflexology. The American Reflexology Certification Board (ARCB) has a three-part examination process that ensures practitioners meet certain standards. Certification by the ARCB requires the completion of a minimum of 110 hands-on training hours. To remain certified by the ARCB, practitioners must pay an annual fee and participate in twelve hours of continuing education every two years. This certification is voluntary and not mandatory to practice reflexology. It is important to remember that certification is not a license to practice reflexology. Licensing laws to perform reflexology, probably categorized as massage, are set at the state and local government levels. Most states do not differentiate between massage therapy and reflexology. To qualify as a professional member of the Reflexology Association of America, practitioners must have a minimum of 300 hours of reflexology training, 60 percent of which must have been taken in a live classroom setting. It is the responsibility of each individual reflexologist to know the current regulatory laws.

People searching for a practitioner of reflexology may find them in a number of different settings. They may open an office both in their own homes or in an office building setting. They may travel to the home of clients or work at a chiropractic office, fitness center, salon, or spa. One of the best ways to locate a practitioner is by a referral from a trusted professional or friend.

A typical reflexology session lasts from thirty minutes to one hour. It may begin with immersing feet in a footbath. After the bath, the client sits in a chair or lies on a massage table while the practitioner applies pressure in a thumb and finger walking pattern to specific zones of the feet and hands. In addition, the practitioner stretches and massages areas of the feet and hands. Doing one foot or hand at a time, they will use mild to moderate pressure and different techniques. Sometimes, people feel so relaxed that they fall asleep; on other occasions, they might experience a rush of emotions as energy moves throughout the body, which is followed by a sense of calm. (For those who wish to informally try this at home, reflexology socks and gloves are sold online.)

While reflexologist charges vary, a thirty-minute session tends to range between $30 and $50, and a one-hour session ranges between $40 and $90. While it is always a good idea to check with insurers, do not assume that insurers will cover the cost of these treatments.

Side Effects and Risks

During reflexology, some people may have minor side effects such as light-headedness, tender feet, and emotional sensitivity. People with sores, acute injuries, athlete's foot, burns, wounds, and/or infections on their feet or hands should avoid reflexology until these are healed. People with blood clots should not allow massage near these clots. It could release these clots into the bloodstream. Massaging may aggravate gout, vascular problems, and epilepsy; people with these conditions should check with a medical provider before scheduling an appointment. Of course, anyone with recent surgery to their feet or hands should not be massaged. And, there is some limited evidence that rubbing the feet could stimulate contractions in pregnant women. So, reflexology should be avoided in the later stages of pregnancy.

It should be parenthetically noted that there is very little research on hand reflexology. While it might not be clear if hand reflexology is useful, it has very few risks or negative health effects. And, there are many anecdotes from people who have found it helpful. At the same time, until more is known, pregnant women should not have hand reflexology.

Research Findings

Foot Reflexology May Help Women with Anxiety and Pain During Brachytherapy for Cervical Cancer

In a trial published in the journal *Oncology Nursing Forum*, researchers from Ohio studied the use of foot reflexology and aromatherapy for anxiety and pain during brachytherapy for cervical cancer. (Brachytherapy is a type of internal radiation therapy in which sealed radiation is placed near the area requiring treatment.) The cohort consisted of forty-one women with locally advanced cervical cancer who had a total of 193 intracavitary brachytherapy treatments. The women were randomized to receive a thirty-minute foot reflexology session and diffused aromatherapy ($n = 22$) during treatment or the usual care ($n = 19$). The women in the intervention groups were asked to evaluate their experience. Both foot reflexology and aromatherapy were rated highly, with foot reflexology being the most helpful in reducing their anxiety. Moreover, the researchers determined that the women in the intervention group had statistically significant lower levels of anxiety and pain, and they used less treatment-related medication than the women in the control group.[2]

Hand Reflexology May Be as Useful as Acupressure for Anxiety in Women with Coronary Artery Diseases

In a randomized, placebo-controlled, double-blinded trial published in the journal *Healthcare*, researchers from Iran, Boseman, Montana, and Norway compared the effectiveness of hand reflexology to acupressure for women with anxiety who were hospitalized for one day in the cardiac care unit. They all had a diagnosis of acute coronary syndrome. The cohort consisted of 135 female patients, with a mean age of 49.77 years, hospitalized in the cardiac care unit. Except for their occupations, there were no statistical differences between the women. They were divided into three groups—hand reflexology, acupressure, and placebo; there were forty-five women in each group. The women in the intervention groups received ten minutes of hand reflexology or acupressure in each hand; the women in the placebo group were randomly touched on their hands. Levels of anxiety were assessed before and after the interventions. The women in the two intervention groups had similar reductions in their levels of anxiety, and there were no reported adverse events.[3]

Foot Reflexology May or May Not Be Useful for Anxiety in Women in Labor

In a retrospective study published in the journal *Acta Medica Iranica*, researchers from Iran examined the use of foot reflexology to treat the anxiety, pain, and outcomes of labor in primigravida women (in labor with their first child). The cohort consisted of eighty women; forty women received forty minutes of foot reflexology—twenty minutes on each foot—when their cervix measured 3 to 4 cm, the beginning of active labor; the practitioners focused on areas of the foot that connect to the pituitary gland, solar plexus, and uterus. Forty women served as controls; they received foot massage on other parts of their feet. Anxiety was measured with the Spielberger State-Trait Anxiety Inventory before and after the intervention in both groups. The researchers determined that reflexology significantly decreased levels of anxiety, pain, and improved outcomes. In fact, while the anxiety levels in the intervention group decreased, the levels in the control group increased. And, the women in the intervention group were more likely to have a vaginal birth than the women in the control group—92.5 percent to 80 percent, respectively. The researchers concluded that "using this non-invasive technique, obstetricians can achieve, to some extent, one of the most important goals of midwifery as pain relief and reducing anxiety during labor and encourage the mothers to have a vaginal delivery."[4]

In an open-label, randomized, controlled trial published in the journal *Complementary Therapies in Clinical Practice*, researchers from Israel evaluated the use of foot reflexology for reducing anxiety and the duration of labor in primiparas with moderate to severe anxiety. The cohort consisted of 189 women with at least moderate levels of anxiety; 99 women received foot reflexology as well as the usual care, and 90 received only the usual care. The researchers found that foot reflexology significantly reduced the level of anxiety immediately after treatment. This was primarily observed in women with professional or academic education and in women admitted with ruptured membranes or post-term pregnancy and less in women with a high school education or were admitted with contractions. However, thirty to ninety minutes after reflexology treatment ended, the level of anxiety worsened in the reflexology group and slightly improved in the control group, particularly among women with academic education. Interestingly, when the women were anxious for the safety of their babies, anxiety was not relieved by reflexology, while when the women's anxiety was related to another factor, such as fear or pain, foot reflexology was more effective, especially during the minutes following administration. Though there were no adverse effects from the reflexology, there is a need for further research to determine how reflexology may be most effectively used during labor.[5]

May Help Adults Dealing with Anxiety, Depression, and Sleep Quality Issues

In a systematic review and meta-analysis published in the journal *Evidence-Based Complementary and Alternative Medicine*, researchers from Taiwan wanted to learn if foot reflexology would be useful for adults dealing with anxiety, depression, and sleep quality problems. They located twenty-six randomized controlled trials with 2,366 subjects that met their criteria. The studies were conducted in Iran, Turkey, Taiwan, South Korea, Japan, and Israel, and published between 2011 and 2020. The sample sizes ranged from 50 to 189 subjects, and the ages ranged from twenty seven to seventy two years. In each study, foot reflexology sessions lasted from ten to sixty minutes; the number of sessions ranged from one to eighteen, and the treatment periods ranged from one to eight weeks. The studies tended to be short term and did not have long-term follow-ups. None of the studies reported any adverse effects. Sixteen of the studies, which were heterogeneous, examined the effect of foot reflexology on anxiety. In general, they found that foot reflexology significantly lowered levels of anxiety. The researchers recommended that future studies focus on specific populations and include more subjects with longer term follow-ups.[6]

May Help Patients with Burn-Related Anxiety

In a randomized, controlled clinical trial published in the journal *Burns*, researchers from Iran, China, and Australia investigated the use of foot reflexology to ease the anxiety and sleep disorders associated with patients hospitalized in the burn intensive care unit. The cohort consisted of fifty-two patients with accidental moderate to severe burns who had mean ages of forty-three years; the vast majority of burns were thermal. Most patients in both groups were male and married, with high school diplomas or higher degrees. Twenty-six were assigned to receive foot reflexology fifteen minutes before wound dressing changes on the third, fourth, and fifth day of hospitalization; twenty-six patients served as controls. Before interventions, the patients tended to have high levels of pain anxiety. Beginning their third day of hospitalization, the patients in the intervention group received twenty minutes of foot reflexology for three consecutive days, ten minutes for each foot, five zones on each foot related to the brain, pituitary gland, kidney, adrenal gland, and solar plexus. After the dressings were changed, levels of pain anxiety were measured and found to be significantly less in the intervention group on their fifth day of hospitalization, while the patients in the control group had significant increases in pain anxiety after dressing changes also on the fifth day of hospitalization. The researchers noted that their findings support the pain anxiety benefits of foot reflexology for these patients. "Due to the easy, low-cost and availability of the interventions applied, this complementary therapy is suggested for the burn patients."[7]

May Be Useful for Older Female Adults with Anxiety and Depression Related to Hospitalization for Acute Coronary Syndrome

In a trial published in the *International Journal of Therapeutic Massage and Bodywork*, researchers from Iran and Norway evaluated the use of foot reflexology to ease the anxiety and depression of women sixty years of age or older who were hospitalized for one day with acute coronary syndrome. Ninety women were randomly assigned to the intervention group or control group; there were forty-five in each group. The women in both groups received routine care; the women in the intervention group received ten minutes of foot reflexology on each foot. No harm or side effects were reported in either group. While the women in both groups had similar demographic characteristics, the women in the intervention group had significant reductions in anxiety and depression. No such reductions were seen in the women in the control group. The researchers concluded that foot reflexology is a "safe and effective non-pharmacological intervention that can be used, along with pharmacological measures, to reduce psychological symptoms and improve quality of care in patients with ACS."[8]

May Be Helpful for Women with Anxiety Following an Abdominal Hysterectomy

In a randomized, controlled trial published in the journal *Complementary Therapies in Medicine*, between September 2013 and September 2014 researchers from Turkey examined the use of foot reflexology for anxiety and pain in women hospitalized in the intensive care unit following an abdominal hysterectomy. The cohort consisted of sixty-three patients; they had an average age of 47.23 years. Thirty-two were placed in the intervention group, and thirty-one were in the control group. There were no statistically meaningful differences between the groups. Though all the women received the standard medications, the women in the intervention group also received foot reflexology on the postoperative first, second, and third days. Reflexology was applied for ten minutes on each foot. Anxiety and pain levels were assessed at baseline, immediately after treatment, and thirty minutes later. The researchers learned that on each of the three days of reflexology, the average level of anxiety experience by the women after the intervention was significantly less than the anxiety in the women in the control group. The researchers concluded that "applying reflexology can be an easy, cheap, effective nursing intervention."[9]

Though They Don't Directly Address Anxiety, Some Researchers Say Reflexology Does Not Work for Any Medical Condition

In a systematic review published in the journal *Maturitas*, researchers from the UK evaluated twenty-three randomly controlled trials on the ability of reflexology to treat a host of different medical conditions and situations, such as diabetes, premenstrual syndrome, cancer patients, multiple sclerosis, and dementia but not anxiety. The researchers found that the methodological quality of the trials was variable and mostly poor. Many of the trials did not adequately control for "non-specific effects," and most had low sample sizes. Numbers of sessions and duration vary from trial to trial. Several studies did not mention the length of follow-up. Eight trials had more than fifty subjects and another eight had less than thirty. Of the four trials with sample sizes of 100 or more, three generated negative results. Of the higher quality trials, five had positive results and nine had negative results. While noting that reflexology is popular, the researchers concluded that "the notion that reflexology is an effective treatment option is currently not based on the evidence from independently replicated, high-quality, clinical trials."[10]

References and Further Readings

Alinia-najjar, Reza, Masoumeh Bagheri-Nesami, Seyed Afshin Shorofi et al. "The Effect of Foot Reflexology Massage on Burn-Specific Pain Anxiety and Sleep Quality and Quantity of Patients Hospitalized in the Burn Intensive Care Unit (ICU)." *Burns* 46 (2020): 1942–51.

Bahrami, Tahereh, Nahid Rejeh, Majideh Heravi-Karimooi et al. "The Effect of Foot Reflexology on Hospital Anxiety and Depression in Female Older Adults: A Randomized Controlled Trial." *International Journal of Therapeutic Massage and Bodywork* 12, no. 3 (September 2019): 16–21.

Blackburn, Lisa, Catherine Hill, Amy L. Lindsey et al. "Effect of Foot Reflexology and Aromatherapy on Anxiety and Pain During Brachytherapy for Cervical Cancer." *Oncology Nursing Forum* 48, no. 3 (May 2021): 265–76.

Ernst, E., P. Posadzki, and M. S. Lee. "Reflexology: An Update of a Systematic Review of Randomised Clinical Trials." *Maturitas* 68, no. 2 (February 2011): 116–20.

Levy, I. S. Attias, T. S. Lavee et al. "The Effectiveness of Foot Reflexology in Reducing Anxiety and Duration of Labor in Primiparas: An Open-Label Randomized Controlled Trial." *Complementary Therapies in Clinical Practice* 38 (February 2020): 101085.

Moghimi-Hanjani, S., Z. Mehdizadeh-Tourzani, and M. Shoghi. "The Effect of Foot Reflexology on Anxiety, Pain, and Outcomes of the Labor in Primigravida Women." *Acta Medica Iranica* 53, no. 8 (2015): 507–11.

Öztürk, Rusen, Ümran Sevil, Asuman Sargin, and M. Sait Yücebilgin. "The Effects of Reflexology on Anxiety and Pain in Patients After Abdominal Hysterectomy: A Randomized Controlled Trial." *Complementary Therapies in Medicine* 36 (2018): 107–12.

Rahmani Vasokolaei, Zohre, Nahid Rajeh, Majideh Heravi-Karimooi et al. "Comparison of the Effects of Hand Reflexology versus Acupressure on Anxiety and Vital Signs in Female Patients with Coronary Artery Diseases." *Healthcare* 7, no. 1 (March 2019): 26.

Take Charge of Your Well-Being. University of Minnesota. https://www.takingcharge .csh.umn.edu/reflexology.

Wang, Wei-Li, Hao-Yuan Hung, Ying-Ren Chen et al. "Effect of Foot Reflexology Intervention on Depression, Anxiety, and Sleep Quality in Adults: A Meta-Analysis and Metaregression of Randomized Controlled Trials." *Evidence-Based Complementary and Alternative Medicine* (2020): Article ID 2654353.

Selective Serotonin Reuptake Inhibitors

Introduction

Selective serotonin reuptake inhibitors (SSRIs) increase levels of serotonin in the brain with minimal effect on the other chemicals in the brain. In so doing, they work to restore the balance of serotonin in the brain. People suffering from anxiety have imbalances of the brain's neurotransmitters, chemicals in the brain such as serotonin that help cells communicate. Serotonin is released from one nerve cell and reaches the next. During the process, the first nerve cell reabsorbs some of the released serotonin. SSRIs block the reabsorption of serotonin back into the nerve cells. The blocking action increases the amount of serotonin available, thus improving the transmission of messages between neurons. SSRIs are called selective because they mainly affect serotonin, not other transmitters. In fact, SSRIs have little effect on other neurotransmitters. And, though they have a long list of potential side effects, after a few weeks on these medications, many people experience notable benefits with few, if any, significant side effects.

The FDA has approved eight SSRIs in the following order—fluoxetine (Prozac), paroxetine (Paxil), sertraline (Zoloft), citalopram (Celexa), escitalopram (Lexapro), fluvoxamine (Luvox), vilazodone (Viibryd), and vortioxetine (Trintellix). While they have many similarities, each of the SSRIs is slightly different. People who are unable to tolerate one type of SSRI may well be able to take another.

Evidence for the role of serotonin for treating depression began to emerge early in the 1970s. The serotonin-based drugs appeared to have fewer side effects than some previously used medication, such as the benzodiazepines. In 1987, fluoxetine was approved by the FDA. One year later, it was marketed as Prozac. The following year, almost 2.5 million Prozac prescriptions were prescribed. Soon, it became evident that Prozac and the seven other SSRIs that emerged over time were also useful for different forms of anxiety, which may or may not be present with a depressive disorder.

Today, SSRIs are commonly prescribed for many anxiety disorders, such as generalized anxiety disorder, obsessive-compulsive disorder, panic disorder, and post-traumatic stress disorder. In the United States, it is believed that one in ten people takes SSRIs. One of every four women in their forties and fifties takes a SSRI.

Regulation, Administration, and Costs

In the United States, all medication dispensed by prescription are regulated by the FDA. No medication may be legally dispensed without FDA authorization. As a result, all eight of the noted SSRIs have been approved by the FDA. When approving a medication, the FDA recommends how it should be used. However, when actually advising patients, medical providers often prescribe medications for another medical problem, a process known as off-label prescribing.

Fluoxetine (Prozac)

The FDA has approved fluoxetine for the anxiety disorders of OCD and panic disorder, and it is prescribed off-label for social anxiety disorder and PTSD. Fluoxetine is sold as a tablet, capsule, solution, and delayed-release capsule. Doses, which vary according to the specific type of anxiety, range from 20 to 80 mg per day. The delayed-release capsule should never be crushed. Insurance may cover all or part of the cost of fluoxetine, which is about $15 per month.

Paroxetine (Paxil)

Though often prescribed to those under the age of eighteen, paroxetine was approved by the FDA in 1992 to treat generalized anxiety disorder, OCD, PTSD, social anxiety disorders, and panic disorders for adults eighteen years and older. Paroxetine is administered as an immediate-release tablet, oral suspension, capsule, and extended-release tablet in doses from 10 to 60 mg per day. Insurance may cover all or part of the cost of paroxetine which is about $20 per month or more depending upon the prescription

Citalopram (Celexa)

In 1998, the FDA approved citalopram for the treatment of depression, not anxiety, in adults. But, it has been used for generalized anxiety disorder, OCD, PTSD, social anxiety disorders, and panic disorders and for people under the age of eighteen years. Citalopram is administered as a capsule, tablet, or solution in doses that range from 10 to 40 mg per day. Insurance may cover all or part of the cost of citalopram, which is only a few dollars per month.

Sertraline (Zoloft)

In 1999, sertraline was approved by the FDA for social anxiety disorder, PTSD, and panic disorder, as well as OCD in adults and children ages six years and older. It is sold as a capsule, tablet, or oral concentrate; daily doses usually range from 50 to 200 mg. When the liquid form of sertraline is used, it should be added to four ounces of liquid immediately before it is taken. Insurance may cover all or part of the cost of this medicine, which is about $20 per month.

Escitalopram (Lexapro)

Escitalopram was approved by the FDA in 2002 for the treatment of generalized anxiety disorder in adolescents and adults twelve years of age and older. Still, it is used off-label for OCD, panic disorder, and PTSD. Escitalopram is sold as a tablet or a solution in doses between 5 and 20 mg per day. Insurance may cover all or part of the cost of escitalopram, which is only a few dollars per month.

Fluvoxamine (Luvox)

In 2007, the FDA approved the use of fluvoxamine for adults and children eight years of age and older for the treatment of obsessive-compulsive disorder. Still, it is used off-label for social anxiety disorder, PTSD, and panic disorder. It is administered as a tablet and extended-release capsule. Doses range from 50 to 200 mg per day. Insurance may cover all or part of the cost, which is between $15 and $25 per month.

Vilazodone (Viibryd)

Approved by the FDA in 2011 to treat depression, vilazodone is a tablet that should be taken with food. Doses range from 20 to 40 mg per day. Though not approved for anxiety disorders, vilazodone may be prescribed for those medical problems. Prices for vilazodone tend to vary from around $40 to $100 per month, which may or may not be covered all or in part by insurance.

Vortioxetine (Trintellix)

Approved in 2013 only for depression in adults, not children, vortioxetine is often used off-label to treat anxiety disorders such as generalized anxiety disorder and OCD and to treat children. It is sold as tablets that are available in doses ranging from 5 to 20 mg. Vortioxetine works a little different than the other SSRIs. It also binds to serotonin receptors and functions much the same way as serotonin. Since vortioxetine is sold only as a brand name, it is much more costly, several hundred dollars per month. Citing the availability of far less expensive options, insurers may refuse to cover any of the costs of this medication.

Side Effects and Risks

It is important to know that a small number of children, adolescents, and young adults, up to the age of twenty-four years, during clinical trials became suicidal after taking SSRIs. They considered harming or killing themselves or actually planned and carried out the suicide. That is why in 2004 the FDA issued a Black Box warning for all SSRIs. This is the most serious warning that the FDA issues. The FDA advised medical providers of children, adolescents, and young adults to compare the benefits of SSRIs to their potential harm for each patient, always remembering that the psychiatric symptoms may increase the risk of suicidality.

Among the many potential side effects of SSRIs are sleep disturbances, weight fluctuations, blurred vision, dry mouth, diarrhea, constipation, nausea, stomach pain, heartburn, light-headedness, irritability, nervousness, dizziness, change in appetite, excessive sweating, flu-like symptoms, and sexual problems. As the body adjusts to the medication, the side effects tend to diminish. On rare occasions, there may be more serious side effects that may require emergency attention. These include difficulty breathing or swallowing, swelling of the face, mouth, or tongue, fast heartbeat, seizures, confusion, rash, hallucinations, stiff muscles, and vomiting.

Further, SSRIs are known to promote bleeding. So, they should not be mixed with other medications that thin blood, such as warfarin and nonsteroidal anti-inflammatory drugs. And, they should not be combined with certain psychiatric and pain medications, drugs that reduce stomach acids, and diuretics. Even taking SSRIs with the supplement St. John's wort may be dangerous. It raises serum levels of serotonin and may cause serotonin syndrome or serotonin toxicity. Before beginning a SSRI, it is best to provide your medical professional with a list of all your medications and supplements.

Women who are pregnant or planning to become pregnant should know that animal research has found adverse effects to the fetus when the animal mothers take SSRI. There are too few studies in humans to know if a similar effect may occur. And, breastfeeding women pass the medication along to their babies. Women who are breastfeeding may be advised to discontinue their medication or stop breastfeeding. Children taking SSRIs are at increased risk for decreased appetite and weight loss. So, they should have their height and weight periodically monitored. And seniors on these drugs may have lowered blood sodium levels, especially if they are also taking a diuretic medication, which may result in a loss of coordination and increase the risk of falling.

Still, SSRIs should never be suddenly discontinued. An abrupt stoppage may trigger side effects such as irritability, agitation, anxiety, high or low mood, restlessness, change in sleep habits, headaches, sweating, nausea, dizziness, electric-shock sensation, shaking, and confusion. To prevent these side effects, the dosage reduction should be supervised by a medical provider.

Research Findings

Though Somewhat Common, the Simultaneous Initiation of SSRIs and Benzodiazepines in Young People with Anxiety Disorders May or May Not Be Advised

In a study published in the *Journal of Clinical Psychiatry*, researchers from New Brunswick, New Jersey, Durham, North Carolina, and New York City examined the benefits and risks of treating anxiety in younger people with a combination of a SSRI and a benzodiazepine. Their cohort included 94,399 adolescents (ten to seventeen years) and 130,971 young adults (eighteen to twenty-four years) who initiated SSRI treatment for anxiety disorders; 4.3 percent of the adolescents and 16.7 percent of the young adults began benzodiazepine treatment on the same day. An additional 4 percent of the adolescents and 7 percent of the young adults started benzodiazepine treatment one to ninety days after beginning their SSRI medication. The highest prevalence of simultaneous initiation was among adolescents (13 percent) and young adults (35 percent) with panic disorder. Psychiatrists and family physicians were more likely to simultaneously prescribe than pediatricians. Yet, the researchers observed an overall decline in the proportion of SSRI initiators simultaneously starting benzodiazepine treatment. And, adolescents and young adults who received psychotherapy prior to SSRI initiation were less likely to have benzodiazepine treatment. The researchers concluded that "given the risks" of benzodiazepines, the potential benefits of adding them to SSRI treatment "must be carefully weighed."[1]

Is an SSRI or a Benzodiazepine Better for Treating Panic Disorder

In a study published in the journal *Expert Opinion on Drug Safety*, researchers from Brazil conducted a literature search to compare the use of SSRIs and benzodiazepines for the treatment of panic disorder. They located twenty-four open or placebo-controlled clinical trials, published between 1997 and 2017, that met their criteria. The researchers learned that SSRIs are often prescribed first. But, they may require weeks of treatment before therapeutic effects are felt, and they may initially worsen the condition. While benzodiazepines may bring quick relief, they may cause tolerance and dependence. Still, both types of medication do help those with panic disorder. Yet, the researchers emphasized that there is a need for more studies directly comparing the risks and benefits of these medications. "Few studies to date have performed head-to-head comparisons of these two drug classes."[2]

SSRI Treatment May Lower Serum Sodium Levels

In a large, population-based trial published in the journal *Medicine*, researchers from Israel wanted to learn if anxiety by itself or in combination with SSRI treatment for anxiety is associated in hyponatremia, low levels of sodium concentrations in blood serum. The subjects were selected from a large electronic database insuring two million Israelis. The researchers assembled a cohort of 3,520 patients with a diagnosis of anxiety who received at least one prescription for a SSRI. The control group consisted of 6,985 age and gender-matched participants who did not have a diagnosis of anxiety. The researchers found that the prevalence of hyponatremia was about 4 percent in the intervention group; that is a small but significantly lower level of serum sodium than was found in the control subjects. "It is the use of SSRIs and not anxiety itself that causes hyponatremia among anxious patients."[3]

Fluoxetine May Help Generalized Anxiety Disorder in Children, Adolescents, and Adults

In a study published in the *Journal of the American Academy of Child & Adolescent Psychiatry*, researchers based in Pittsburgh, Pennsylvania, evaluated the efficacy and tolerability of fluoxetine for the acute treatment of children and adolescents with generalized anxiety disorder, separation anxiety disorder, and/or social phobia. The cohort consisted of seventy-four "anxious youths with significant functional impairment." Fifty-four percent were female, and 96 percent were white and middle class. Seventy percent of the subjects had two anxiety disorder and 26 percent had three. Thirty-two percent had other nonanxiety psychiatric disorders. Overall, the duration of the anxiety disorder was 62.7 months. About 60 percent of the youths had parents and/or siblings with lifetime anxiety and/ or mood disorders. For twelve weeks, the children and teens, between the ages of seven and seventeen years, with a mean age of 11.8 years, were randomized to first take 10 mg per day and then 20 mg per day of fluoxetine ($n = 37$) or a placebo ($n = 37$). Two experienced psychiatric research nurses screened and interviewed all of the subjects, and all of the diagnoses were confirmed by a child psychiatrist. The subjects were offered follow-up assessments every four months for one year at no cost. Fifty-nine subjects (80 percent) completed the entire trial. The researchers found that fluoxetine was "efficacious and well tolerated" for the acute treatment of these children and teens. Approximately, 61 percent of the patients treated with fluoxetine and 35 percent of those on placebo showed "very much and much improvement." Poorer functional responses were seen in those with more severe illness at intake and a positive family history for anxiety disorders. The subjects tolerated the fluoxetine well, with only a few patients experiencing mild transient headaches and gastrointestinal symptoms. The researchers concluded that fluoxetine "is useful and well tolerated for the acute treatment of anxious youths."[4]

In a literature review published in *Neuropsychiatric Disease and Treatment*, researchers from China and St. Louis, Missouri, examined the efficacy and safety of fluoxetine for treating generalized anxiety disorder in Chinese patients. The researchers identified fifteen randomized, open-label, head-to-head clinical trials comparing fluoxetine with other anxiolytics without a placebo arm, except for one study which investigated the efficacy of fluoxetine with a different schedule. All of the studies had adults diagnosed with generalized anxiety disorder and included evaluations of treatment and reports on the safety and tolerability of fluoxetine. The researchers found that fluoxetine brought relief quickly, within one to two weeks, and seemed effective in maintenance treatment. It was generally well-tolerated with the most often side effects of dry mouth and nausea, followed by insomnia, drowsiness, constipation, and agitation. Adverse events related to active treatment tended to be mild to moderate in severity and resolved with continued treatment. The researchers found that the response rate of the patients to short-term treatment was more than 70 percent and the recovery rate was between 30 and 50 percent. Nevertheless, the researchers noted that their studies had a high risk of bias, overall small sample sizes, and the lack of placebo control groups. Without those, they were unable to recommend fluoxetine as a reliable first-line treatment in Chinese patients with generalized anxiety disorder. "Trials with larger sample sizes, better quality, longer duration, and more clinically meaningful outcomes are needed in future research."[5]

Fluoxetine May Be Useful for Obsessive-Compulsive Disorder in Children and Adolescents

In a seven-year randomized controlled trial published in *JAMA*, researchers from Australia and London investigated the use of fluoxetine for OCD behaviors in 146 children and adolescents between the ages of 7.5 and 18 years, 85 percent male, with autism spectrum disorders. They wanted to learn if fluoxetine would reduce the frequency and severity of their OCD behaviors in these children and teens, 30 percent of whom had intellectual disability. For sixteen weeks, the children and adolescents randomly received fluoxetine ($n = 75$) every morning or a placebo ($n = 71$). The subjects receiving fluoxetine began with a dose of 4 or 8 mg per day and titrated to a maximum dose of 20 or 30 mg per day. No further increases were made after week four of the trial. At the end of the study, the medication was tapered under the supervision of a physician. Assessments were conducted weekly or biweekly. Forty-five percent of the fluoxetine group and 42 percent of the placebo group had adverse events such as mood disturbance, particularly irritability, gastrointestinal problems, such as nausea and diarrhea, and sleep disorders. Thirty-one subjects in the fluoxetine group and twenty-one in the placebo group did not complete the trial. Still, upon first analyzing their data, the researchers determined that the subjects in the fluoxetine group had significantly lower scores for OCD behaviors. But, further analyses found no significant differences between the groups. And, there were additional problems, including the fact that the subjects in the placebo group had a comparatively more severe behavioral phenotype than the subjects in the fluoxetine group and a high dropout rate. The researchers acknowledged that their interpretation of the data was therefore "limited."[6]

Paroxetine May Be Useful for Panic Disorders in Adults

In a meta-analysis of multicenter, randomized, parallel-group controlled trials published in the journal *Frontiers in Pharmacology*, researchers from China explored the short-term efficacy and tolerability of paroxetine in the treatment of panic disorder in adults. Focusing on how paroxetine compared to placebos in reducing the total number of full panic attacks, the researchers located thirteen randomized controlled trials, conducted between 1994 and 2007, that met their criteria. There were a total of 2,654 subjects; of these, 1,329 were in intervention groups and 1,325 were in placebo groups. Mean ages ranged from 34.7 to 45.0 years. Six studies had a fixed dose of paroxetine, and seven studies had a flexible dose. The maximum dosage reached 75 mg; and, the course of treatments ranged from nine to twelve weeks. The researchers learned that the subjects who received paroxetine experienced more improvement in the frequency of panic attacks than those on placebos. There were no evident differences in withdrawal rates due to adverse events between the intervention and placebo groups. Still, the incidence of adverse events was higher in the treatment groups. Among the most common were nausea, diarrhea, dry mouth, sleepiness, sexual problems, and insomnia. The researchers concluded that "paroxetine was effective and well-tolerated in the short-term treatment of adults with PD [panic disorder]."[7]

Paroxetine May Be Helpful for Those with Anxiety Disorders

In a meta-analysis published in *PLoS ONE*, researchers from Detroit, Michigan, and Boston, Massachusetts, tested the efficacy of paroxetine and a placebo in treating anxiety and depression. The researchers included thirty-nine published and unpublished GlaxoSmithKline trials on paroxetine that included changes in scores on the Hamilton Rating Scale for Anxiety (HRSA) and/or the Hamilton Rating Scale for Depression (HRSD); all of the trials were double-blind randomized interventions with a placebo group and at least one group receiving paroxetine. There were twelve trials that evaluated changes in HRSA in adults, and their duration ranged from eight to twelve weeks. Seven trials evaluated panic disorder and five were on generalized anxiety disorder. Flexible dose adjustment was permitted in nine of the twelve studies, and eight of the studies were published in peer-review journals. The researchers determined that for the treatment of anxiety, the efficacy difference between paroxetine and placebo was modest and independent of the baseline severity of anxiety. The overall change in placebo-treated subjects was 79 percent of the magnitude of the paroxetine response. Efficacy was far better for the treatment of panic disorder than for generalized anxiety disorder, but the overall response to both paroxetine and placebo was larger for generalized anxiety disorder. The researchers noted a limitation of their findings was that the studies were only conducted by GlaxoSmithKline, and there were no studies completed by independent researchers. Nevertheless, the researchers concluded that paroxetine "provided only a modest benefit over placebo in treating symptoms of anxiety based on available evidence."[8]

Paroxetine May Relieve the Symptoms of Social Anxiety Disorder

In a meta-analysis published in the journal *Medicine*, researchers from China and Canada evaluated the efficacy and tolerability of paroxetine in adults with social anxiety disorder. The researchers located eleven articles, published between 1998 and 2016, that described thirteen multicenter, randomized placebo-controlled trials that met their criteria. The researchers were primarily looking at measurements of fear and avoidance of public and social situations, as well as responses to treatments and remission rates. The trials included a total of 2,593 subjects with social anxiety disorder; 1,281 were placed on paroxetine and 1,312 took placebos. Most of the trials continued for twelve weeks, although one trial lasted for eight weeks and one for twenty-four weeks. Six trials administered fixed doses of paroxetine at 20, 40, and 60 mg per day; five trials administered flexible doses at 20 to 50 mg per day; one trial administered a flexible dose of 20 to 60 mg per day; and the final trial administered a flexible dose of 12.5 to 37.5 mg per day. The researchers found that the subjects taking paroxetine had significantly greater improvement than those taking the placebos, and their response and remission rates were higher. Discontinuation rates because of adverse effects were higher in the paroxetine group, and discontinuation rates because of a lack of efficacy were higher in the placebo group. The researchers concluded that "paroxetine was effective in reliving the symptoms of fear and avoidance and improving social participation" and was generally well-tolerated.[9]

Sertraline Is Useful for Childhood and Adolescent Anxiety, with or without Cognitive Behavioral Therapy

In a randomized, controlled, two-phase trial published in the *New England Journal of Medicine*, researchers from multiple locations in the United States but based in Baltimore, Maryland, evaluated the use of sertraline for childhood anxiety with and without cognitive behavioral therapy. During the first phase of the trial, the researchers assigned 488 children and adolescents between the ages of seven and seventeen years who had a primary diagnosis of separation anxiety disorder, generalized anxiety disorder, or social phobia, to receive sertraline at a dose of up to 200 mg per day, or 14 sixty-minute cognitive behavioral therapy sessions, or a combination of both, or a placebo for a total of twelve weeks. There were no significant differences in the groups with respect to baseline demographics and clinical characteristics; they had nearly equal numbers of males and females, and 78.9 percent were white. Anxiety levels were assessed at baseline and at weeks four, eight, and twelve. At baseline, most subjects had moderate to severe anxiety. There were fourteen withdrawals because of an adverse event. The researchers learned that the highest rate of improvement (80.7 percent) was seen in the children and adolescents on combination therapy; there was a 54.9 percent improvement for sertraline alone and a 59.7 percent improvement for cognitive behavioral therapy alone. All types of therapy were better than a placebo, which only had a 23.7 percent improvement rate. The researchers commented that "all three of the treatment options may be recommended, taking into consideration the family's treatment preferences, treatment availability, cost, and time burden."[10]

Sertraline May Be Useful for PTSD

In a multisite, randomized trial published in the *Journal of Traumatic Stress*, researchers from Seattle, Washington, and Cleveland, Ohio, compared the use of sertraline to prolonged exposure to treat PTSD. (Prolonged exposure is a type of cognitive behavior therapy which teaches people to confront their fears through gradually approaching their traumatic memories.) The cohort consisted of 200 men and women between the ages of eighteen and sixty-five years who had a primary diagnosis of PTSD. The average time since the trauma was twelve years, which means that improvement without some sort of intervention was not likely to occur. The subjects who received sertraline took doses between 12.5 and 300 mg per day, with the average final dose of 115 mg per day. They also had ten weekly sessions with board-certified psychiatrists, which included assessments of symptoms and side effects. The prolonged exposure group had ten sessions with master's or doctoral-level clinicians that included psychoeducation, a breathing technique to manage anxiety, a gradual approach to trauma memory through imaginal exposure, gradual in vivo exposure to previously avoided trauma reminders, the processing of trauma-related thoughts and feelings, and between-session homework. Both groups were followed for twenty-four months. The researchers determined that improvement in the sertraline group was slower than the pace of improvement in the prolonged exposure group, but the subjects in both groups made "substantial improvements across various indices of social functioning, stretching beyond symptoms reduction to concrete and highly protective social benefits." And this progress was maintained over the course of the follow-up. The researchers noted that "clinicians can expect that PE (prolonged exposure) and sertraline will improve multiple aspects of social functioning, especially among individuals who begin treatment with more difficulties, with gains achieved during treatment and maintained up to at least two years."[11]

In a ten-week, randomized, double-blind, placebo-controlled trial published in *Psychological Medicine*, researchers from Iran examined the use of sertraline to treat combat-related PTSD in Iranian veterans. Seventy Iranian veterans with PTSD received either flexibly dosed sertraline (50 to 200 mg per day) or a placebo. Though the groups were not significantly different in terms of age, occupation, education, and the presence of chemical injury, the sertraline group had a longer duration of PTSD. Although there were initially thirty-five subjects in each group, thirty-two subjects in the sertraline group and thirty in the placebo group completed the trial. The subjects were seen every two weeks by a psychiatrist to review drug doses and adverse events. The researchers determined that the veterans on sertraline experienced significant improvement in a variety of different problems associated with their PTSD. Further, sertraline was safe and well-tolerated. Only 6 percent discontinued the medication because of adverse reactions.[12]

Citalopram May Help the Anxiety of Seriously Ill People

In a randomized controlled trial published in the *Iranian Journal of Kidney Diseases*, researchers from Iran studied the ability of citalopram and psychological training to treat anxiety and depression in hemodialysis patients. A total of forty-four end-stage renal disease (ESRD) hemodialysis patients with anxiety and depression were randomly allocated to receive citalopram, 20 mg per day, for three months or to attend six one-hour sessions of psychological training. The pre-intervention anxiety and depression scores between the two groups were not significantly different. The researchers learned that there were no significant differences between the two interventions in reductions of anxiety and depression. So, the pharmacological citalopram intervention worked as well as the psychological intervention. As a result, positive psychological interventions were obtained by both methods.[13]

Citalopram May Be Useful for Panic Disorder

In a clinical trial published in the *Journal of Clinical Pharmacology*, researchers from Turkey studied the use of citalopram for the treatment of pregnant women with panic disorder. The cohort consisted of twenty-two pregnant women with panic disorder who were examined between January 2008 and December 2018. They had a mean age of 33.09 years, and the mean duration of gestation at the first and last assessments were 17.82 weeks and 28.27 weeks. The 20 mg daily dose of citalopram was initiated during the first trimester in seven women, the second trimester in eleven women, and the third trimester in four women. The data were retrospectively collected from clinical registers; as a result, the researchers did not interfere in any way with the treatment of the patients. The researchers learned that citalopram was effective in reducing panic disorder in these pregnant women. Though their findings were promising, the researchers commented that there is a need for controlled studies "to provide more robust evidence on the efficacy of citalopram in this patient population."[14]

Citalopram May Help Children and Adolescents in the Reappraisal of Their Anxiety

In a pilot study published in the *Journal of Child and Adolescent Psychopharmacology*, researchers from Israel evaluated the emotional reactivity and regulation (also known as reappraisal) following citalopram therapy in children and adolescents with anxiety disorders. The cohort included seventy children and adolescents (thirty-eight males and thirty-two females) between the ages of ten and seventeen years. They were divided into three groups. Thirty-five of the subjects with an anxiety disorder were treated with citalopram for eight weeks; fifteen untreated subjects with anxiety disorders were placed on a waiting list for cognitive behavioral therapy after refusing treatment with citalopram; and twenty subjects, who did not have an anxiety disorder, served as controls. Thus, the subjects were not randomly placed in their groups, a potential limitation of the trial. Starting dose for the citalopram was 10 mg per day for the first week. It was then increased to 20 mg per day for the remainder of the trial. The subjects were evaluated for emotional reactivity and regulation at baseline and after eight weeks. The researchers determined that the citalopram-treated subjects had significantly greater improvement in reappraisal ability, or the ability to reappraise threatening images, than the youth waiting for cognitive behavioral therapy, though they also had reductions in symptoms. The ability to reappraise was significantly correlated with decreases in anxiety. Further, there was a decrease in negative emotional reactivity between assessments, which was positively correlated with clinical improvement.[15]

Escitalopram May Be Useful for Phobias

In a double-blind study published in the *Journal of Psychopharmacology*, researchers from Durham, North Carolina, assessed the efficacy and safety of escitalopram in treating specific phobias, such as enclosed spaces, flying, heights, snakes, and animals. The cohort consisted of thirteen subjects between the ages of eighteen and sixty-five years. All of the subjects had been diagnosed with a specific phobia; some had two phobias. For twelve weeks, they were randomly placed on either escitalopram (n = 6) or a placebo (n = 7). One subject failed to return after randomization and a second subject was lost to follow-up. For five days, the treatment subjects received 5 mg per day; the dose was then increased to 10 mg per day for eighteen days, and up to 20 mg per day through the twelfth week of treatment. Using various measurement tools, subjects were evaluated for their phobias at baseline and at weeks 1, 2, 4, 8, and 12. At each meeting, the subjects rated their fear, avoidance, and state of the phobia(s). In cases where the subjects had no exposure to their specific phobia since their last visit, they were asked how they would feel if they were exposed. Subjects who had two main phobias were asked to rank both. The final analyses were completed with five subjects in the treatment group and six in the placebo group. The sample was predominantly female, white, married, with a mean age of 42.8 years, a homogenous group. Two people in the treatment group reported nausea. The researchers found that escitalopram was very effective in the treatment of phobias. Though noting that their sample size was small, the effects were "strong." And, they concluded that escitalopram may be useful for the treatment of specific phobias.[16]

Escitalopram May Help in the Treatment of the Fear of Learning

In a case summary published in *Neuropsychopharmacology Reports*, a physician from Japan summarized the symptoms of a fifteen-year-old male adolescent. At the age of fourteen, he began to experience a host of different symptoms when he studied. These included anxiety and feelings of panic, shortness of breath, tightness in his chest, and palpitations. Soon, he was avoiding situations which required him to study, a phobia known as sophophobia (fear of learning). Earlier, another physician prescribed lorazepam (Ativan) but that did not resolve his symptoms. Although the adolescent recognized that his fear was irrational, it persisted. Under the direction of his physician, the teen was taught guided relaxation techniques and placed on 10 mg per day of escitalopram, which was increased to 15 mg. Although he initially improved, his level of improvement seemed to plateau and then stop. So, another medication, perospirone (an atypical antipsychotic), was also added. Thanks to combination of these two medications, after four weeks his fear had decreased significantly and did not interfere with his daily studying. He and his family reported increased feelings of calmness and relaxation.[17]

Escitalopram Appears Promising for People with Social Anxiety Disorder

In a multicenter, randomized, double-blind, placebo-controlled study published in the journal *Current Medical Research and Opinion*, researchers from Japan compared the efficacy and tolerability of 10 mg or 20 mg per day of escitalopram in patients with social anxiety disorder. The cohort consisted of 587 patients, between the ages of eighteen and sixty-four years, recruited from eighty-six medical institutions. The patients had a mean age of thirty-three years, and approximately 56 percent were women. Following a one-week screening period, for twelve weeks, patients were assigned to receive one of the doses of escitalopram per day or a placebo. There were 198 patients in the 10 mg group, 193 in the 20 mg group, and 196 in the placebo group. Patients in the 20 mg group began with a one-week dose of 10 mg before switching to 20 mg. Patients were seen at baseline and at weeks 1, 2, 4, 6, 8, and 12. An additional safety review was scheduled for two weeks after completion of the study or after withdrawal from the study. Using the Japanese version of the Liebowitz Social Anxiety Scale, a commonly used measure of anxiety, trained raters, who were all psychiatrists or psychologists, assessed the effect of escitalopram versus placebo. It is notable that during the course of the entire study, about 70 percent of the patients in each treatment group had one or more treatment-emergent adverse events. The most common adverse events reported by at least 5 percent of patients were somnolence, nausea, and ejaculation disorder. Most were mild or moderate. Adverse events were the primary reason that some patients left the study. Still, the researchers concluded that escitalopram was "efficacious, safe, and well-tolerated."[18]

Fluvoxamine May Be Useful in the Treatment of Moderate to Severe Obsessive-Compulsive Disorder

In a retrospective chart review published in the *Journal of the Canadian Academy of Child and Adolescent Psychiatry*, researchers from British Columbia, Canada, studied the use of a combination of fluvoxamine and clomipramine, a tricyclic antidepressant, for the treatment of moderate to severe obsessive-compulsive disorder in children and adolescents. They conducted their research with children, eighteen years or younger, with OCD at a tertiary hospital; between January 2010 and August 2017, six adolescents were treated with this combination therapy. A total of thirty-five sets of serum concentrations were included, with approximately 60 percent of the data from two patients. The median peak daily doses of fluvoxamine and clomipramine were 112.5 mg and 87.5 mg, respectively. The combination therapy with this cohort appeared to be well-tolerated with no severe or life-threatening adverse effects and no adverse effects requiring dose reductions. The combination medication permitted a lower dose of clomipramine than is normally used and appeared to be a safe alternative for children and adolescents with OCD. The researchers noted that their findings are limited by a small sample size, and data for all patients were not available at all point of therapy. Some of the data were available only for the initiation of treatment and others had data available for up to nine months of treatment. Further, three patients were eighteen years of age at initiation and had few serum concentrations analyzed prior to leaving pediatric care and being lost to follow-up. And, as a retrospective chart review, the study could only use information that was documented in the charts. The researchers noted that this combination therapy appeared safe and well tolerated, which is important "given the limited pharmacologic options for severe, refractory OCD."[19]

Fluvoxamine May Reduce the Symptoms of Social Anxiety Disorder

In a double-blind, placebo-controlled trial published in the *International Journal of Neuropsychopharmacology*, researchers from Japan investigated the use of fluvoxamine for the treatment of social anxiety disorder. The trial, which was conducted at fifty-four centers in Japan, included 271 subjects with generalized anxiety disorder. Only people between the ages of eighteen and sixty-five years were eligible to be part of the trial. For ten weeks, the subjects received either fluvoxamine or a placebo. Those taking fluvoxamine dosage of 50 mg per day increased their dosage weekly for a maximum of 150 or 300 mg per day. The fluvoxamine group included 182 subjects, with 93 taking 150 mg per day and 89 taking 300 mg per day. There were eighty-nine subjects in the placebo group. The mean age of the subjects in the fluvoxamine group was 39.3 years, and the mean age of the subjects in the placebo group was 37.9 years. The subjects were evaluated during nine visits, at baseline and weeks 1, 2, 3, 4, 5, 6, 8, 10. The overall incidence of reported adverse events was 88.5 percent in the fluvoxamine group and 66.3 percent in the placebo group. In the fluvoxamine group, the most commonly reported adverse events were somnolence and nausea. The incidence of adverse events was 91.4 percent in the 150 mg per day group and 85.4 percent in the 30 mg per day group. Dehydration and acute renal failure were observed in one fluvoxamine subject taking 300 mg per day and serotonin syndrome was seen in another 300 mg per day recipient. Though these were classified as serious adverse drug reactions, they disappeared within two weeks after the drug was discontinued. Compared to the subjects on the placebo, the subjects taking fluvoxamine had a statistically superior improvement of their symptoms of social anxiety disorder. "Treatment with fluvoxamine was well tolerated and was associated not only with improvement in symptoms but also the improvement in functional measures."[20]

In a meta-analysis published in the journal *Medicine*, researchers from China reviewed the efficacy and tolerability of fluvoxamine in adults with social anxiety disorder. They found five randomized placebo-controlled trials, conducted between 1999 and 2007, that met their criteria. The duration of three studies was twelve weeks, one lasted ten weeks, and the fifth study continued twenty-four weeks. Three studies had flexible doses between 100 and 300 mg per day, and two trials had flexible doses of 50 to 300 mg per day. The researchers found that the symptoms of social anxiety disorder improved far more in the intervention subjects, and their response rate was higher. Because they had a higher rate of adverse events, the discontinuation rates of the subjects in the fluvoxamine group were higher than the placebo groups. The most frequent adverse events were nausea, somnolence, insomnia, sexual problems, and headache, though the incidence of headache was not significantly different between the groups. The researchers concluded that "fluvoxamine was found to be an effective and well-tolerated treatment option in adults with SAD [social anxiety disorder]."[21]

Vilazodone May Help People with Generalized Anxiety Disorder

In a randomized, placebo-controlled, parallel-group, multicenter study published in the *Journal of Clinical Psychiatry*, researchers from Jersey City, New Jersey, and Tampa, Florida, evaluated the efficacy, safety, and tolerability of vilazodone for the treatment of generalized anxiety disorder. For eight weeks, 400 subjects with generalized anxiety disorder were placed on doses of vilazodone or a placebo; each group had 200 subjects. Seventy-six percent of the subjects completed the study. The treatment group had at least twice as many adverse events as the placebo group; these included nausea, diarrhea, dizziness, and fatigue. The researchers observed statistically significant improvements in all measures of anxiety and functional impairment in the treatment group. And, they concluded that "vilazodone was generally well tolerated, and no new safety concerns were noted."[22]

Vilazodone May Not Be Useful for PTSD and Comorbid Depression

In a twelve-week, prospective, double-blind, placebo-controlled trial published in the online journal *Primary Care Companion for CNS Disorders*, researchers from Nebraska, California, and Arizona investigated the usefulness of vilazodone for the treatment of chronic PTSD and comorbid mild to moderate depression in veteran. The trial, which was conducted between February 2013 and September 2015 at two sites, included fifty-nine primarily white, outpatient men ($n = 57$) and women ($n = 2$) between the ages of eighteen and fifty-five years. While they began at lower doses and flexible dosing was allowed, twenty-nine subjects took up to 40 mg of vilazodone and thirty took a placebo. Twelve subjects discontinued or were lost to follow-up, leaving forty-seven treatment completers. The study schedule included multiple visits and a tapering of medication at the end of the trial. Vilazodone was well tolerated, and there were few reported side effects, such as gastrointestinal upset, sexual and sleep problems, headaches, and irritability. One patient who exhibited self-destructive behavior was eliminated from the trial. Still, no significant differences were observed between the treatment and placebo groups in the primary and secondary outcome measures. Vilazodone did not appear to alleviate the symptoms of PTSD, which is similar to other studies on the use of SSRIs for combat-related PTSD.[23]

Vilazodone May Have Efficacy in Adult Separation Anxiety Disorder

In a randomized, controlled pilot trial published in the journal *Depression and Anxiety*, researchers from New York City studied the ability of vilazodone to help adults with separation anxiety disorder. The initial cohort consisted of twenty-four adults between the ages of eighteen and sixty. For twelve weeks, thirteen were placed on vilazodone (10 or 20 mg) and eleven took a placebo. While the subjects began with a low dose, doses could be increased to 40 mg. The sample was about two-thirds female with a mean age in the thirties. Fifty-eight percent had comorbid psychiatric disorders. The researchers learned that across all time points, the vilazodone group had greater improvements in several measures. "The findings of greater response to vilazodone on several outcome measures remain suggestive of clinical potential for this treatment." Yet, they cautioned that the small sample size makes their findings "preliminary."[24]

Vortioxetine May or May Not Be Useful for Generalized Anxiety Disorder

In a systematic review and meta-analysis published in the *Journal of Psychiatric Research*, researchers from Korea, Italy, Durham, North Carolina, and New York City studied the effectiveness of vortioxetine in reducing generalized anxiety disorder. The researchers found four short-term randomized controlled trials that met their criteria. All four of the studies were multicentered; three were conducted in the United States. Each study had 150 or more subjects per treatment arm, and all of the subjects had a primary diagnosis of generalized anxiety disorder, and the length of follow-up was eight weeks. The subjects had inadequate responses to previous SSRI and SNRI treatments. Among the 1,831 subjects, 1,068 took vortioxetine, 609 took placebos, and 154 were on duloxetine 60 mg per day, a medication for anxiety and depression. The doses of vortioxetine were 2.5, 5, and 10 mg per day. Two of the studies had different doses of vortioxetine (2.5 to 10 mg per day), and the other studies had one fixed dose (5 mg per day). All studies had larger number of women, with percentiles ranging from 61.6 percent to 72.4 percent. All of the studies were financially supported by the manufacturer. Only one study, conducted outside the United States, showed that vortioxetine was effective in treating generalized anxiety disorder; in the other three studies, there was not a significant difference between vortioxetine and the placebos. Across all of the studies, the most frequent reported adverse events were nausea, headache, dizziness, and dry mouth. Early withdrawal rates were higher in the vortioxetine groups than the placebo groups. Those taking higher doses of vortioxetine were more likely to withdraw. The researchers concluded that the "definite clinical efficacy of vortioxetine for the short-term control of GAD symptoms remain to be further elucidated with subsequent clinical trials to confirm the practical utility."[25]

In a multinational, randomized, placebo-controlled, fixed-dose trial published in the journal *CNS Spectrums*, researchers from Denmark and Ontario, Canada, examined the use of vortioxetine to treat generalized anxiety disorder in subjects who were working and/or pursuing an education. The cohort consisted of 301 subjects with generalized anxiety disorder; there were men and women between the ages of eighteen and sixty-five years; sixty percent of the subjects noted that they were working or pursuing either a full-time or part-time education. Seventy-one subjects were in the professional group, thirty-eight were in the associate professional group, and sixty-five were in the skilled laborer group. For eight weeks, the subjects took daily doses of either 5 mg vortioxetine or a placebo. Subjects were excluded if they had any psychiatric problems other than generalized anxiety disorder. The researchers found that vortioxetine appeared to be more effective in treating generalized anxiety disorder in subjects who were working; it also improved their "global functioning" and quality of life. And the strongest effects were seen in those working in professional or associate professional positions. The researchers suggested that the medication may be more effective in those with "a higher internal focus of control," as well as those "who are higher in the organizational structure." The researchers concluded that their findings may "be relevant for further research into the clinical value and cost-effectiveness of targeted interventions."[26]

Vortioxetine Appears to Be Useful for Anxious Depression

In a study published in the journal *Neuropsychiatric Disease and Treatment*, researchers reanalyzed data from a multicenter, randomized, double-blind, placebo-controlled, parallel-group phase 3 trial of the safety and efficacy of vortioxetine in Japanese patients with major depressive disorder. In this investigation, the subjects were between the ages of twenty and seventy-five years and had a primary diagnosis of major depressive disorder, with the current major depressive disorder having lasted three to twelve months. Subjects with symptoms of anxiety were eligible to participate, though those with a formal diagnosis of an anxiety disorder were excluded. Data were available on 489 subjects, who were assigned to take vortioxetine 10 mg ($n = 165$), vortioxetine 20 mg ($n = 163$), or a placebo for eight weeks (161). Of these subjects, 282 had anxious depression or depression with anxiety symptoms (57.7 percent) and 207 had non-anxious depression (42.3 percent). Was vortioxetine also useful for the subjects with anxious depression? The researchers commented that major depressive disorder is often comorbid with anxiety disorders. And, they found that vortioxetine was "a viable option" for treating major depressive patients with anxious depression. This is important because people with major depressive disorder who also have symptoms of anxiety have "consistently [been] associated with poor treatment outcomes." The researchers concluded that "further research is warranted to investigate these effects in a real-world clinical setting."[27]

References and Further Readings

Alamy, Sayed, Wei Zhang, Indu Varia et al. "Escitalopram in Specific Phobia" Results in Placebo-Controlled Pilot Trial." *Journal of Psychopharmacology* 22, no. 2 (2008): 157–61.

Asakura, Satoshi, Osamu Tajima, and Tsukasa Koyama. "Fluvoxamine Treatment of Generalized Social Anxiety Disorder in Japan: A Randomized Double-Blind, Placebo-Controlled Study." *International Journal of Neuropsychopharmacology* 10, no. 2 (2007): 263–74.

Asakura, Satoshi, Taiji Hayano, Atsushi Hagino, and Tsukasa Koyama. "A Randomized, Double-Blind, Placebo-Controlled Study of Escitalopram in Patients with Society Anxiety Disorder in Japan." *Current Medical Research and Opinion* 32, no. 4 (2016): 749–57.

Birmaher, Boris, David A. Axelson, Kelly Monk et al. "Fluoxetine for the Treatment of Childhood Anxiety Disorders." *Journal of the American Academy of Child & Adolescent Psychiatry* 42, no. 4 (April 2003): 415–23.

Bushnell, Greta A., Moira A. Rynn, Stephen Crystal et al. "Simultaneous Benzodiazepine and SSRI Initiation in Young People with Anxiety Disorders." *Journal of Clinical Psychiatry* 82, no. 6 (November–December 2021): 20m13863.

Carthy, Tal, Noa Benaroya-Milshtein, Avi Valevski, and Alan Apter. "Emotional Reactivity and Regulation Following Citalopram Therapy in Children and Adolescents with Anxiety Disorders." *Journal of Child and Adolescent Psychopharmacology* 27, no. 1 (2017): 43–51.

Christensen, M. C., H. Loft, I. Florea, and R. S. McIntyre. "Efficacy of Vortioxetine in Working Patients with Generalized Anxiety Disorder." *CNS Spectrums* 24(2019): 249–57.

Durgam, Suresh, Carol Gommoll, Giovanna Forero et al. "Efficacy and Safety of Vilazodone in Patients with Generalized Anxiety Disorder: A Randomized, Double-Blind, Placebo-Controlled, Flexible-Dose Trial." *Journal of Clinical Psychiatry* 77, no. 12 (2016): 1687–94.

Fung, Ryan, Dean Elbe, and Evelyn Stewart. "Retrospective Review of Fluvoxamine-Clomipramine Combination Therapy in Obsessive-Compulsive Disorder in Children and Adolescents." *Journal of the Canadian Academy of Child and Adolescent Psychiatry* 30, no. 3 (August 2021): 150–5.

Gilboa, M. G. Koren, R. Katz et al. "Anxiolytic Treatment But Not Anxiety Itself Causes Hyponatremia Among Anxious Patients." *Medicine* 98, no. 5 (February 2019): e14334.

Graham, Belinda, Natalie M. Garcia, Hannah E. Bergman et al. "Prolonged Exposure and Sertraline Treatments for Posttraumatic Stress Disorder Also Improve Multiple Indicators of Social Functioning." *Journal of Traumatic Stress* 33, no. 4 (August 2020): 488–99.

Inoue, Takeshi, Shinji Fujimoto, Tatsuro Marumoto et al. "Therapeutic Potential of Vortioxetine for Anxious Depression: A Post Hoc Analysis of Data from a Clinical Trial Conducted in Japan." *Neuropsychiatric Disease and Treatment* 17 (2021): 3781–90.

Li, Xinyuan, Yanbo Hou, Yingying Su et al. "Efficacy and Tolerability of Paroxetine in Adults with Social Anxiety Disorder." *Medicine* 99, no. 14 (2020): e19573.

Liu, Xue, Xinyuan Li, Congxiao Zhang et al. "Efficacy and Tolerability of Fluvoxamine in Adults with Social Anxiety Disorder: A Meta-Analysis." *Medicine* 97, no. 28 (2018): e11547.

Miyazaki, Kensuke. "Perospirone Augmentation of Escitalopram in the Treatment of an Adolescent Sophophobia (Fear of Learning) Patient." *Neuropharmacology Reports* First Published May 4, 2022.

Pae, Chi-Un, Sheng-Min Wang, Changsu Han et al. "Vortioxetine, a Multimodel Antidepressant for Generalized Anxiety Disorder: A Systematic Review and Meta-Analysis." *Journal of Psychiatric Research* 64 (2015): 88–98.

Panahi, Y., B. Rezazadeh Moghaddam, A. Sahebkar et al. "A Randomized, Double-Blind, Placebo-Controlled Trial on the Efficacy and Tolerability of Sertraline in Iranian Veterans with Post-Traumatic Stress Disorder." *Psychological Medicine* 41 (2011): 2159–66.

Quagliato, Laiana, Rafael C. Freire and Antonio E. Nardi. "Risks and Benefits of Medications for Panic Disorder: A Comparison of SSRIs and Benzodiazepines." *Expert Opinion on Drug Safety* 17, no. 3 (March 2018): 315–24.

Ramaswamy, Sriram, David Driscoll, Christopher Reist et al. "A Double-Blind, Placebo-Controlled Randomized Trial of Viazodone in the Treatment of Posttraumatic Stress Disorder and Comorbid Depression." *Primary Care Companion for CNS Disorders* 19, no. 4 (2017): 17m02138.

Reddhough, Dinah S., Catherine Marraffa, Anissa Mouti et al. "Effect of Fluoxetine on Obsessive-Compulsive Behaviors in Children and Adolescents with Autism Spectrum Disorders." *JAMA* 322, no. 16 (October 22, 2019): 1561–9.

Sayed Hamzeh, Hosseini, Fatemeh Espahbodi, and Sayed Mohammad Mehdi Mirzadeh Goudarzi. "Citalopram Versus Psychological Training for Depression and Anxiety Symptoms in Hemodialysis Patients." *Iranian Journal of Kidney Diseases* 6 (2012): 446–51.

Schneier, Franklin R., Danielle M. Moskow, Tse-Hwei Choo et al. "A Randomized Controlled Pilot Trial of Vilazodone for Adult Separation Anxiety Disorder." *Depression and Anxiety* 34, no. 12 (December 2017): 1085–95.

Sugarman, Michael A., Amy M. Loree, Boris B. Baltes et al. "The Effect of Paroxetine and Placebo on Treating Anxiety and Depression: A Meta-Analysis of Change on the Hamilton Rating Scales." *PLoS ONE* 9, no. 8 (August 27, 2014): e106337.

Uguz, Faruk. "Citalopram in Treatment of Pregnant Women with Panic Disorder: A Retrospective Study." *Journal of Clinical Psychopharmacology* 40, no. 6 (November/December 2020): 615–17.

Walkup, John T., Anne Marie Albano, John Piacentini et al. "Cognitive Behavioral Therapy, Sertraline, or a Combination in Childhood Anxiety." *New England Journal of Medicine* 359, no. 26 (December 25, 2008): 2753–66.

Zhang, Beilin, Chao Wang, Lexiang Cui et al. "Short-Term Efficacy and Tolerability of Paroxetine Versus Placebo for Panic Disorder: A Meta-Analysis of Randomized Controlled Trials." *Frontiers in Pharmacology* 11 (March 2020): Article 275.

Zou, Chuan, Xiang Ding, Joseph H. Flaherty, and Birong Dong. "Clinical Efficacy and Safety of Fluoxetine in Generalized Anxiety Disorder in Chinese Patients." *Neuropsychiatric Disease and Treatment* 9 (2013): 1661–70.

Serotonin and Norepinephrine
Reuptake Inhibitors

Introduction

Serotonin and norepinephrine reuptake inhibitors comprise a class of medications that have been approved by the US Food and Drug Administration primarily to treat depression. But, they are sometimes used to treat other medical problems, such as anxiety disorders and chronic pain, especially nerve pain. At present, there are five serotonin and norepinephrine reuptake inhibitors (SNRIs) that are FDA approved; they are desvenlafaxine (Pristiq), duloxetine (Cymbalta), levomilnacipran (Fetzima), milnacipran (Savella), and venlafaxine (Effexor). However, only duloxetine and venlafaxine extended release have been approved for anxiety, and there are only a few peer-reviewed studies on the association between the other SNRIs and anxiety disorders. So, this entry will only discuss duloxetine and venlafaxine.

The SNRIs, which all work in similar ways, affect neurotransmitters, or chemical messengers, that are used to communicate between brain cells. They trigger changes in brain chemistry, which help to regulate mood, relieve depression, ease anxiety, and reduce pain. How does that occur? SNRIs block the brain's reabsorption or reuptake of the neurotransmitters serotonin and norepinephrine, thus making them more abundant and available for use.

Like SSRIs, SNRIs may take several weeks to begin working. In fact, it may take as long as two months to feel the full effects.

Regulation, Administration, and Costs

Since SNRIs are sold only by prescription, they are regulated by the FDA. Duloxetine is available in 20, 30, and 40 mg; the starting dose is usually between 30 and 60 mg, with a maintenance dose of 60 mg. It is taken once daily. The monthly generic price is around $236, and the brand price is around $337.

Venlafaxine extended-release tablets and capsules, which are also taken once daily, are sold in 25, 37.5, 50, 75, 100, 112.5, 150, and 225 mg. The starting dose is usually between 37.5 and 75 mg, with a maintenance dose of 75 to 225 mg. The monthly generic price is around $60, and the brand price is around $657. Medical insurance should cover most of the cost of these medicines, at least in the generic forms.

Side Effects and Risks

While many people taking SNRIs do not have any side effects, there are several associated with these medications; these include nausea, dry mouth, dizziness, headache, excessive sweating, tiredness, constipation, insomnia, loss of appetite, and changes in sexual function. After a few weeks of treatment, they tend to diminish. To reduce the risk of side effects, it is best to take these medications with food. People who are unable to tolerate the side effects of one SNRI may wish to try another one.

For certain people, SNRIs may be risky. Venlafaxine may raise blood pressure, and duloxetine may worsen liver problems. In addition, they may interact with other medications or supplements. It is important to list your other medications and supplements for your medical provider. For example, if people who take medicine that thins blood take SNRIs, they are at increased risk for bleeding. Even something as simple as ibuprofen may be problematic. And, SNRIs should never be combined with other medications or products that raise levels of serotonin. This may cause serotonin syndrome, with symptoms such as anxiety, agitation, high fever, sweating, confusion, tremors, restlessness, lack of coordination, changes in blood pressure, and rapid heart rate. Severe cases of serotonin syndrome may have symptoms such as confusion, delirium, fever, seizures, and loss of consciousness. Before taking any SNRI, discuss pregnancy or breastfeeding status with a medical provider.

And, SNRIs may trigger suicidal thoughts in children, adolescents, and young adults. That is why in 2004 the FDA issued a Black Box warning for all SNRIs. This is the most serious warning that the FDA issues. The FDA advised medical providers of children, adolescents, and young adults to compare the benefits of SNRIs to their potential harm for each patient, always remembering that the psychiatric symptoms may increase the risk of suicidality.

While SNRIs are not addictive, they should not be abruptly discontinued. The sudden withdrawal may trigger withdrawal-like symptoms, also known as discontinuation syndrome, characterized by dizziness, headache, flu-like symptoms such as tiredness, chills, muscle aches, irritability, agitation, insomnia or sleep disturbances, and diarrhea.

Research Findings

Duloxetine Seems Useful for Generalized Anxiety Disorder

In a ten-week, double-blind, flexible dose, progressive titration, placebo-controlled trial published in the journal *Depression and Anxiety*, researchers from Philadelphia, Pennsylvania, Indianapolis, Indiana, and Boston, Massachusetts, evaluated the efficacy, safety, and tolerability of duloxetine for 327 adults with generalized anxiety disorder. Recruited from twenty-seven outpatient treatment centers across the United States, 168 subjects were placed on 60 to 120 mg per day of duloxetine and 159 were placed on a placebo. At baseline, both groups had similar demographic characteristics; 61.7 percent of the total sample was female, with a mean age of 41.6 years. Levels of anxiety were measured with the Hamilton Anxiety Scale. Study visits were conducted during weeks one, two, four, seven, and ten. At the end of the trial, the subjects were tapered off their medication. Citing adverse events and other factors, only 62 percent of the subjects completed the entire trial. The most common adverse event was mild to moderate nausea. Because of adverse events, many more duloxetine-treated patients (20.2 percent) than placebo-treated patients (8.2 percent) discontinued. The researchers determined that within the first two weeks of beginning treatment with duloxetine, the subjects began to experience relief from their GAD and improvement in their overall functioning. And, the researchers concluded that "if the findings from this study are replicated, duloxetine could provide an additional SNRI pharmacological intervention for addressing the treatment needs of the GAD population."[1]

In a randomized, double-blind, placebo-controlled, flexible-dose, phase IV trial published in the *International Journal of Geriatric Psychiatry*, researchers from several locations in the United States, Canada, and Europe tested the use of duloxetine on GAD in subjects who were at least sixty-five years old and dealing with GAD. The cohort included 151 elders in the duloxetine group and 140 in the placebo group; the subjects came from forty-seven sites across nine countries—Argentina, Austria, Canada, Germany, Mexico, Poland, Spain, the United Kingdom, and the United States. For ten weeks, the seniors in the treatment group took duloxetine; they began with a dose of 30 mg that was increased in many but not all cases up to 60 to 120 mg. They were evaluated on weeks two, four, seven, and ten. The treatment time was following by a two-week tapering period. The other seniors took the placebo. The two groups had similar demographic characteristics. One hundred and fifteen duloxetine patients and 105 placebo patients completed the trial. Levels of anxiety were measured with the Hamilton Anxiety Rating Scale. The researchers learned that patients treated with duloxetine had significantly greater baseline to endpoint improvement in their anxiety scores than those on the placebo. Adverse events, especially dry mouth, constipation, and somnolence, occurred at twice the rate in those on duloxetine. While four subjects on duloxetine and five on the placebo had suicidal ideation, there were no suicide attempts. The researchers concluded that their findings "demonstrated that duloxetine treatment was efficacious in the improvement of illness severity, functioning, and enjoyment of life for older adult patients with GAD."[2]

Duloxetine May Be Useful for Resistant Obsessive-Compulsive Disorder

In an eight-week, double-blind, controlled trial published in the *Journal of Clinical Psychopharmacology*, researchers from Iran evaluated the ability of duloxetine to relieve the symptoms of resistant obsessive-compulsive disorder. The forty-six patients had all failed to respond to at least twelve weeks of treatment with one of three selective serotonin reuptake inhibitors—fluoxetine, citalopram, or fluvoxamine. The patients were randomly assigned to receive duloxetine or sertraline (a SSRI) in addition to their current OCD regimen; there were twenty-four patients in the duloxetine group, with a mean age of 43.3 years, and twenty-two patients in the sertraline group, with a mean age of 41.1 years. Both groups were about 60 percent female. While the patients on duloxetine were initially treated with 20 mg per day, the goal was to raise the dose to 60 mg per day. Levels of OCD were measured with the Yale-Brown Obsessive Compulsive Scale. The researchers determined that duloxetine was as effective as sertraline in reducing obsessions and compulsions of patients with resistant OCD. However, the researchers underscored that their findings are "preliminary and larger double-blind studies are necessary to confirm the results."[3]

Venlafaxine May Also Be Useful for OCD

In a twelve-week, randomized, double-blind, single center trial published in the *Journal of Psychopharmacology*, researchers from the Netherlands compared the efficacy and tolerability of treatment of OCD with venlafaxine to treatment with paroxetine, a SSRI. The cohort consisted of 150 patients with primary OCD; they were divided into two groups of seventy-five subjects. Both groups had similar baseline demographic characteristics. The subjects in one group began with 75 mg per day of venlafaxine and gradually increased to 300 mg per day at week seven; the seventy-five subjects in the other group began with a dose of 15 mg per day of paroxetine and increased to 60 mg per day at week seven. The subjects were evaluated at baseline and during weeks one, three, five, eight, ten, and twelve. Symptoms of OCD were measured with the Yale-Brown Obsessive Compulsive Scale, and anxiety was measured with the Hamilton Anxiety Scale. One hundred and thirty-four subjects completed the study. While the venlafaxine group experienced a significant improvement in OCD symptoms in the third week, the subjects in the paroxetine group did not have significant improvement until the fifth week. After that, both groups had significant improvement until week ten when improvement stopped. Both groups had similar improvements in anxiety. All but five of the subjects reported at least one adverse event; the most frequent were somnolence, sweating, insomnia, dry mouth, and nausea. The researchers noted that venlafaxine appeared be as effective as paroxetine for the symptoms of OCD. And, they concluded that "venlafaxine is a safe, effective, and well-tolerated treatment of OCD."[4]

People with Refractory Post-Traumatic Stress Disorder May Benefit from Duloxetine

In an eight-week, open-label trial published in the journal *Pharmacopsychiatry*, researchers from West Haven, Connecticut, evaluated the effectiveness and tolerability of duloxetine for the treatment of post-traumatic stress disorder and comorbid major depressive disorder. The cohort consisted of twenty-one treatment refractory male patients with combat-related PTSD and comorbid major depressive disorder; they were recruited from the Veterans Affairs Connecticut Healthcare System. All of the men had failed at least two antidepressant trials. The men started treatment at 30 mg per day of duloxetine; that was followed by 60 mg per day for two weeks. After that, the dose was gradually increased up to 120 mg per day. The patients who had positive responses to duloxetine continued treatment when the trial ended. The PTSD Checklist, a seventeen-item assessment tool, was used to measure PTSD symptoms at baseline and at eight weeks. Twenty patients completed the trial; at that point, one patient was taking 60 mg, five were taking 90 mg, and fourteen were on 120 mg per day. Adverse events were mostly mild and transient. The results were very favorable. The men tended to improve quickly, and the improvement was sustained throughout the trial. The researchers commented that there is a need for larger trials on duloxetine "comparing its effects to placebo and active comparators, as well as proof of concept studies linking together the neurobiology of PTSD with the mechanism of action of this novel antidepressant."[5]

People with Anxiety Without Depression
May Benefit from Venlafaxine XR

In a twenty-eight-week, randomized, double-blind, placebo-controlled, parallel-group trial published in *JAMA*, researchers from Tucson, Arizona, Charleston, South Carolina, and Philadelphia, Pennsylvania, tested the longer-term use of venlafaxine XR for people with anxiety who are also not dealing with depression. The initial cohort consisted of 251 subjects from fourteen outpatient clinics in the United States; 124 subjects, with a mean age of forty-one years, were assigned to receive either 75, 150, or 225 mg of venlafaxine XR per day, and 127 subjects, with a mean age of thirty-eight years, took placebos. All of the patients on medication began with 75 mg per day and were increased up to 225 mg per day. The subjects were seen frequently during the first months of the trial and less often thereafter. Anxiety levels were periodically measured with the Hamilton Rating Scale for Anxiety and the Clinical Global Impressions Scale. A follow-up visit took place four to ten days after the medication was tapered. Large numbers of subjects in both groups withdrew. Only sixty subjects in the venlafaxine group and forty-four in the placebo group completed the trial. Still, the researchers observed that during the weeks six through twenty-eight response rates in the venlafaxine XR group were 69 percent or higher compared to rates of 42 to 46 percent in the placebo group. The most common adverse events were nausea, somnolence, and dry mouth. The researchers concluded that "venlafaxine XR is a safe, effective treatment for outpatients with GAD."[6]

Venlafaxine Seems to Be a Better Choice Than Citalopram for Generalized Anxiety Disorder

In a twelve-week trial published in the journal *Experimental and Therapeutic Medicine*, researchers from China compared venlafaxine XR to citalopram (the SSRI Celexa) for treating GAD. The cohort consisted of 100 outpatients, 58 females and 42 males, with GAD. Fifty patients were assigned to take venlafaxine; for the first seven days, they took 75 mg per day of venlafaxine and 50 mg per day of sulpiride, an antipsychotic medication. After that, they took 150 mg once per day. The patients in the citalopram group began with 10 mg citalopram and 50 mg sulpiride once per day. On the eighth day, they began 20 mg citalopram. At the end of weeks two, four, and twelve, the researchers evaluated the efficacy of the treatments with the Hamilton Anxiety Scale and recorded adverse reactions. Before the treatments began, both groups had similar anxiety scores. However, after two weeks, the patients in the venlafaxine group had better improvement than those in the citalopram group. During the four and twelve-week assessment, venlafaxine was significantly better than citalopram. After twelve weeks, 94 percent of those on the venlafaxine treatment were considered "cured." That is a sharp contrast to the 70 percent in the citalopram treatment that were thought to be "cured." The Hamilton Anxiety Scale scores for the two groups were significantly different during the second, fourth, and twelfth weeks of treatment. In the venlafaxine group, twenty-eight patients had adverse reactions, such as gastrointestinal discomfort, nausea, high blood pressure, dizziness, sleepiness, and physical fatigue. In the citalopram group, twenty-six patients had reactions, such as dizziness, body fatigue, drowsiness, gastrointestinal discomfort, and nausea. The researchers concluded that "venlafaxine is more cost-effective than citalopram in the treatment of outpatients with GAD."[7]

Venlafaxine May Help Ease the Symptoms of Panic Disorder

In a randomized, double-blind, placebo-controlled, parallel-group flexible-dose trial published in the *British Journal of Psychiatry*, researchers from Canada, Finland, South Africa, France, and Collegeville, Pennsylvania, examined the efficacy, safety, and tolerability of venlafaxine ER for treating panic disorder. The cohort consisted of 361 adult outpatients with panic disorder, with or without agoraphobia, who were treated at fifty sites in Canada, Europe, and South Africa; 181 patients were placed on venlafaxine and 180 were placed on a placebo. For the first four days of treatment, the patients in the intervention group took

37.5 mg per day. That was then increased to 75 mg. If clinically indicated, it could be increased to a maximum of 225 mg per day. Doses decreased to 75 mg per day were permitted. The primary assessments were conducted with the Panic and Anticipatory Anxiety Scale. A total of 265 patients completed all ten weeks of the trial. Treatment emergent adverse events, especially anorexia, nausea, insomnia, and sweating, were the most common reasons for withdrawal of the subjects in the venlafaxine group, and lack of efficacy was the most common reason for withdrawal from the placebo group. At the final on-therapy evaluation, 55 percent of the patients on venlafaxine XR and 53.4 percent of the placebo patients were free from full-symptom panic attacks, a nonsignificant difference. However, a number of other areas of concern showed improvement. For example, the median reduction from baseline in full-symptoms panic frequency was significantly greater in the venlafaxine XR group, and a significantly higher proportion of the venlafaxine XR group responded to treatment beginning week three and experienced remission beginning week six. The researchers concluded that venlafaxine XR was superior to placebo in most outcome measures. "The favorable safety and tolerance profile of venlafaxine XR suggests that it is a viable treatment option for panic disorder."[8]

Venlafaxine Appears to Be Useful for PTSD

In a six-month, double-blind, placebo-controlled trial published in the journal *Archives of General Psychiatry*, researchers based in Durham, North Carolina, examined the ability of venlafaxine ER to treat people with PTSD at fifty-six international outpatient psychiatric clinics in Argentina, Chile, Colombia, Denmark, Finland, Mexico, Norway, Portugal, South Africa, Spain, Sweden, and the UK. The initial cohort consisted of 329 adult outpatients with a primary diagnosis of PTSD; they had all been ill with PTSD for at least six months. The patients were randomly assigned to receive 37.5 mg per day of venlafaxine ER ($n = 161$) that could be increased up to 300 mg per day or a placebo ($n = 168$). (Unlike most researchers, these researchers abbreviate extended as ER not XR.) The mean age of the venlafaxine ER group was 42.2 years, with seventy-two men and eighty-nine women, and the mean age of the placebo group was 40.5 years, with seventy-nine women and eighty-nine men. The most common type of trauma was nonsexual abuse followed by accidental injury. Other frequently cited types of abuse were unexpected death, combat, and adult sexual assault. In both groups, only 112 patients (68 percent) completed the entire trial; the primary reason for withdrawal was adverse events, such as mild to severe nausea and dizziness, and unsatisfactory responses. The researchers learned that in almost all of the symptoms measured, the patients taking venlafaxine ER had significantly greater improvement than those taking the placebo. The researchers questioned whether this was caused by the inability of SNRIs "to adequately control the full range of PTSD symptoms" or was it "a deficiency in the rating scale itself." Still, the researchers concluded that "venlafaxine ER was effective and well tolerated in short-term and continuation treatment of patients with posttraumatic stress disorder."[9]

Duloxetine and Venlafaxine XR Both Appear to Be Useful for Generalized Anxiety Disorder

In a ten-week double-blind, placebo-controlled, multicenter trial published in the journal *Psychological Medicine*, researchers from Mexico City, Mexico, Ottawa, Canada, and Indianapolis, Indiana, examined the usefulness of 20 mg or 60–120 mg once daily of duloxetine or 75 to 225 once daily venlafaxine XR for GAD. The randomized cohort consisted of 581 adults; 84 were assigned to take 20 mg per day of duloxetine, 158 to take 60 to 120 mg per day of duloxetine, 169 to take 75 to 225 mg per day of venlafaxine XR, and 170 to take a placebo. There were 332 women and 249 men with a mean age of 42.8 years, and the trial took place in eight countries—Australia, Argentina, Belgium, Canada, Mexico, Russia, Taiwan, and the UK. The majority of the subjects were Caucasian. Anxiety levels were measured with the Hamilton Anxiety Rating Scale; at baseline, the subjects tended to have moderate to severe levels of generalized anxiety disorder. Compared to the placebo group, the subjects in the other three groups all had significant improvement in their anxiety scores. The researchers concluded that these medications were "effective and similarly tolerated for patients with GAD compared with placebo."[10]

Withdrawal from Duloxetine and Venlafaxine and Other SNRIs May Trigger Significant Symptoms

In a systematic review published in the journal *Psychotherapy and Psychosomatics*, researchers from Italy, Buffalo, New York, and Schuylkill Haven, Pennsylvania, conducted a systematic review to identify the occurrence, frequency, and features of withdrawal from SNRIs. The researchers located sixty-one English-language studies that met their criteria. There were twenty-two double-blind randomized controlled trials, six studies in which patients were treated in an open fashion and then randomized to a double-blind controlled phase, eight open trials, one prospective naturalistic study, one retrospective study, and twenty-three case reports. The researchers determined that withdrawal symptoms may occur after discontinuation of any SNRI. While the prevalence of withdrawal symptoms was variable, it was highest after the discontinuation of venlafaxine. The rates of withdrawal symptoms from both randomized controlled trials and open trials ranged from 6 to 55 percent after duloxetine and 23 to 78 percent after venlafaxine. On average, studies found that the withdrawal symptoms began a few days after drug discontinuation and lasted a few weeks. But, there were also episodes of longer duration. The researchers noted an extensive list of withdrawal symptoms ranging from headache, fatigue, and sweating to visual sensations and/or hallucinations, electric-shock sensations, coordination problems, and unsteady gait. The researchers wrote that clinicians are familiar with the withdrawal symptoms associated with alcohol, benzodiazepines, barbiturates, opioids, and stimulants. "They need to add SNRI to the list of drugs potentially inducing withdrawal phenomena, as found to be the case with SSRI."[11]

References and Further Readings

Bradwejn, Jacques, Antti Ahokas, Dan J. Stein et al. "Venlafaxine Extended-Release Capsules in Panic Disorder." *British Journal of Psychiatry* 187 (2005): 353–9.

Davidson, Jonathan, David Baldwin, Dan J. Stein et al. "Treatment of Posttraumatic Stress Disorder with Venlafaxine Extended Release: A 6-Month Randomized Controlled Trial." *Archives of General Psychiatry* 63, no. 10 (2006): 1158–65.

Fava, Giovanni A., Giada Benasi, Marcella Lucente et al. "Withdrawal Symptoms After Serotonin-Noradrenaline Reuptake Inhibitor Discontinuation: Systematic Review." *Psychotherapy and Psychosomatics* 87 (2018): 195–203.

Gelenberg, A. J., R. B. Lydiard, R. L. Rudolph et al. "Efficacy of Venlafaxine Extended-Release Capsules in Nondepressed Outpatients with Generalized Anxiety Disorder: A 6-Month Randomized Controlled Trial." *JAMA* 283, no. 23 (June 21, 2000): 3082–8.

NIcolini, H., D. Bakish, H. Duenas et al. "Improvement of Psychic and Somatic Symptoms in Adult Patients with Generalized Anxiety Disorder: Examination from a Duloxetine, Venlafaxine Extended-Release and Placebo-Controlled Trial." *Psychological Medicine* 39 2008): 267–76.

Walderhaug, S., D. Aikins Kasserman et al. "Effects of Duloxetine in Treatment-Refractory Men with Posttraumatic Stress Disorder." *Pharmacopsychiatry* 43, no. 2 (March 2010): 45–9.

Zhang, Jingjing, Hongbing Xu, and Zhiqing Chen. "Pharmacoeconomic Evaluation of Venlafaxine Compared with Citalopram in Generalized Anxiety Disorder." *Experimental and Therapeutic Medicine* 5 (2013): 840–4.

Tai Chi

Introduction

A type of traditional Chinese medicine, tai chi is a gentle mind-body exercise that consists of slow, deliberate movements, meditation, and deep breathing. Created centuries ago by a Chinese martial artist, tai chi attempts to balance the body, mind, and spirit. First introduced to the United States in the early 1970s, tai chi had grown widely in popularity.

Tai chi is believed to improve fitness, coordination, balance, sleep, and agility. It is thought to foster better posture, flexibility, muscle tone, coordination, range of motion, balance, and mental alertness. And, some say that it is beneficial for a host of different medical concerns, such as chronic pain, gout, heart disease, metabolic disorder, chronic obstructive pulmonary disease, hypertension, arthritis, osteoporosis, diabetes, headaches, fibromyalgia, and anxiety. In fact, according to tai chi supporters, the combination of controlled movements, meditative thoughts, and deep breathing are useful for almost any chronic medical problem, and they certainly promote overall health and well-being.

Central to tai chi, which is also known as tai chi chuan, and other types of traditional Chinese medicine is the belief that "qi" or "chee," or life energy, flows throughout the body. In order to achieve or maintain good health, *qi* must be able to move freely. The purpose of tai chi is to encourage *qi* to flow strongly, but smoothly, throughout the body.

Tai chi involves low-impact, weight-bearing exercises that strengthen bones and may slow bone loss. These movements help stretch, rotate, and twist the body's muscles, tendons, and ligaments. This, in turn, releases and reduces tension, thus lowering levels of anxiety. While there are many variations of tai chi, they all involve exercises combined with meditation and deep breathing. They use the mind to initiate the movements, moving with relaxed and loose joints. They synchronize circular body movements and maintain a continuous flow. There are five main tai chi styles. The oldest type of tai chi, chen incorporates elements of martial arts, with kicks, punches, and jumps. Yang has slower, more graceful movements, focusing on balance. Wu is characterized by softness. It includes more forward and backward-leaning movements. Sun includes more dance-like styles, and hao, which requires far more advanced skills, is rarely practiced today.

According to the market data company Statisca, in 2018, about 3.76 million people, six years and older, practiced tai chi in the United States.[1] Though most of them were middle aged or older, increasing numbers of younger people are beginning to include tai chi movements into their physical activity routines.

Regulation, Administration, and Costs

There are no national or state regulations regarding tai chi and no licensing of instructors. Obviously, some instructors are better trained than others. It is best to do a little research and ask friends for suggestions. You may be able to locate a tai chi instructor who has training in a medical field or has more knowledge about dealing with mental health issues, especially anxiety. It is also possible to find one who has personal experience with using tai chi for the symptoms of anxiety.

While one may easily take tai chi classes online, many people chose to begin their tai chi study with an on-site class or a personal instructor. These classes may be held in a wide variety of settings, from a fairly pricey private club or vacation spa to a religious or community center. Instructors who offer personal sessions may offer them in the home.

Tai chi classes usually begin with a warm-up exercise. Then, the instructor will lead the class through a series of tai chi movements that together comprise a "form." The forms are a series of connected movements executed continuously from beginning to end. The classes usually end with a wind-down exercise. In addition to on-site classes, tai chi instructors recommend that students practice fifteen to twenty minutes, twice daily, at home.

The costs associated with tai chi instruction and classes tend to be a function of location. Online classes, which one may watch at home or in another informal setting, are inexpensive or free. Classes held in more expensive settings, such as private gyms or with a private instructor, will probably cost at least $100. Those held in more modest settings cost about $15 to $25 per class. Of course, prices vary. Classes in a major city cost more than a less expensive suburb. In-person classes may not be available in rural areas.

Side Effects and Risks

There are very few side effects and risks associated with tai chi. Since it involves movement and minimal stress on muscles and joints, there is at least the potential of falls. Though tai chi is often recommended even for the most elderly and the most physically challenged, falls are relatively unlikely to occur. And, of course, the movements may be easily modified to meet the needs of almost anyone. Thus, for those unable to stand, there are tai chi movements designed for those in chairs or wheelchairs. It is probably safe for most women who are pregnant to practice tai chi. Nevertheless, before practicing tai chi or enrolling in any classes, people who are concerned about their readiness for tai chi should check with their healthcare provider.

Research Findings

Tai Chi Seems to Have Anxiety-Reducing Properties in People with Elevated Blood Pressure

In a randomized, controlled trial published in the *Journal of Alternative and Complementary Medicine*, researchers from Taiwan and Hong Kong examined the use of tai chi to reduce anxiety in people with mildly elevated blood pressure or stage 1 hypertension. The cohort consisted of seventy-six healthy subjects with mildly elevated blood pressure; thirty-seven, with an average age of 51.6 years, were placed in a tai chi group, and thirty-nine, with an average age of 50.5 years, were in a sedentary control group. At baseline, the groups had similar demographic characteristics, and they had almost equal numbers of males and females. For twelve weeks, the subjects in the tai chi group had three practices per week. Each session consisted of a ten-minute warm-up, thirty minutes of tai chi, and a ten-minute cooldown. At the end of the trial, in addition to reductions in blood pressure and lipid levels, the subjects in the tai chi group reported lower levels of both state and trait anxiety. The subjects in the control group had increases in blood pressure and no improvements in lipid or anxiety levels. The researchers commented that their findings indicated that "by using this nonpharmacologic method of blood pressure reduction in treating mild hypertensive patients will avoid many side effects of drugs."[2]

Tai Chi Appears to Have Anti-Anxiety Properties

In a systematic review published in the *Journal of Evidence-Based Complementary & Alternative Medicine*, researchers from Jackson, Mississippi, and New York City reviewed quantitative studies published between 1989 and March 2014 on the use of tai chi to reduce anxiety. The cohort consisted of seventeen peer-reviewed studies that met their criteria; eight were from the United States, two each from Australia, Japan, and Taiwan, and one each from Canada, Spain, and China. Intervention durations ranged from one day to one year; the majority of the studies ranged from eight to twelve weeks. The length of the interventions ranged from a one-minute session to sixty-minute classes held three times per week. The majority of the studies utilized hour-long sessions. The mean total instruction time was thirty hours. While there were a few problems with the studies, such as the fact that several did not have randomized controlled designs, the sample sizes tended to be smaller, often under thirty, and the tai chi interventions were not standardized. Twelve of the studies did have statistically significant results. The researchers concluded that "tai chi is a promising modality for anxiety management."[3]

Tai Chi Seems to Offer Physically Healthy Adolescents Some Improvement to Their Anxiety

In a systematic review and meta-analysis published in the journal *Frontiers in Psychology*, researchers from China and the UK reviewed the effects of tai chi and qigong on psychological issues, such as anxiety, in adolescents. The researchers identified four randomized controlled trials and six non-randomized comparison studies, with a total of 1,244 adolescents between the ages of twelve and eighteen years, that met their criteria. All of the studies compared adolescents participating in tai chi or qigong to adolescents on a wait-list or participating in another form of exercise. The ten studies were published between 2009 and 2018; the majority were conducted in China, Hongkong, and Taiwan, the remainder in Portugal, Sweden, and Korea. All of the studies included physically healthy adolescents. Sample sizes ranged from 16 to 312; 776 subjects were in the tai chi or qigong groups and 468 were in controls. Mean ages ranged from 11.75 to 18.4 years; the duration of interventions ranged from seven weeks to one year, with tai chi or qigong sessions lasting from twenty-five to ninety minutes. Sessions were held from one to seven times per week. The researchers learned that in the studies that addressed anxiety, the subjects participating in tai chi or qigong perceived lower levels of anxiety than those in the control groups. Unfortunately, those participating in qigong had more improvement than those in tai chi; and the difference in improvement between qigong and tai chi was significant. So, for teens hoping to achieve relief from their anxiety, qigong would be a better choice than tai chi. Of course, these teens would still achieve relief with tai chi, and they would clearly benefit from both. The researchers commented that "Tai Chi and Qigong exercise—both short and long-term—appears to have potential mental health benefits in improving psychological symptoms (i.e. depression, anxiety)."[4]

Tai Chi May Be Useful for Outpatient Psychiatric Patients with Anxiety and Depression

In a trial published in the journal *Integrative Medicine Reports*, researchers from Canada evaluated the use of tai chi and qigong for outpatient psychiatry patients with anxiety and depression. Sixty-six adult outpatient psychiatric patients with a mean age of 50.19 years, were initially recruited for the study; each of the patients had a diagnosis of anxiety and/or depression. The patients, who were provided with thirteen weeks of classes that combined tai chi and qigong movements, described their symptoms before the program began and within two weeks after it ended. The General Anxiety Disorder-7 scale was used to measure levels of anxiety. Only thirty-one patients, with a mean age of 47.83 years, completed all aspects of the trial. Of these, 74.2 percent were female and 93.5 percent used psychotropic medication. The researchers learned that the patients who completed the trial had significant reductions in their symptoms of anxiety. And, they concluded that "it may be appropriate to establish and implement these programs in psychiatric settings as treatment adjuncts."[5]

Combination of Tai Chi and Yoga Sessions May Improve Anxiety

In a trial published in *Complementary Therapies in Clinical Practice*, researchers from Florida, California, and Alabama wanted to learn if brief classes that combined tai chi and yoga would help alleviate anxiety. The cohort consisted of thirty-eight clinicians and staff of a medical facility; the group, which had a mean age of forty-one years, was 95 percent female, 57 percent Caucasian, 14 percent Hispanic, 14 percent Asian, and 5 percent Black. A notable 72 percent of the sample had never participated in tai chi or yoga sessions. Using the State Anxiety Inventory measure, anxiety levels were assessed before and after a single twenty-minute tai chi/yoga session. Ten minutes of tai chi were followed by ten minutes of yoga. The researchers commented that their data "suggest the value of this short routine of combined tai chi and yoga."[6]

Tai Chi May Be Useful for the Anxiety Associated with Some Serious Medical Problems

In a systematic review and meta-analysis published in a different issue of *Complementary Therapies in Clinical Practice*, researchers from China evaluated the use of tai chi for anxiety and depression in people with breast cancer, stroke, heart failure, and chronic obstructive pulmonary disease (COPD). The cohort consisted of twenty-five English or Chinese randomized controlled trials with 1,819 participants; of these, 921 subjects participated in tai chi. The trials were conducted in China, the United States, the United Kingdom, Japan, and Australia, and they used a variety of scales to measure anxiety, such as Self-Rating Anxiety Scale, Hospital Anxiety and Depression Scale-Anxiety, and the Hamilton Anxiety Scale. Five trials addressed breast cancer, ten dealt with stroke, five on heart failure, and five on COPD. Though the intervention group always participated in tai chi, the types of tai chi varied from trial to trial, as did the frequency and duration of exercise. The control groups in the included studies received either the usual care or exercise training. Trial durations ranged from five to twenty-four weeks, with most around twelve weeks. The quality of the included studies was medium, with most having low or uncertain bias. The researchers learned that in both stroke and breast cancer, the differences in levels of anxiety symptoms between the tai chi and control groups were statistically significant. However, that was not true for heart failure or COPD. The researchers concluded that tai chi is a useful treatment for anxiety, especially for those with breast cancer and stroke. But, it should not be considered a substitute for psychiatric treatment. Still, because it is safe, it may be used as "an adjuvant or initial therapy for those who receive psychiatric treatment unconditionally, are unwilling to receive psychiatric treatment, or have mild psychiatric symptoms."[7]

Tai Chi May Have a Limited Ability to Reduce the Anxiety of Patients with Systematic Heart Failure

In a randomized controlled pilot trial published in the *Postgraduate Medical Journal*, researchers from the UK evaluated the use of tai chi and qigong to treat the symptoms associated with stable symptomatic heart failure, including anxiety. The initial cohort consisted of sixty-five patients; they were divided into two groups. The intervention group, which had thirty-two subjects, twenty-six men and six women with a mean age of 68.4 years, participated in sixteen weeks of twice weekly fifty-five-minute tai chi and qigong classes; the control group, which had thirty-three subjects, twenty-seven men and six women and a mean age of 67.9 years, received standard medical care without tai chi and qigong rehabilitation. On Mondays and Fridays, the patients attended the classes that were led by a trained tai chi insturctor, and they were encouraged to practice at home. Over the weeks, the program increased in intensity until it reached its maximum level on the eighth week. Fifty-two subjects completed the entire program; there were forty-two men with a mean age of 68.9 years and ten women with a mean age of seventy years. No adverse effects occurred in the intervention group. The researchers learned that both groups had significant reductions in anxiety scores. However, this reduction was even greater in the intervention group.[8]

When Compared to Reducing Anxiety and Other Forms of Mental and Emotional Stress with Brisk Walking, Medication, and Reading, Tai Chi Does Not Fare Well

In a trial published in the *Journal of Psychosomatic Research*, a researcher from Australia compared the use of tai chi, brisk walking, meditation, and reading for reducing anxiety and other forms of mental and emotional stress. The cohort consisted of forty-eight healthy males, with an average age of 34.6 years, and forty-eight healthy females, with an average age of 37.8 years, who were recruited from tai chi clubs in Melbourne, Australia. The men and women came from "different walks of life" and various ethnic backgrounds. The males had an average of 46.4 months of tai chi practice; the women had an average of 36.4 months. At baseline, both the males and the females had similar trait anxiety scores. During the trial, the subjects were initially subjected to different mental and emotional stressors. Then, they were divided into four groups that separately participated in one of four different activities designed to reduce anxiety. These were tai chi, brisk walking, meditation, or reading. After these activities, which each took an hour, the subjects completed several tests and two forms measuring anxiety, stress, and other factors. Although the researchers determined that the subjects in the tai chi group had a greater reduction in anxiety than those in the reading group, they suggested that this finding may have been "partially accounted for by the subjects' high expectations about gains from Tai Chi."[9]

Tai Chi Decreased Levels of Anxiety in Patients with Scleroderma

In a randomized, controlled parallel trial published in a different issue of *Complementary Therapies in Clinical Practice*, researchers from Turkey investigated the use of tai chi for a number of problems, including anxiety in people with scleroderma. The cohort consisted of thirty-four men and women with scleroderma. Seventeen patients, with an average age of 53.35 years, were assigned to a tai chi group, and the other seventeen, with an average age of 52.64 years, were assigned to home exercise. The baseline demographics for each group were similar; except for two patients in the tai chi group, all of the patients were male. For ten weeks, the patients in the tai chi group met for one hour in an outpatient hospital setting. After fifteen minutes of warm-up exercises, they practiced tai chi for thirty minutes and had another fifteen minutes for cool-down exercises. All of the movements were performed slowly, and no side effects were observed. At home, these patients were asked only to practice the tai chi they learned in the sessions. The patients in the other group were given an one-hour home exercise program which they were told to practice two days per week. The practices began with fifteen minutes of warm-up exercises and ended with fifteen minutes of cool-down exercises. Fourteen patients in each group completed the trial. At the end of the trial, the researchers determined that the patients who participated in the tai chi group had far better results in all but one of the parameters studied, including lowering anxiety. Because tai chi had such a positive effect in so many parameters, the researchers advised that it be included in rehabilitation programs designed for people with scleroderma.[10]

References and Further Readings

Barrow, D. E., A. Bedford, G. Ives et al. "An Evaluation of the Effects of Tai Chi Chuan and Chi Kung Training in Patients with Symptomatic Heart Failure: A Randomised Controlled Pilot Study." *Postgraduate Medical Journal* 83 (2007): 717–21.

Cai, Qian, Shu-bin Cai, Jian-kun Chen et al. "Tai Chi for Anxiety and Depression Symptoms in Cancer, Stroke, Heart Failure, and Chronic Obstructive Pulmonary Disease: A Systematic Review and Meta-Analysis." *Complementary Therapies in Clinical Practice* 46 (2022): 101510.

Cetin, S. Y., B. B. Calik, and A. Ayan. "Investigation of the Effectiveness of Tai Chi Exercise Program in Patients with Scleroderma: A Randomized Controlled Study." *Complementary Therapies in Clinical Practice* 40 (2020): 101181.

Field, Tiffany, Miguel Diego, and Maria Hernandez-Reif. "Tai Chi/Yoga Effects on Anxiety, Heartrate, EEG, and Math Computations." *Complementary Therapies in Clinical Practice* 16 (2010): 235–8.

Jin, Putai. "Efficacy of Tai Chi, Brisk Walking, Meditation, and Reading in Reducing Mental and Emotional Stress." *Journal of Psychosomatic Research* 36, no. 4 (1992): 361–70.

Liu, Xuan, Ru Li, Jiabao Cui et al. "The Effects of Tai Chi and Qigong Exercise on Psychological Status in Adolescents: A Systematic Review and Meta-Analysis." *Frontiers in Psychology* 12 (November 2021): Article 746975.

Novelli, Julia, Karin Cinalioglu, Angela Potes et al. "Tai Chi/Qigong in Adults with Depression and Anxiety: A Pilot Retrospective Study." *Integrative Medicine Reports* 1, no. 1 (August 2022): 131–9.

Sharma, Manoj and Taj Haider. "Tai Chi as an Alternative and Complementary Therapy for Anxiety: A Systematic Review." *Journal of Evidence-Based Complementary & Alternative Medicine* 20, no. 2 (April 2015): 143–53.

Tsai, Jen-Chen, Wei-Hsin Wang, Paul Chan et al. "The Beneficial Effects of *Tai Chi Chuan* on Blood Pressure and Lipid Profile and Anxiety Status in a Randomized Controlled Trial." *Journal of Alternative and Complementary Medicine* 9, no. 5 (2003): 747–54.

Vitamin D

Introduction

Vitamin D is a nutrient the body needs to absorb calcium, a primary building block for strong bones. Working together with calcium, vitamin D helps prevent the weakening and thinning of bones. It helps muscles move and enables nerves to carry messages between the brain and the body. It supports the immune system and may play a role in reducing anxiety.

Unlike the B vitamins and vitamin C, which are water soluble vitamins that dissolve in water-based fluids and are quickly eliminated from the body, vitamin D is a fat-soluble vitamin. It dissolves in fats and oils and may be stored in the body for longer periods of time.

For those who live in sunny climates, the easiest way to obtain vitamin D is through exposure to ultraviolet rays from the sun. When exposed to these rays, vitamin D is produced from the 7-hydrioxycholesterol in the skin. Sitting in the sun for ten to thirty minutes a few times a week is all that is needed. After that time has passed, it is important to remember to use sunscreen. For those who live in less sunny areas or have long winters, it is essential to obtain vitamin D from food, specifically fatty fish and eggs, fortified foods, such as fortified milk and cereal, and supplements. Others who should supplement their diets with vitamin D include elders, those with darker skin tones, people with conditions that limit fat absorption, such as Crohn's disease, cystic fibrosis, celiac disease, and those with obesity or who have undergone gastric bypass surgery, and people living in areas with skies that are often filled with clouds and/or smog.

Still, vitamin D deficiency remains a serious public health problem throughout the world. Vitamin D deficiency is known to affect children, adults, and seniors. It has been estimated that worldwide, about one billion people are deficient. In the United States, statistics vary. But, one may easily say that at least 35 percent of the adult population is deficient. Many sources suggest much higher numbers, especially among children. Why is this an important component to a discussion of anxiety? Since it is known that vitamin D plays a role in the functioning of the nervous system, a vitamin D deficiency may easily increase the risk of anxiety and other psychiatric problems. At the same time, adding vitamin D foods and/ or vitamin D supplementation to the diet has the potential to improve anxiety and related problems.

Following ingestion, vitamin D is converted into twenty-five hydroxyvitamin D (calcidiol) in the liver, the storage form of the vitamin. Then, it is converted into dihydroxyvitamin D (calcitriol), primarily in the kidneys; this is the active form of vitamin D. Dihydroxyvitamin D interacts with the vitamin D receptor (VDR) found in almost every cell of the body.

Regulation, Administration, and Costs

Since the US Food and Drug Administration does not regulate supplements, vitamin D supplements are not regulated. There are two main types of vitamin D. Also known as ergocalciferol, vitamin D2 is found in some plants, mushrooms, and yeasts, and vitamin D3, which is also known as cholecalciferol, is found in animal foods, like fatty fish, cod liver oil, beef liver, and egg yolks. Of the two types, vitamin D3 is almost twice as effective as increasing blood levels of vitamin D than vitamin D2. As a result, for those who are not vegetarian or vegan, it is the preferable alternative. Vitamin D is found in most multivitamins and is sold by itself in many forms, such as tablets, capsules, softgels, and liquids. It is best to take vitamin D with a meal or a snack with a little fat. The recommended daily dose for vitamin D is 400 IU for infants, zero to twelve months, 600 IU for children and adults one to seventy years, and 800 IU for older adults. While a vitamin D blood level of 20 ng/ml is considered normal, it is not uncommon for providers to recommend blood levels of 30 ng/ml or higher. A blood level under 12 ng/ml is considered deficient. While some people take prescription vitamin D to obtain high doses, most people are told not to exceed a total intake of 4,000 IU per day. Vitamin D supplementation tends to be relatively inexpensive.

Side Effects and Risk

It is somewhat difficult to overdose on vitamin D. Overdoses tend to occur only when high doses of supplemental vitamin D are used for an extended period of time without the proper monitoring by a medical professional. Symptoms of vitamin D toxicity (hypervitaminosis D) include confusion, headaches, lack of concentration, excessive urination and thirst, kidney stones, drowsiness, depression, vomiting, abdominal pain, constipation, and high blood pressure. Symptoms of extreme toxicity include kidney failure, unsteady gait, irregular heartbeat, and death.

Supplemental vitamin D may interact with several medications. One of the most common interactions include the weight loss medication orlistat. It may reduce the amount of vitamin D the body absorbs from food and supplements. High levels of vitamin D reduce the ability of statin medications to lower cholesterol. Steroids bring down blood levels of vitamin D, and thiazide diuretics may raise blood levels of calcium. To avoid problems, have a medical provider or pharmacist review the list of medications being used.

Research Findings

Low Levels of Serum Calcidiol Seem to Be Associated with Anxiety Disorders

In a trial published in the journal *Physiological Research*, researchers from the Czech Republic analyzed the relationship between low levels of serum calcidiol and anxiety disorders. The cohort consisted of twenty men and twenty women with several different types of anxiety disorders. The researchers compared their levels of calcidiol to healthy subjects, twelve males and twenty-four women. Using the Mini-International Neuropsychiatric Interview, an independent clinical psychiatrist confirmed the diagnoses. The researchers found that levels of calcidiol were significantly lower in the subjects with anxiety disorders; this was true for both males and females. The researchers concluded that "affective disorders are associated with significantly lower levels of calcidiol, the precursor of the active hormone calcitriol."[1]

Vitamin D Supplementation Improves Anxiety in Subjects with Vitamin D Deficiency

In a six-month trial published in the journal *Brain and Behavior*, researchers from China evaluated the ability of vitamin D supplementation to improve anxiety and depression in people with those disorders, as well as low levels of serum 25-hydroxyvitamin D. The initial cohort consisted of 158 subjects; at baseline, all of the subjects were screened by an experienced psychiatrist. Using various tools, such as the Hamilton Anxiety Rating Scale and the Hamilton Depression Rating Scale, all of the subjects were diagnosed with both anxiety and depression. Seventy-nine subjects were assigned to take 1,600 IU vitamin D supplementation per day and seventy-nine subjects served as controls. The baseline demographic characteristics of both groups were similar. Follow-ups were conducted in the third and sixth months. Sixty-two subjects in the vitamin D group and forty-four in the control group completed the entire trial; the average age of the vitamin D subjects was 46.3 years and the control subjects was 43.3 years. Similar anxiety and depression measurements were conducted at the end of the trial. While the researchers found no improvement in levels of depression, the vitamin D supplementation significantly improved levels of anxiety. The researchers concluded that they found "a clear relationship between low VD [vitamin D] levels and high levels of anxiety."[2]

High Doses of Vitamin D Supplementation Ameliorates the Severity of Generalized Anxiety Disorder

In a trial published in the journal *Metabolic Brain Disease*, researchers from Saudi Arabia and Boston, Massachusetts, examined the use of high-dose vitamin D supplementation to ameliorate the symptoms of generalized anxiety disorder. The cohort consisted of thirty adult patients from Saudi Arabia with vitamin D deficiency and generalized anxiety disorder. The seventeen male and thirteen female subjects had a mean age of forty years. The majority of the subjects had moderate to severe levels of anxiety. The researchers divided the subjects into two groups of fifteen, both with about equal levels of anxiety and about the same vitamin D serum levels. For three months, the subjects in one group received the usual care plus 50,000 IU per week of vitamin D; the subjects in the second group received the usual care. Levels of anxiety were measured using the Generalized Anxiety Disorder-7. At the end of the trial, the anxiety scores of the group that received vitamin D were significantly lower, and there were no significant changes in the anxiety levels of the other group. The researchers underscored the need for a larger scale, placebo-controlled, clinical trial to verify their findings.[3]

Sun Avoidance and Low Intake of Vitamin D Are Correlated with Generalized Anxiety Disorder Among College Women

In a trial published in the journal *Nutrients*, researchers from several locations but based in the United Arab Emirates studied the association between dietary intake of vitamin D, sun exposure, and generalized anxiety disorder among university students. The initial cohort consisted of 425 subjects. They completed questionnaires about their levels of anxiety, their previous four-week intake of dietary vitamin D, and their sun exposure and avoidance. They were also asked if they had been diagnosed with vitamin D deficiency or had taken vitamin D supplementation within the previous twelve weeks. Because some of the subjects did not complete all aspects of the trial, the final analyses included 386 subjects. Of these, 88 percent were twenty-five years old or younger; 58 percent took vitamin D supplementation, but 65 percent reported that they were deficient in vitamin D. A notable 67 percent had anxiety. The researchers determined that the younger subjects who had a history of vitamin D deficiency, less vitamin D in their diets, and greater sun avoidance had a clinically significant higher risk of anxiety symptoms. The researchers concluded that "rectifying vitamin D levels may be a convenient, cost-effective, and low-risk method to improve anxiety and mental health status in general."[4]

Lower Levels of Vitamin D May Increase the Risk of Panic Attacks

In a case-controlled study published in the *Asian Journal of Psychiatry*, researchers from China examined the relationship between serum levels of vitamin D to panic attacks. The cohort consisted of sixty men and sixty women. Sixty subjects were diagnosed with panic attacks and sixty were healthy individuals. The average age of the subjects with panic attacks was 43.03 years, and the average age of the healthy controls was 38.85 years. In order to measure levels of vitamin D, blood samples were obtained from each of the subjects, and each subject with panic attacks completed anxiety questionnaires. The researchers learned that the average concentration of vitamin D levels was 15.75 ng/ml in the subjects with panic attacks and 20.68 ng/ml in the controls. The number of subjects with serum vitamin D levels under 20.0 ng/ml were significantly higher in the subjects with panic attacks. Those with the highest levels of vitamin D were far less likely to have panic attacks and those with the lowest levels were far more likely to have panic attacks. They concluded that "it is necessary to perform well-designed, double-blind, randomized and controlled studies with a sufficient number of subjects to shed light on this problem."[5]

Children, Teens, and Adults with Obsessive-Compulsive Disorder Tend to Have Low Levels of Serum Vitamin D

In a trial published in the journal *CNS Spectrums*, researchers from Italy, Brazil, and Australia reviewed the relationship between low levels of serum vitamin D and obsessive-compulsive disorder. The cohort consisted of fifty male and female outpatients with OCD with a mean age of 31.84 years; half of the subjects were unemployed. Only twelve subjects did not have a psychiatric comorbidity; thirty-four were taking a psychiatric medication. The severity of OCD was assessed with the Yale-Brown Obsessive Compulsive Scale. The vitamin D values in the total sample were 15.88, with no significant difference between the two sexes. Thirty-six subjects had insufficient levels; eleven had critical deficiency; and two had severe critical levels. Only one subject had an optimal level of vitamin D. The researchers commented that "further studies are urgently needed to evaluate the potential benefits of vitamin D supplementation either as an augmenting agent or as an alternative treatment for patients with OCD."[6]

In a trial published in the journal *Psychiatry Research*, researchers from Turkey investigated whether children and adolescents with OCD had inadequate levels of serum vitamin D, vitamin B12, folic acid, and homocysteine, an amino acid. The initial cohort consisted of fifty-two children and adolescents with obsessive-compulsive disorder and thirty healthy controls; the OCD group had twenty-six males and twenty-six females, and the control group had fourteen males and sixteen females. The mean age of the OCD group was 14.7 years, and the mean age of the control group was 14.2 years. At baseline, all of the subjects completed laboratory tests and several different psychological assessments, such as the Yale-Brown Obsessive Compulsive Scale. The researchers found that the children and adolescents with OCD had higher levels of anxiety and statistically significant lower levels of vitamin D than the control group. And, they concluded that "vitamin D deficiency may be a risk factor for development of OCD."[7]

Vitamin D Supplementation Improves Anxiety in People with Rheumatoid Arthritis

In a trial published in the journal *Clinical Rheumatology*, researchers from China wanted to determine the association between vitamin D, anxiety, and depression in people with rheumatoid arthritis. They noted that the general prevalence of rheumatoid arthritis in China ranges from 0.2 to 0.37 percent, and the incidence of anxiety with this disorder ranges from 21 to 70 percent. The cohort consisted of 161 people with rheumatoid arthritis; there were 123 women and 38 men, with a mean age of 47.15 years. The mean duration of illness was 78.85 months. At recruitment, they were all taking about 800 IU per day of vitamin D. Levels of anxiety were measured using the Hamilton Anxiety Scale, and blood samples were taken after one-night fast. Serum levels of vitamin D3 ranged from 5.32 to

45.24 ng/ml, with a mean level of 19.91 ng/ml. Since vitamin D deficiency was defined as below 20 ng/ml, seventy-six subjects had vitamin D deficiency. More than half of the subjects had both anxiety and depressions; 15.53 percent had moderate anxiety and 7.45 percent had severe anxiety. The researchers found an association between low levels of vitamin D3 and the severity of anxiety. The researchers underscored the need for clinicians treating patients with rheumatoid arthritis to check levels of serum vitamin D3.[8]

Increased Intake of Vitamin D May Reduce Anxiety in Athletes

In a trial published in the journal *PeerJ*, researchers from Japan evaluated the ability of an increased intake of vitamin D to reduce anxiety. The cohort consisted of forty-one female intercollege-level track and field athletes and sixty-six international-level rowing athletes between the ages of fifteen and twenty-four years. After the athletes submitted lists and photographs of food intake, the food was analyzed by dietitians. Levels of anxiety were measured with the State-Trait Anxiety Inventory. (State anxiety is anxiety that is a reaction to a particular situation; trait anxiety is more of a tendency to respond with concerns and worries.) Sixty-seven subjects exhibited state anxiety, and seventy-five had trait anxiety. Thirty-five had both types. Their values were "much higher than those observed in the general population." The researchers learned that higher intake of vitamin D was associated with lower levels of anxiety. And, they concluded that "future longitudinal studies will provide a more accurate interpretation of data from this study."[9]

Vitamin D Alleviates Anxiety in Elders with Prediabetes

In a twelve-month, open-label trial published in the journal *Metabolites*, researchers from Greece investigated the effect of vitamin D supplementation on anxiety and depression in elderly people with prediabetes. The cohort consisted of ninety subjects over the age of sixty years. Forty-five subjects, with a mean age of 73.10 years, were randomly assigned to take a weekly dose of an oral solution of 25,000 IU of vitamin D, and forty-five, with a mean age of 74.03 years, were not given any vitamin D. The subjects in both groups, who had similar baseline characteristics, were told to participate in aerobic exercise at least 150 minutes per week and to lose weight by following the Mediterranean diet. The subjects were periodically assessed by a physician and dietitian. Anxiety levels were measured with the Spielberger Inventory of State-Trait Anxiety

Self-Esteem Scale. While all of the subjects in the vitamin D group completed the trial, only thirty-five in the control group finished. No adverse effects were observed. At the end of the trial, the percentage of vitamin D-deficient subjects in the intervention group decreased from 92.86 to 52.39 percent; meanwhile, the percentage of vitamin D-deficient subjects in the control group decreased from 97.14 to 82.86 percent. At the same time, the anxiety levels of the vitamin D group were significantly lower than the anxiety levels of the control group. And, the elders who were deficient in vitamin D at baseline appeared to obtain the most benefits from the supplementation. The researchers concluded that their findings "showed that in a high-risk population, a weekly vitamin D supplementation scheme was effective in reducing anxiety and depression levels."[10]

People with Lipedema May Have Lower Levels of Serum Vitamin D and an Increased Risk of Anxiety

In a trial published in the journal *Hormone Molecular Biology and Clinical Investigation*, researchers from Jordan and Italy studied the relationship between lipedema, low levels of serum vitamin D, and anxiety. The cohort consisted of forty female patients with lipedema; they had a mean age of 43.35 years and an average lipedema duration of 5.58 years. (Lipedema is the accumulation of excess fat in the lower part of the body.) Blood samples were obtained from all of the subjects and tested for levels of vitamin D. Anxiety levels were measured with the Hamilton Anxiety Scale. About 77.5 percent of the subjects had vitamin D levels that were below normal; the mean serum concentration of vitamin D was 20.05 ng/ml. There was a significant inverse association between mean serum levels of vitamin D and severity of anxiety; the higher the levels of vitamin D, the lower the intensity of anxiety. The researchers concluded that their findings suggest a strong correlation between vitamin D and anxiety in people with lipedema.[11]

Symptomatic Vitamin D Toxicity Is Rare

In a retrospective study published in the journal *Laboratory Medicine*, researchers from Iowa wanted to learn more about elevated levels of serum/plasma 25(OH)D and vitamin D toxicity. That is why they reviewed sixteen years of patient records. During this time period, 127,932 measurements of 25(OH)D were performed on 73,779 individual patients. The researchers identified 1,068 samples from 780 patients with 25(OH)D concentrations levels greater than 80 ng per ml, which they defined as elevated; eighty-nine patients had concentration levels that exceeded 120 ng per ml. Specimens with elevated levels of 25(OH)D comprised only 0.8 percent of the total and 1.1 percent of the patients tested. The age range of those affected was 0.3 to 100.6 years, with a mean age of 49.0 years. Eighty-six patients were younger than eighteen years. The results from the female patients ranged from 81 to 480 ng per ml, and the results from the male patients ranged from 81 to 805 ng per ml. From the patient records, it appeared that seventeen patients were taking 50,000 IU tablets, four were taking 20,000 IU tablets, six were taking 10,000 IU tablets, eleven were taking 5,000 IU tablets, and six were taking 1,000 IU tablets. In addition, seven were taking liquid formulations with varying concentrations. Eighteen patients had no vitamin D supplementation recorded in their medical record. Still, only four patients showed symptoms of vitamin D toxicity; the two patients with the most severe symptoms were pediatric. Three of the four cases involved inadvertent misdosing of liquid formations. The researchers concluded "that symptomatic vitamin toxicity is quite rare."[12]

References and Further Readings

Al Anouti, F., W. B. Grant, J. Thomas et al. "Associations Between Dietary Intake of Vitamin D, Sun Exposure, and Generalized Anxiety Among College Women." *Nutrients* 14 (2022): 5327.

Al-Wardat, Mohammed, Nuha Alwardat, Gemma Lou De Santis et al. "The Association Between Serum Vitamin D and Mood Disorders in a Cohort of Lipedema Patients." *Hormone Molecular Biology and Clinical Investigation* 42, no. 4 (July 29, 2021): 351–5.

Bičíková, M., M. Dušková, J. Vítku et al. "Vitamin D in Anxiety and Affective Disorders." *Physiological Research* 64, no. Suppl 2 (2015): S101–S103.

Eid, Alaa, Sawsan Khoja, Shareefa AlGhamdi et al. "Vitamin D Supplementation Ameliorates Severity of Generalized Anxiety Disorder (GAD)." *Metabolic Brain Disease* 34 (2019): 1781–6.

Esnafoglu, Erman and Elif Yaman. "Vitamin B12, Folic Acid, Homocysteine and Vitamin D Levels in Children and Adolescents with Obsessive Compulsive Disorder." *Psychiatry Research* 254 (2017): 232–7.

Lee, John P., Michael Tansey, Jennifer G. Jetton, and Matthew D. Krasowski. "Vitamin D Toxicity: A 16-Year Retrospective Study at an Academic Medical Center." *Laboratory Medicine* 49, no. 2 (May 2018): 123–9.

Liu, Chen, Weiqing Jiang, Mingzhu Deng et al. "Lower Vitamin D Levels in Panic Attacks in Shanghai: A Case-Control Study." *Asian Journal of Psychiatry* 51 (2020): 101948.

Marazziti, Donatella, Filippo M. Barberi, Leonardo Fontenelle et al. "Decreased Vitamin D Levels in Obsessive-Compulsive Disorder Patients." *CNS Spectrums* 28, no. 5 (2023): 606–13.

Miyamoto, Mana, Yuko Hanatani, and Kenichi Shibuya. "Increased Vitamin D Intake May Reduce Psychological Anxiety and the Incidence of Menstrual Irregularities in Female Athletes." *PeerJ* 10 (November 21, 2022): e14456.

Pu, Dan, Jing Luo, Yanhua Wang et al. "Prevalence of Depression and Anxiety in Rheumatoid Arthritis Patients and Their Associations with Serum Vitamin D Level." *Clinical Rheumatology* 37 (2018): 179–84.

Zaromytidou, Evangelia, Theocharis Koufakis, Georgios Dimakopoulos et al. "Vitamin D Alleviates Anxiety and Depression in Elderly People with Prediabetes: A Randomized Controlled Study." *Metabolites* 12 (2022): 884.

Zhu, Cuizhen, Yu Zhang, Ting Wang et al. "Vitamin D Supplementation Improves Anxiety But Not Depression Symptoms in Patients with Vitamin D Deficiency." *Brain and Behavior* 10 (2020): e01760.

Notes

Introduction to Anxiety Disorders

1 https://www.nimh.nih.gov/health/topics/anxiety-disorders.

Acupressure

1 Su-Ru Chen, Wen-Hsian Hou, Jung-Nien Lai et al., "Effects of Acupressure on Anxiety: A Systematic Review and Meta-Analysis," *Journal of Integrative and Complementary Medicine* 28, no. 1 (January 2022): 25–35.

2 Doreen W. Au, Hector W. Tsang, Paul, P. Ling et al., "Effects of Acupressure on Anxiety: A Systematic Review and Meta-Analysis," *Acupuncture in Medicine* 33, no. 5 (October 2015): 353.

3 Foziyeh Abadi, Faezeh Abadi, Zhila Fereidouni et al., "Effect of Acupressure on Preoperative Cesarean Section Anxiety," *Journal of Acupuncture and Meridian Studies* 11, no. 6 (2018): 361–6.

4 Hsing-Chi Hsu, Kai-Yu Tseng, Hsin-Yuan Fang et al., "The Effects of Acupressure on Improving Health and Reducing Cost for Patients Undergoing Thoracoscopic Surgery," *International Journal of Environmental Research and Public Health* 19 (2022): 1869.

5 U. Erappa, S. Konde, M. Agarwal et al., "Comparative Evaluation of Efficacy of Hypnosis, Acupressure and Audiovisual Aids in Reducing the Anxiety of Children During Administration of Local Anesthesia," *International Journal of Clinical Pediatric Dentistry* 14, no. S-2 (2021): S186–S192.

6 N. T. T. Hmwe, P. Subramanian, L. P. Tan, and W. K. Chong, "The Effects of Acupressure on Depression, Anxiety and Stress in Patients with Hemodialysis: A Randomized Controlled Trial," *International Journal of Nursing Studies* 52 (2015): 509–18.

7 F. Mohaddes Ardabili, S. Purhajari, T. Najafi Ghzeljeh, and H. Haghani, "The Effect of Shiatsu Massage on Underlying Anxiety in Burn Patients," *World Journal of Plastic Surgery* 4, no. 1 (January 2015): 36–9.

8 Aleksandra K. Macznik, Anthony G. Schneiders, Josie Athens, and S. John Sullivan, "Does Acupressure Hit the Mark? A Three-Arm Randomized Placebo-Controlled Trial of Acupressure for Pain and Anxiety Relief in Athletes with Acute

Musculoskeletal Sports Injuries," *Clinical Journal of Sport* Medicine 27, no. 4 (July 2017): 338–43.

9 Y. Honda, A. Tsuda, S. Horiuchi, and S. Aoki, "Baseline Anxiety Level as Efficacy Moderator for Self-Administered Acupressure for Anxiety Reduction," *International Journal of Prevention and Treatment* 2, no. 3 (2013): 41–5.

Acupuncture

1 Jia Cui, Shaobai Wang, Jiehui Ren et al., "Use of Acupuncture in the USA: Changes over a Decade (2002–2012)," *Acupuncture in Medicine* 35, no. 3 (June 2017): 200–7.

2 Diogo Amorim, Irma Brito, Armando Caseiro et al., "Electroacupuncture and Acupuncture in the Treatment of Anxiety—A Double Blinded Randomized Parallel Clinical Trial," *Complementary Therapies in Clinical Practice* 46 (2022): 101541.

3 Jing-qi Fan, Wei-jing Lu, Wei-qiang Tan et al., "Effectiveness of Acupuncture for Anxiety Among Patients with Parkinson Disease: A Randomized Clinical Trial," *JAMA Network Open* 5, no. 9 (2022): e2232133.

4 Brenda Leung, Wendy Takeda, and Victoria Holec, "Pilot Study of Acupuncture to Treat Anxiety in Children and Adolescents," *Journal of Paediatrics and Child Health* 54, no. 8 (August 2018): 881–8.

5 Jakub K. Wunsch, Catharina Klausenitz, Henriette Janner et al., "Auricular Acupuncture for Treatment of Preoperative Anxiety in Patient Scheduled for Ambulatory Gynaecological Surgery: A Prospective Controlled Investigation with a Non-Randomised Arm," *Acupuncture in Medicine* 36, no. 4 (August 2018): 222–7.

6 M. D. Wiles, J. Mamdani, M. Pullman, and C. Andrzejowski, "A Randomised Controlled Trial Examining the Effect of Acupuncture at the EX-HN3 (Yintang) Point on Pre-Operative Anxiety Levels in Neurosurgical Patients," *Anaesthesia* 72, no. 3 (March 2017): 335–42.

7 Young-Dae Kim, In Heo, Byung-Cheul. Shin et al., "Acupuncture for Posttraumatic Stress Disorder: A Systematic Review of Randomized Controlled Trials and Prospective Clinical Trials," *Evidence-Based Complementary and Alternative Medicine* (2013): Article ID 615857.

8 Arthur Dun-Ping Mak, Vincent Chi Ho Chung, Suet Ying Yuen et al., "Noneffectiveness of Electroacupuncture for Comorbid Generalized Anxiety Disorder and Irritable Bowel Syndrome," *Journal of Gastroenterology and Hepatology* 34, no. 10 (October 2019): 1736–42.

9 Guo-juan Dong, Di Cao, Yue Dong et al., "Scalp Acupuncture for Sleep Disorder Induced by Pre-Examination Anxiety in Undergraduates," *World Journal of Acupuncture* 28, no. 3 (September 2018): 156–60.

10 Catharina Klausenitz, Henriette Hacker, Thomas Hesse et al., "Auricular Acupuncture for Exam Anxiety in Medical Students—A Randomized Crossover Investigation," *PLoS ONE* 11, no. 12 (2016): e0168338.

11 Jia-Yu Ye, Yi-Jing He, Ming-Jie Zhan, and Fan Qu, "Effects of Acupuncture on the Relief of Anxiety and/or Depression During *in vitro* Fertilization: A Systematic Review and Meta-Analysis," *European Journal of Integrative Medicine* 42 (2021): 101287.

12 Charles C. Engel, Elizabeth H. Cordova, David M. Benedek et al., "Randomized Effectiveness Trial of a Brief Course of Acupuncture for Posttraumatic Stress Disorder," *Medical Care* 52, No. 12 Supplement 5 (December 2014): S57–S64.

Animal Therapy

1 Dasha Grajfoner, Emma Harte, Lauren M. Potter, and Nicola McGuigan, "The Effect of Dog-Assisted Intervention on Student Well-Being, Mood, and Anxiety," *International Journal of Environmental Research and Public Health* 14, no. 5 (2017): 483.

2 Dorota Wolyńczyk-Gmaj, Aleksandra Ziólkowska, Piotr Rogala et al., "Can Dog-Assisted Intervention Decrease Anxiety Level and Autonomic-Agitation in Patients with Anxiety Disorders?" *Journal of Clinical Medicine* 10 (2021): 5171.

3 Katherine Hinic, Mildred Ortu Kowalski, Kristin Holtzman, and Kristi Mobus, "The Effect of Pet Therapy and Comparison Intervention on Anxiety in Hospitalized Children," *Journal of Pediatric Nursing* 46 (2019): 55–61.

4 Sandra B. Barker, Janet S. Knisely, Christine M. Schubert et al., "The Effect of an Animal-Assisted Intervention on Anxiety and Pain in Hospitalized Children," *Anthrozoös* 28, no. 1 (March 2015): 101–12.

5 Amanda Bulette Coakley, Christine Donahue Annese, Joanne Hughes Empoliti, and Jane M. Flanagan, "The Experience of Animal Assisted Therapy on Patients in an Acute Care Setting," *Clinical Nursing Research* 30, no. 4 (May 2021): 401–05.

6 Kimberly Hoagwood, Aviva Vincent, Mary Acri et al., "Reducing Anxiety and Stress Among Youth in a CBT-Based Equine-Assisted Adaptive Riding Program," *Animals* 12, no. 19 (September 20, 2022): 24911.

7 Della Anderson and Stephanie Brown, "The Effect of Animal-Assisted Therapy on Nursing Student Anxiety: A Randomized Controlled Study," *Nurse Education in Practice* 52 (March 2021): 103042.

8 Jeffrey A. Coto, Erika K. Ohlendorf, Andrea E. Cinnamon et al., "A Correlational Study Exploring Nurse Work Anxiety and Animal-Assisted Therapy," *Journal of Nursing Administration* 52, no. 9 (September 2022): 498–502.

9 B. Berget, Ø. Ekeberg, I. Pedersen, and B. Braastad, "Animal-Assisted Therapy with Farm Animals for Persons with Psychiatric Disorders: Effects on Anxiety and Depression, a Randomized Controlled Trial," *Occupational Therapy in Mental Health* 27 (2011): 50–64.

10 Megan K. Mueller, Eric C. Anderson, Erin K. King, and Heather L. Urry, "Null Effects of Therapy Dog Interaction on Adolescent Anxiety During Laboratory-Based Social Evaluative Stressor," *Anxiety, Stress, & Coping* 34, no. 4 (2021): 365–80.

Benzodiazepines

1 Carlos Blanco, Beth Han, Christopher M. Jones et al., "Prevalence and Correlates of Benzodiazepine Use, Misuse, and Use Disorders Among Adults in the United States," *Journal of Clinical Psychiatry* 79, no. 6 (October 16, 2018): 18m12174.

2 Jeannette Y. Wick, "The History of Benzodiazepines," *The Consultant Pharmacist* 28, no. 9 (September 2013): 538–48.

3 Carlos Blanco, Beth Han, Christopher M. Jones et al., "Prevalence and Correlates of Benzodiazepine Use, Misuse, and Use Disorders Among Adults in the United States," *Journal of Clinical Psychiatry* 79, no. 6 (October 16, 2018): 18m12174.

4 Aarti Gupta, Gargi Bhattacharya, Syeda Arshiya Farheen et al., "Systematic Review of Benzodiazepines for Anxiety Disorders in Late Life," *Annals of Clinical Psychiatry* 32, no. 2 (May 2020): 114–26.

5 Lauren B. Gerlach, Donovan T. Maust, Shirley H. Leong et al., "Factors Associated with Long-Term Benzodiazepine Use Among Older Adults," *JAMA Internal Medicine* 178, no. 11 (2018): 1560–2.

6 Great A. Bushnell, Tobias Gerhard, Stephen Crystal, and Mark Offson, "Benzodiazepine Treatment and Fracture Risk in Young Persons with Anxiety Disorders," *Pediatrics* 146, no. 1 (July 2020): 20193478.

7 Angelina F. Gomez, Abigail L. Barthel, and Stefan G. Hofmann, "Comparing the Efficacy of Benzodiazepines and Serotonergic Anti-Depressants for Adults with Generalized Anxiety Disorder: A Meta-Analytic Review," *Expert Opinion on Pharmacotherapy* 19, no. 8 (June 2018): 883–94.

8 Babette Bais, Nina M. Molenaar, Hilmar H. Bijma et al., "Prevalence of Benzodiazepines and Benzodiazepine-Related Drugs Exposure Before, During and After Pregnancy: A Systematic Review and Meta-Analysis," *Journal of Affective Disorders* 269 (May 15, 2020): 18–27.

9 Hyunji Lee, Jae-Whoan Koh, Young-Ah Kim et al., "Pregnancy and Neonatal Outcomes After Exposure to Alprazolam in Pregnancy," *Frontiers in Pharmacology* 13 (April 2022): Article 854562.

10 J. B. Cohn and C. S. Wilcox, "Long-Term Comparison of Alprazolam, Lorazepam and Placebo in Patients with an Anxiety Disorder," *Pharmacotherapy* 4, no. 2 (March–April 1984): 93–8.

11 Robert Elie and Yves Lamontagne, "Alprazolam and Diazepam in. the Treatment of Generalized Anxiety," *Journal of Clinical Psychopharmacology* 4, no. 3 (June 1984): 125–9.

12 Antonio E. Nardi, Rafael C. Freire, Marina D. Mochcovitch et al., "A Randomized, Naturalistic, Parallel-Group Study for the Long-Term Treatment of Panic Disorder with Clonazepam or Paroxetine," *Journal of Clinical Psychopharmacology* 32, no. 1 (February 2012): 120–6.

13 Daniela Z. Knijnik, Carlos Blanco, Giovanni Abrahãon Salum et al., "A Pilot Study of Clonazepam Versus Psychodynamic Group Therapy Plus Clonazepam in the Treatment of Generalized Social Anxiety Disorder," *European Psychiatry* 23, no. 8 (December 2008): 567–74.

14 M. W. Van Laar, E. R. Volkerts, and A. P. P. van Willigenburg, "Therapeutic Effects and Effects on Actual Driving Performance of Chronically Administered Buspirone and Diazepam in Anxious Outpatients," *Journal of Clinical Psychopharmacology* 12, no. 2 (April 1992): 86–95.

15 Toshiya Inada, Shoko Nozaki, Ataru Inagaki, and Toshiaki A. Furukawa, "Efficacy of Diazepam as an Anti-Anxiety Agent: Meta-Analysis of Double-Blind, Randomized Controlled Trials Carried Out in Japan," *Human Psychopharmacology* 18, no. 6 (August 2003): 483–7.

16 J. E. McCall, C. G. Fischer, G. Warden et al., "Lorazepam Given the Night Before Surgery Reduces Preoperative Anxiety in Children Undergoing Reconstructive Burn Surgery," *Journal of Burn Care & Rehabilitation* 20, no. 2 (March–April 1999): 151–4.

17 Jayne E. Clarkson, Ann Marie Gordon, and Barry K. Logan, "Lorazepam and Driving Impairment," *Journal of Analytical Toxicology* 28 (September 2004): 475–80.

18 Nunzio Pomara, Sang Han Lee, Davide Bruno et al., "Adverse Performance Effects of Acute Lorazepam Administration in Elderly Long-Term Users: Pharmacokinetic and Clinical Predictors," *Progress in Neuro-Psychopharmacology & Biological Psychiatry* 56 (2015): 129–35.

Beta-Blockers

1 Cody Armstrong and Michelle R. Kapolowicz, "A Preliminary Investigation on the Effects of Atenolol for Treating Symptoms of Anxiety," *Military Medicine* 185 (November/December 2020): e1954–e1960.

2 P. Saul, B. P. Jones, K. G. Edwards, and J. A. Tweed, "Randomized Comparison of Atenolol and Placebo in the Treatment of Anxiety: A Double-Blind Study," *European Journal of Clinical Pharmacology* 28 (1985): 109–10.

3 Michael J. Elman, Joel Sugar, Richard Fiscella et al., "The Effect of Propranolol Versus Placebo on Resident Surgical Performance," *Transactions of the American Ophthalmology Society* 96 (1998): 283–91.

4 C. O. Brantigan, T. A. Brantigan, and N. Joseph, "Effect of Beta Blockade and Beta Stimulation on Stage Fright," *The American Journal of Medicine* 72 (January 1982): 88–94.

5 Guillaume Valva, François Ducrocq, Karine Jezequel et al., "Immediate Treatment with Propranolol Decreases Posttraumatic Stress Disorder Two Months After Trauma," *Biological Psychiatry* 54, no. 9 (November 1, 2003): 947–9.

6 Lorenzo Tarsitani, Vincenzo De Santis, Martino Mistrette et al., "Treatment with Beta-blockers and Incidence of Post-Traumatic Stress Disorder After Cardiac Surgery: A Prospective Observational Study," *Journal of Cardiothoracic and Vascular Anesthesia* 26, no. 2 (April 2012): 265–9.

7 Laura Rosenberg, Marta Rosenberg, Sherri Sharp et al., "Does Acute Propranolol Treatment Prevent Posttraumatic Stress Disorder, Anxiety, and Depression in Children with Burns," *Journal of Child and Adolescent Psychopharmacology* 28, no. 2 (March 2018): 117–23.

8 Serge A. Steenan, Naichuan Su, Roos van Westrhenen et al., "Perioperative Propranolol Against Dental Anxiety: A Randomized Controlled Trial," *Frontiers in Psychiatry* 13 (February 2022): Article 842353.

9 S. G. Kilminster, M. J. Lewis, and D. M. Jones, "Anxiolytic Effects of Acebutolol and Atenolol in Healthy Volunteers with Induced Anxiety," *Psychopharmacology* 95 (1998): 245–9.

10 Serge Al Steenen, Arjen J. van Wijk, Geert JMG van der Heijden et al., "Propranolol for the Treatment of Anxiety Disorders: Systematic Review and Meta-Analysis," *Journal of Psychopharmacology* 30, no. 2 (February 2016): 128–39.

11 Sandra E. File and R. G. Lister, "A Comparison of the Effects of Lorazepam and Those of Propranolol on Experimentally-Induced Anxiety and Performance," *British Journal of Clinical Pharmacology* 19 (1985): 445–51.

Buspirone

1 M. Lader and J. C. Scotto, "A Multicentre Double-Blind Comparison of Hydroxyzine, Buspirone and Placebo in Patients with Generalized Anxiety Disorder," *Psychopharmacology* 139, no. 4 (October 1998): 402–6.

2 Naghmeh Mokhber, Mahmoud Reza Azarpazhooh, Mohammad Khajehdaluee et al., "Randomized, Single-Blind, Trial of Sertraline and Buspirone for Treatment

of Elderly Patients with Generalized Anxiety Disorder," *Psychiatry and Clinical Neuroscience* 64 (2010): 128–33.

3   John J. Sramek, Edyta J. Frackiewicz, and Neal R. Cutler, "Efficacy and Safety of Two Dosing Regimes of Buspirone in the Treatment of Outpatients with Persistent Anxiety," *Clinical Therapeutics* 19, no. 3 (1997): 498–506.

4   G. Laakmann, C. Schüle, G. Lorkowski et al., "Buspirone and Lorazepam in the Treatment of Generalized Anxiety Disorder in Outpatients," *Psychopharmacology* 136 (1998): 357–66.

5   T. A. Ceranoglu, Janet Wazniak, Ronna Fried et al., "A Retrospective Chart Review of Buspirone for the Treatment of Anxiety in Psychiatrically Referred Youth with High-Functioning Autism Spectrum Disorder," *Journal of Child and Adolescent Psychopharmacology* 29, no. 1 (2019): 28–33.

6   Ruth B. Schneider, Peggy Auinger, Chistopher G. Tarolli et al., "A Trial of Buspirone Parkinson's Disease: Safety and Tolerability," *Parkinsonism and Related Disorders* 81 (2020): 69–74.

7   Jean Cottraux, Ivan-Druon Note, Charley Cungi et al., "A Controlled Study of Cognitive Behavior Therapy with Buspirone or Placebo in Panic Disorder with Agoraphobia," *British Journal of Psychiatry* 167 (1995): 635–41.

8   Moira Rynn, Felipe Garcia-Espana, David Greenblatt et al., "Imipramine and Buspirone in Patients with Panic Disorder Who Are Discontinuing Long-Term Benzodiazepine Therapy," *Journal of Clinical Psychopharmacology* 23, no. 5 (October 2003): 505–8.

9   P. H. Thomsen and H. U. Mikkelsen, "The Addition of Buspirone to SSRI in the Treatment of Adolescent Obsessive-Compulsive Disorder: A Study of Six Cases," *European Child & Adolescent Psychiatry* 8 (1999): 143–8.

Cannabis and CBD

1   Marc-Antoine Crocq, "History of Cannabis and the Endocannabinoid System," *Dialogues in Clinical Neuroscience* 22, no. 3 (September 2020): 223–8.

2   https://www.singlecare.com/blog/news/cbd-statistics/#:~:text=16%25%20of %20people%20ages%2030,65%20and%20older%20use%20CBD.

3   https://drugabusestatistics.org/marijuana-addiction.

4   Tory R. Spindle, Dennis J. Sholler, Edward J. Cone et al., *JAMA Network Open* 5, no. 7 (2022): e2223019.

5   Scott Shannon, Nicole Lewis, Heather Lee, and Shannon Hughes, "Cannabidiol in Anxiety and Sleep: A Large Case Series," *The Permanente Journal* 23 (2019): 18–41.

6   Maximus Berger, Emily Li, Simon Rice et al., "Cannabidiol for Treatment-Resistant Anxiety Disorder in Young People: An Open-Label Trial," *Journal of Clinical Psychiatry* 83, no. 5 (August 2022): 21m14130.

7   Toni Spinella, Sherry H. Stewart, Julia Naugler et al., "Evaluating Cannabidiol (CBD) Expectancy Effects on Acute Stress and Anxiety in Health Adults: A Randomized Crossover Study," *Psychopharmacology* 238 (2021): 1965–77.

8   Pablo Roitmaan, Raphael Mechoulam, Rena Cooper-Kazaz, Arieh Shalev, "Preliminary, Open-Label, Pilot Study of Add-On Oral Delta 9-Tetrahydrocannabinol in Chronic Post-Traumatic Stress Disorder," *Clinical Drug Investigation* 34 (2014): 587–91.

9   Emily M. LaFrance, Nicholas C. Glodosky, Marcel Bonn-Miller, and Carrie Cuttler, "Sort and Long-Term Effects of Cannabis on Symptoms of Post-Traumatic Stress Disorder," *Journal of Effective Disorders* 274 (2020): 298–304.

10 Marcel O. Bonn-Miller, Sus Sisley, Paula Riggs et al., "The Short-Term Impact of Smoke Cannabis Preparations Versus Placebo on PTSD Symptoms: A Randomized Cross-Over Clinical Trial," *PLoS ONE* 16, no. 3 (2021): e0246990.

11 Yih-Ing Hser, Larissa J. Mooney, David Huang et al., "Reductions in Cannabis Use Are Associated with Improvements in Anxiety, Depression, and Sleep Quality, But Not Quality of Life," *Journal of Substance Abuse Treatment* 81 (October 2017): 53–8.

12 Julia D. Buckner, Marcel O. Bonn-Miller, Michael J. Zvolensky, and Norman B. Schmidt, "Marijuana Use Motives and Social Anxiety Among Marijuana-Using Young. Adults," *Addictive Behaviors* 32 (2007): 2238–52.

13 Conal D. Twomey, "Association of Cannabis Use with the Development of Elevated Anxiety Symptoms in the General Population: A Meta-Analysis," *Journal of Epidemiology & Community Health* 71, no. 8 (August 2017): 811–16.

Cognitive Behavioral Therapy

1   Joseph K. Carpenter, Leigh A. Andrews, Sara M. Witcraft et al., "Cognitive Behavioral Therapy for Anxiety and Related Disorders: A Meta-Analysis of Randomized Placebo-Controlled Trials," *Depression and Anxiety* 35, no. 6 (June 2018): 502–14.

2   Z. Wang, S. P. H. Whiteside, L. Sim et al., "Comparative Effectiveness and Safety of Cognitive Behavioral Therapy and Pharmacotherapy for Childhood Anxiety Disorders: A Systematic Review and Meta-Analysis," *JAMA Pediatrics* 171, no. 11 (November 2017): 1049–56.

3   Gretchen A. Brenes, Suzanne C. Danhauer, Mary F. Lyles et al., "Telephone-Delivered Cognitive Behavioral Therapy and Telephone-Delivered Nondirective Supportive Therapy for Rural Older Adults with Generalized Anxiety Disorder: A Randomized Clinical Trial," *JAMA Psychiatry* 72, no. 10 (October 2015): 1012–20.

4 Michelle Rozenman, John Piacentini, Joseph O'Neill et al., "Improvement in Anxiety and Depression Symptoms Following Cognitive Behavior Therapy for Pediatric Obsessive Compulsive Disorder," *Psychiatry Research* 276 (2019): 115–23.

5 Arne Kodal Krister Fjermestad, Ingvar Bjelland et al., "Long-Term Effectiveness of Cognitive Behavioral Therapy for Youth with Anxiety Disorders," *Journal of Anxiety Disorders* 53 (2018): 58–67.

6 Jingjing Li, Zhu Cai, Xiaoming Li et al., "Mindfulness-Based Therapy Versus Cognitive Behavioral Therapy for People with Anxiety Systems: A Systematic Review and Meta-Analysis of Random Controlled Trials," *Annals of Palliative Medicine* 10, no. 7 (July 2021): 7596–612.

7 Truls Bilet, Torbjørn Olsen, John Roger Andersen, and Egil W. Martinsen, "Cognitive Behavioral Group Therapy for Panic Disorder in a General Cohort Setting: A Prospective Cohort Study with 12 to 31 Years Follow-Up," *BMC Psychiatry* 20 (2020): 259.

8 Gene Efron and Bethany M. Wooten, "Remote Cognitive Behavioral Therapy for Panic Disorder: A Meta-Analysis," *Journal of Anxiety Disorders* 79 (2021): 102385.

9 Tine Nordgreen, Rolf Gjestad, Gerhard Andersson et al., "The Effectiveness of Guided-Internet Based Cognitive Behavioral Therapy for Social Anxiety Disorder in a Routine Care Setting," *Internet Interventions* 13 (2018): 24–9.

10 Marie-Louise Schermuly-Haupt, Michael Linden, and A. John Rush, "Unwanted Events and Side Effects in Cognitive Behavioral Therapy," *Cognitive Therapy and Research* 42, no. 3 (June 2018): 219–29.

Exercise

1 Matthew P. Herring, Marni L. Jacob, Cynthia Suveg et al., "Feasibility of Exercise Training for Short-Term Treatment of Generalized Anxiety Disorder: A Randomized Controlled Trial," *Psychology and Psychosomatics* 81, no.1 (December 2011): 21–8.

2 Ana M. Abrantes, David R. Strong, Amy Cohn et al., "Acute Changes in Obsessions and Compulsions Following Moderate-Intensity Aerobic Exercise Among Patients with Obsessive-Compulsive Disorder," *Journal of Anxiety Disorders* 23, no. 7 (October 2009): 923–7.

3 B. S. Hale and J. S. Raglin, "State Anxiety Responses to Acute Resistance Training and Step Aerobic Exercise Across Weeks of Training," *Journal of Sports Medicine and Physical Fitness* 42, no. 1 (March 2002): 108–12.

4 Dafna Merom, Philayrath Phongsavan, Renate Wagner et al., "Promoting Walking as an Adjunct Intervention to Group Cognitive Behavioral Therapy for Anxiety

Disorders—A Pilot Group Randomized Trial," *Journal of Anxiety Disorders* 22 (2008): 959–68.

5 Rebecca A. Johnson, David L. Albright, James R. Marzolf et al., "Effects of Therapeutic Horseback Riding on Post-Traumatic Stress Disorder in Military Veterans," *Military Medical Research* 5 (2018): 3.

6 Camillo Pérez-Chaparro, Maria Kangas, Phillip Zech et al., "Recreational Exercise Is Associated with Lower Prevalence of Depression and Anxiety and Better Quality of Life in German People Living with HIV," *AIDS Care* 34, no. 2 (2022): 182–7.

7 S. Córdoba-Torrecilla, V. A. Aparicio, A. Soriano-Maldonado et al., "Physical Fitness Is Associated with Anxiety Levels in Women with Fibromyalgia: The Al-Ándalus Project," *Quality of Life Research* 25 (2016): 1053–8.

8 Diego Munguía-Izquierdo and Alejandro Legaz-Arrese, "Assessment of the Effects of Aquatic Therapy on Global Symptomatology in Patients with Fibromyalgia Syndrome: A Randomized Controlled Trial," *Archives of Physical Medicine Rehabilitation* 89 , no. 12 (December 2009) 2250–7.

9 Rachel Blacklock, Ryan Rhodes. Chris Blanchard, and Catherine Gaul, "Effects of Exercise Intensity and Self-Efficacy on State Anxiety with Breast Cancer Survivors," *Oncology Nursing Forum* 37, no. 2 (March 2010):206–12.

10 Goran Kuvačić, Patrizia Fratini, Johnny Padulo, and Antonio Dello Iacono, "Effectiveness of Yoga and Educational Intervention on Disability, Anxiety, Depression, and Pain in People with CLBP: A Randomized Controlled Trial," *Complementary Therapies in Clinical Practice* 31 (2018): 262–7.

Gabapentin

1 Jill E. Lavigne, Karen Mustian, Jennifer L. Matthews et al., "A Randomized, Controlled, Double-Blinded Clinical Trial of Gabapentin 300 mg versus 900 mg versus Placebo for Anxiety Symptoms in Breast Cancer Survivors," *Breast Cancer Research and Treatment* 136, no. 2 (November 2012): 479–86.

2 Fernanda de-Paris, Marcia K. Sant' Anna, Monica R. M. Vianna et al., "Effects of Gabapentin on Anxiety Induced by Simulated Public Speaking," *Journal of Psychopharmacology* 17, no. 2 (2003): 184–8.

3 Hance Clarke, Kyle R. Kirkham, Beverley A. Orser et al., "Gabapentin Reduces Preoperative Anxiety and Pain Catastrophizing in High Anxious Patients Prior to Major Surgery: A Blinded Randomized Placebo-Controlled Trial," *Canadian Journal of Anesthesia* 60 (2013): 432–43.

4 Hance Clarke, Joseph Kay, Beverley A. Orser et al., "Gabapentin Does Not Reduce Preoperative Anxiety When Given Prior to Total Hip Arthroplasty," *Pain Medicine* 11 (2010): 966–71.

5 Tim Thomas Joseph, Handattu Mahabaleswara Krishna, and Shyamsunder Kamath, "Premedication with Gabapentin, Alprazolam or a Placebo for Abdominal Hysterectomy: Effect on Pre-Operative Anxiety, Post-Operative Pain and Morphine Consumption," *Indian Journal of Anaesthesia* 58, no. 6 (November–December 2014): 693–9.

6 Atul C. Pande, Jonathan R. T. Davidson, James W. Jefferson et al., "Treatment of Social Phobia with Gabapentin: A Placebo-Controlled Study," *Journal of Clinical Psychopharmacology* 19, no. 4 (August 1999): 341–8.

7 Maria R. Urbano, David R. Spiegel, Nena Laguerta et al., "Gabapentin and Tiagabine for Social Anxiety: A Randomized Double-Blind, Crossover Study of 8 Adults," *Primary Care Companion to the Journal of Clinical Psychiatry* 11, no. 3 (2009): 123.

8 Atul C. Pande, Mark H. Pollack, Jerri Crockatt et al., "Placebo-Controlled Study of Gabapentin Treatment of Panic Disorder," *Journal of Clinical Psychopharmacology* 20, no. 4 (2000): 467–71.

9 Mark B. Hamner, Peter S. Brodrick, and Lawrence A. Labbate, "Gabapentin in PTSD: A Retrospective, Clinical Series of Adjunctive Therapy," *Annals of Clinical Psychiatry* 13, no. 3 (September 2001): 141–6.

10 Emin Önder, Ümit Tural, and Mehmet Gökbakan, "Does Gabapentin Lead to Early Symptom Improvement in Obsessive-Compulsive Disorder," *European Archives of Psychiatry and Clinical Neuroscience* 258 (2008): 319–23.

Herbal Medicine

1 https://craighospital.org/resources/herbs-herbal-medicine.

2 https://www.fda.gov/food/dietary-supplements/dietary-supplement-ingredient-directory.

3 Jun J. Mao, Sharon X. Xie, John R. Keefe et al., "Long-Term Chamomile (Matricaria chamomilla L.) Treatment for Generalized Anxiety Disorder: A Randomized Clinical Trial," *Phytomedicine* 23, no. 14 (December 15, 2016): 1735 -1742.

4 Solmaz Heidari-Fard, Sedighe Amir Ali-Akbari, Abulhasan Rafiei et al., "Investigating the Effect of Chamomile Essential oil on Reducing Anxiety in Nulliparous Women During the First Stage of Childbirth," *International Journal of Biology, Pharmacy and Allied Sciences* 6, no. 5 (2017): 828–42.

5 Forough Rafit, Farzaneh Ameri, Hamid Haghani, and Ali Ghobadi, "The Effect of Aromatherapy Massage with Lavender and Chamomile Oil on Anxiety and Sleep Quality of Patients with Burns," *Burns* 46 (2020): 164–71.

6 U. Malsch and M. Kiser, "Efficacy of Kava-Kava in the Treatment of Non-Psychotic Anxiety Following Pretreatment with Benzodiazepines," *Psychopharmacology* 157 (2001): 277–83.

7 Jerome Sarris, Gerard J. Byrne, Chand A. Bousman et al., "Kava for Generalised Anxiety Disorder: A 16-Week Double-Blind, Randomised, Placebo-Controlled Study," *Australian & New Zealand Journal of Psychiatry* 53, no. 3 (March 2020): 288–97.

8 Jerome Sarris and David J. Kavanagh, "Kava and St. John's Wort: Current Evidence for Use in Mood and Anxiety Disorders," *Journal of Alternative and Complementary Medicine* 15, no. 8 (2009): 827–36.

9 Azizeh Farshbaf-Khalili, Mahin Kamalifard, and Maahsa Namadian, "Comparison of the Effect of Lavender and Bitter Orange on Anxiety in Postmenopausal Women: A Triple-Blind, Randomized, Controlled Clinical Trial," *Complementary Therapies in Clinical Practice* 31 (2018): 132–8.

10 Myoungsuk Kim, Eun Sook Nam, Yongmi Lee, and Hyun-Ju Kang, "Effects of Lavender on Anxiety, Depression, and Physiological Parameters," *Asian Nursing Research* 15 (2021): 279–90.

11 S. Akhondzadeh, H. R. Naghavi, M. Vazirian et al., "Passionflower in the Treatment of Generalized Anxiety: A Pilot Double-Blind Randomized Controlled Trial with Oxazepam," *Journal of Clinical Pharmacy and Therapeutics* 26 (2001): 363–7.

12 Liliane-Poconé Dantas, Artur de Oliveira-Ribeiro, Liane-Maciel de Almeida-Souza, and Francisco-Carlos Groppo, "Effect of *Passiflora incarnata* and Midazolam for Control of Anxiety in Patients Undergoing Dental Extraction," *Medicina Oral Patologia Oral y Cirugia Bucal* 22, no. 1 (January 1, 2017): e95–e101.

13 Mohsen Mazidi, Maryam Shemshian, Seyed Hadi Mousavi et al., "A Double-Blind, Randomized and Placebo-Controlled Trial of Saffron (*Crocus sativus* L.) in the Treatment of Anxiety and Depression," *Journal of Complementary and Integrative Medicine* 13, no. 2 (June 1, 2016): 195–9.

14 Adrian L. Lopresti, Peter D. Drummond Antonio M. Inarejos-García, and Marin Prodanov, Affron, a Standarized Extract from Saffron (*Crocus sativus* L.) for the Treatment of Youth Anxiety and Depressive Symptoms: A Randomised, Double-Blind, Placebo-Controlled Study," *Journal of Affective Disorders* 232 (2018): 349–57.

15 Ehsan Moazen-Zadeh, Seyed Hesameddin Abbasi, Hamideh Safi-Aghdam et al., "Effects of Saffron on Cognition, Anxiety, and Depression in Patients Undergoing Coronary Artery Bypasss Grafting: A Randomized Double-Blind Placebo-Controlled Trial," *Journal of Alternative and Complementary Medicine* 24, no. 4 (2018): 361–8.

16 Kenneth A. Kobak, Leslie V. H. Taylor, Gemma Warner, and Rise Futterer, "St. John's Wort versus Placebo in Social Phobia," *Journal of Clinical Psychopharmacology* 25, no. 1 (February 2005): 51–8.

17 Diethard Müller, T. Pfeil, and V. von den Driesch, "Treating Depression Comorbid with Anxiety—Results of an Open, Practice-Oriented Study with St. John's Wort WS 5572 and Valerian Extract in High Doses," *Phytomedicine* 10, no. Supplement 4 (2003): 25–30.

Hydroxyzine

1 T. Darcis, M. Ferreri, J. Natens et al., "A Multicentre Double-Blind Placebo-Controlled Study Investigating the Anxiolytic Efficacy of Hydroxyzine in Patients with Generalized Anxiety," *Human Psychopharmacology* 10 (1995): 181–7.

2 Malxolm Lader and Jean-Claude Scotto, "A Multicentre Double-Blind Comparison of Hydroxyzine, Buspirone and Placebo in Patients with Generalized Anxiety Disorder," *Psychopharmacology* 139 (1998): 402–6.

3 Pierre-Michel Llorca, Christian Spadone, Oliver Sol et al., "Efficacy and Safety of Hydroxyzine in the Treatment of Generalized Anxiety Disorder: A 3-Month Double-Blind Study," *Journal of Clinical Psychiatry* 63, no. 11 (2002): 1020–27.

4 Charles-Henri Houze-Cerfon, Frédéric Balen, Vanessa Houze-Cerfon et al., "Hydroxyzin Study," *American Journal of Emergency Medicine* 50 (December 2021): 753–7.

5 Esther Aleo, Amanda López Picado, Belén Joyanes Abancens et al., "Evaluation of the Effect of Hydroxyzine on Preoperative Anxiety and Anesthetic Adequacy in Children: Double Blind Randomized Clinical Trial," *BioMed Research International* (November 11, 2021): 7394042.

6 J. H. Boon and D. Hopkins, "Hydroxyzine Premedication—Does It Provide Better Anxiolysis Than a Placebo?" *SAMJ* 86, no. 6 (June 1996): 661–4.

7 George Wallace and Leonard J. Mindlin, "A Controlled Double-Blind Comparison of Intramuscular Lorazepam and Hydroxyzine as Surgical Premedicants," *Anesthesia & Analgesia* 63 (1984): 571–6.

8 Sujata Chaudhary, Reena Jindal, Gautam Girota et al., "Is Midzolam Superior to Triclofos and Hydroxyzine as Premedicant in Children?" *Journal of Anaesthiology Clinical Pharmacology* 30, no. 1 (January 2014): 53–8.

9 A. Pouliquen, E. Boyer, J.-L. Sixou et al., "Oral Sedation in Dentistry: Evaluation of Professional Practice of Oral Hydroxyzine in the University Hospital of Rennes, France," *European Archives of Paediatric Dentistry* 22, no. 5 (October 2021): 801–11.

10 Joseph W. Iskander, Benjamin Griffeth, and Christian Rubio-Cespedes, "Successful Treatment with Hydroxyzine of Acute Exacerbation of Panic Disorder in a Healthy Male: A Case Report," *Primary Care Companion for CNS Disorders* 13, no. 3 (2011): PCC.10l01126.

11 Hans J. Gober, Kathy H. Li, Kevin Yan et al., "Hydroxyzine Use in Preschool Children and Its Effect on Neurodevelopment: A Population-Based Longitudinal Study," *Frontiers in Psychiatry* 12 (January 2022): Article 721875.

Hypnosis

1 Heide Glaesmer, Hendrik Geupel, and Rainer Haak, "A Controlled Trial on the Effect of Hypnosis on Dental Anxiety in Tooth Removal Patients," *Patient Education and Counseling* 98, no. 9 (September 2015): 1112–15.

2 P. Sabherwal, N. Kaira, R. Tyagi et al., "Hypnosis and Progressive Muscle Relaxation for Anxiolysis and Pain Control During Extraction Procedure in 8–12-Year-Old Children: A Randomized Controlled Trial," *European Archives of Paediatric Dentistry* 22 (2021): 823–32.

3 Pauline Courtois-Amiot, Anaïs Cloppet-Fontaine, Aurore Poissonnet et al., "Hypnosis for Pain and Anxiety Management in Cognitively *Impair14, no. 3 June 2017 ed* Older Adults Undergoing Scheduled Lumbar Punctures: A Randomized Controlled Pilot Study," *Alzheimer's Research & Therapy* 14 (2022): 120.

4 Hossein Jafarizadeh, Mojgan Lotfi, Fardin Ajoudani et al., "Hypnosis for Reduction of Background Pain and Pain Anxiety in Men with Burns: A Blinded, Randomised, Placebo-Controlled Study," *Burns* 44 (2018): 108–17.

5 Marie-Christine Frenay, Marie-Elisabeth Faymonville, Sabine Devlieger et al., "Psychological Approaches During Dressing Changes of Burned Patients: A Prospective Randomised Study Comparing Hypnosis Against Stress Reducing Strategy," *Burns* 27 (2001): 793–9.

6 Pei-Ying Chen, Ying-Mei Liu, and Mei-Ling Chen, "The Effect of Hypnosis on Anxiety in Patients with Cancer: A Meta-Analysis," *Worldviews on Evidence-Based Nursing* 14, no. 3 (June 2017): 223–36.

7 R. Lynae Roberts, Joshua R. Rhodes, and Gary R. Elkins, "Effect of Hypnosis on Anxiety: Results from a Randomized Controlled Trial with Women in Postmenopause," *Journal of Clinical Psychology in Medical Settings* 28 (2022): 868–81.

8 Hernán Anlió, Bertrand Herer, Agathe Delignières et al., "Hypnosis for the Management of Anxiety and Dyspnea in COPD: A Randomized, Sham-Controlled Crossover Trial," *International Journal of Chronic Obstructive Pulmonary Disease* 15 (2020): 2609–20.

9 Laura Abensur Vuillaume, Charles Gentilhomme, Sandrine Weber et al., "Effectiveness of Hypnosis for the Prevention of Anxiety During Coronary Angiography (HYPCOR Study): A Prospective Randomized Study," *BMC Complementary Medicine and Therapies* 22, no. 1 (November 29, 2022): 315.

10 Maria Paola Brugnoli, Giancarlo Pescue, Emaniela Pasin et al., "The Role of Clinical Hypnosis and Self-Hypnosis to Relief Pain and Anxiety in Severe Chronic Diseases in Palliative Care: A Two-Year Long-Term Follow-up of Treatment in a Nonrandomized Clinical Trial," *Annals of Palliative Medicine* 7, no. 1 (January 2018): 17–31.

11 Floriane Rousseaux, Nadia Dardenne, Paul B. Massion et al., "Virtual Reality and
    Hypnosis for Anxiety and Pain Management in Intensive Care Units," *European
    Journal of Anaesthesiology* 39 (2022): 58–66.

Magnesium

1 Sara Saba, Fakhrudin Faizi, Mojtaba Sepandi, and Batool Nehrir, "Effect of Short-
   term Magnesium Supplementation on Anxiety, Depression and Sleep Quality in
   Patients After Open-Heart Surgery," *Magnesium Research* 35, no. 2 (2022): 62–70.
2 Michel Hanus, Jacqueline Lafon, and Marc Mathieu, "Double-Blind,
   Randomised, Placebo-Controlled Study to Evaluate the Efficacy and Safety of a
   Fixed Combination Containing Two Plant Extracts *Crataegus oxyacantha* and
   Eschscholtzia californica in Mild-to-Moderate Anxiety Disorders," *Current Medical
   Research and Opinion* 20, no. 1 (2004): 63–71.
3 M. C. De Souza, A. F. Walker, P. A. Robinson, and K. Bolland, "A Synergictic Effect
   of a Daily Supplement for 1 Month of 200 mg Magnesium Plus 50 mg Vitamin B6
   for the Relief of Anxiety-Related Premenstrual Symptoms: A Randomized, Double-
   Blind, Crossover Study," *Journal of Women's Health & Gender-Based Medicine* 9
   (November 2, 2000): 131–9.
4 Javad Anjom-Shoae, Omid Sadeghi, Ammar Hassanzadeh Keshteli et al., "The
   Association Between Dietary Intake of Magnesium and Psychiatric Disorders
   Among Iranian Adults: A Cross-Sectional Study," *British Journal of Nutrition* 120,
   no. 6 (September 2018): 693–702.
5 Nagihan Kircali Haznedar and Pelin Bilgiç, "Evaluation of Dietary Magnesium
   Intake and Its Association with Depression, Anxiety and Eating Behaviors,"
   International Journal of Human Sciences 16, no. 1 (2019): 345–54.
6 Felice N. Jacka, Simon Overland, Robert Stewart et al., "Association Between
   Magnesium Intake and Depression and Anxiety in Community-Dwelling Adults:
   the Hordaland Health Study," *Australian and New Zealand Journal of Psychiatry* 43
   (2009): 45–52.
7 Vildan Manav, Cemre Büsra Türk, Asude Kara Polat et al., "Evaluation of the
   Serum Magnesium and Vitamin D Levels and the Risk of Anxiety in Primary
   Hyperhidrosis," *Journal of Cosmetic Dermatology* 21 (202): 373–9.
8 F. E. Fard, M. Mirghafourvand, S. Mahammad-Alizadeh et al., "Effects of
   Zinc and Magnesium Supplements on Postpartum Depression and Anxiety:
   A Randomized Controlled Clinical Trial," *Women & Health* 57, no. 9 (2017):
   1115–28.

9 Engin Yilirim and Hakan Apaydin, "Zinc and Magnesium Levels of Pregnant Women with Restless Leg Syndrome and Their Relationship with Anxiety: A Case-Control Study," *Biological Trace Element Research* 199 (20): 1674–85.

10 Hasanuzzaman Shohag, Ashik Ulllah, Shalahuddin Qusar et al., "Alteration of Serum Zinc, Copper, Manganese, Iron, Calcium, and Magnesium Concentrations and the Complexity of Interelement Relations in Patients with Obsessive-Compulsive Disorder," *Biological Trace Elements Research* 148 (2012): 275–80.

Melatonin

1 Tushar Patel and Madhuri S. Kurdi, "A Comparative Study Between Oral Melatonin and Oral Midazolam on Preoperative Anxiety, Cognitive, and Psychomotor Functions," *Journal of Anaesthesiology Clinical Pharmacology* 31, no. 1 (January–March 2015): 37–43.

2 A. Samarkandi, M. Niaguib, W. Riad et al., "Melatonin vs. Midazolam Premedication in Children: A Double-Blind, Placebo-Controlled Study," *European Journal of Anaesthesiology* 22, no. 3 (March 2005): 189–96.

3 Aysun Caglar Torun and Ezgi Yüceer, "Should Melatonin Be Used as an Alternative Sedative and Anxiolytic Agent in Mandibular Third Molar Surgery," *Journal of Oral and Maxillofacial Surgery* 77 (2019): 1790–5.

4 Sunanda Gooty, Davi Sai R. Priyanka, Ravikanth Pula et al., "A Comparative Study of Effect of Oral Melatonin versus Oral Midazolam as Premedicant in Children Undergoing Surgery Under General Anesthesia," *Journal of Cellular & Molecular Anesthesia* 7, no. 3 (2022): 160–7.

5 Arvind Khare, Beena Thada, Neena Jain et al., "Comparison of Effects of Oral Melatonin with Oral Alprazolam Use as a Premedicant in Adult Patients Undergoing Various Surgical Procedures Under General Anesthesia: A Prospective Randomized Placebo-Controlled Study," *Anesthesia Essays and Researches* 12, no. 3 (July–September 2018): 657–62.

6 Maurizia Capuzzo, Barbara Zanardi, Elisa Schiffino et al., "Melatonin Does Not Reduce Anxiety More than Placebo in the Elderly Undergoing Surgery," *Anesthesia & Analgesia* 103, no. 1 (July 2006): 121–3.

7 Rahman Abbasivash, Sohrab Salimi, Behzad Ahsan et al., "The Effect of Melatonin on Anxiety and Pain of Tourniquet in Intravenous Regional Anesthesia," *Advanced Biomedical Research* 8 (November 27, 2019): 67.

8 Edwin Seet, Chen Mei Liaw, Sylvia Tay, and Chang Su, "Melatonin Premedication versus Placebo in Wisdom Teeth Extraction: A Randomised Controlled Trial," *Singapore Medical Journal* 56, no. 12 (2015): 666–71.

9 Salah A. Ismail and Hany A. Mowafi, "Melatonin Provides Anxiolysis, Enhances Analgesia, Decreases Intraocular Pressure, and Promotes Better Operation Conditions During Cataract Surgery Under Topical Anesthesia," *Anesthesia & Analgesia* 108, no. 4 (April 2009): 1146–51.

10 Marzieh Khezri and Hamid Merate, "The Effects of Melatonin on Anxiety and Pain Scores of Patients, Intraocular Pressure, and Operating Conditions During Cataract Surgery Under Topical Anesthesia," *Indian Journal of Ophthalmology* 61, no. 7 (2013): 319–24.

11 Lauren A. E. Erland and Praveen K. Saxena, "Melatonin Natural Health Products and Supplements: Presence of Serotonin and Significant Variability of Melatonin Content," *Journal of Clinical Sleep Medicine* 13, no. 2 (2017): 275–81.

12 Peter A. Cohen, Bharathi Avula, Yan-Hong Wang et al., "Quantity of Melatonin and CBD in Melatonin Gummies in the US," *JAMA: Journal of the American Medical Association* 329, no. 16 (2023): 1401–2.

13 Hope M. Foley and Amie E. Steel, "Adverse Events Associated with Oral Administration of Melatonin: A Critical Systematic Review of Clinical Evidence," *Contemporary Therapies in Medicine* 42 (2019): 65–81.

Mindfulness Meditation

1 https://www.cdc.gov/nchs/pressroom/nchs_press_releases/2018/201811_Yoga_Meditation.htm.

2 Holger Cramer, Helen Hall, Matthew Leach et al., "Prevalence, Patterns, and Predictors of Meditation Use Among US Adults: A Nationally Representative Survey," *Scientific Reports* 6 (2016): 36760.

3 Matthew S. Burgstahler and Mary C. Stenson, "Effects of Guided Mindfulness Meditation on Anxiety and Stress in a Pre-Healthcare College Student Population: A Pilot Study," *Journal of American College Health* 68, no. 6 (August–September, 2020): 666–72.

4 Maria Komariah, Kusman Ibrahim, Tuti Pahria et al., "Effect of Mindfulness Breathing Meditation on Depression, Anxiety, and Stress: A Randomized Controlled Trial Among University Students," *Healthcare* 11 (2023): 26.

5 Alba Torné-Ruiz, Mercedes Reguant, and Judith Roca, "Mindfulness for Stress and Anxiety Management in Nursing Students in a Clinical Simulation: A Quasi-Experimental Study," *Nurse Education in Practice* 66 (2023): 103533.

6 Severin Ladenbauer and Josef Singer, "Can Mindfulness-Based Stress Reduction Influence the Quality of Life, Anxiety, and Depression of Women Diagnosed with Breast Cancer?—A Review," *Current Oncology* 29 (2022): 7779–3.

7 Sapna Oberoi, Jiayu Yang, Roberta L. Woodgate et al., "Association of Mindfulness-Based Interventions with Anxiety Severity. In Adults with Cancer," *JAMA Network Open* (August 2020): e2012598.

8 Xiaoyu Liu, Pengcheng Yi, Lijun Ma et al., "Mindfulness-Based Interventions for Social Anxiety Disorder: A Systematic Review and Meta-Analysis," *Psychiatry Research* 300 (2021): 113935.

9 Elizabeth A. Hoge, Eric Bui, Mihriye Mete et al., "Mindfulness-Based Stress Reduction vs Escitalopram for the Treatment of Adults with Anxiety Disorders: A Randomized Clinical Trial," *JAMA Psychiatry* 80, no. 1 (January 2023): 13–21.

10 Katarzyna Odgers, Nicole Dargue, Cathy Creswell et al., "The Limited Effect of Mindfulness-Based Interventions on Anxiety in Children and Adolescents: A Meta-Analysis," *Clinical Child and Family Psychology Review* 23 (2020): 407–26.

11 Zoë Thomas, Marta Novak, Susanna Gabriela et al., "Brief Mindfulness Meditation for Depression and Anxiety Symptoms in Patients Undergoing Hemodialysis," *Clinical Journal of the American Society of Nephrology* 12, no. 12 (December 7, 2017): 2008–15.

Mirtazapine

1 M. Sarchiapone, M. Amore, S. De Risio et al., "Mirtazapine in the Treatment of Panic Disorder: An Open-Label Trial," *International Clinical Psychopharmacology* 18, no. 1 (2003): 35–8.

2 L. Ribeiro, J. V. Busnello, M. Kauer-Sant'Anna et al., "Mirtazapine versus Fluoxetine in the Treatment of Panic Disorder," *Brazilian Journal of Medical and Biological Research* 34, no. 10 (October 2019): 1303–7.

3 Sara I. J. Schutters, Harold J. G. M. Van Megan, Jantien Frederieke Van Veen et al., "Mirtazapine in Generalized Social Anxiety Disorder: A Randomized, Double-Blind, Placebo Controlled Study," *International Clinical Psychopharmacology* 25 (2010): 302–4.

4 Christine Mrakotsky, Bruce Masek, Joseph Biederman et al., "Prospective Open-Label Pilot Trial of Mirtazapine in Children and Adolescents with Social Phobia," *Journal of Anxiety Disorders* 22 (2008): 88–97.

5 Franklin R. Schneier, Raphael Campeas, Jaime Carcamo et al., "Combined Mirtazapine and SSRI Treatment of PTSD: A Placebo-Controlled Trial," *Depression and Anxiety* 32 (2005): 570–9.

6 Won Kim, Chi-Un Pae, Jeong-Ho Chae et al., "The Effectiveness of Mirtazapine in the Treatment of Post-Traumatic Stress Disorder: A 24-Week Continuation Therapy," *Psychiatry and Clinical Neurosciences* 59, no. 6 (December 2005): 743–7.

7 Wei-Han Chou, Feng-Sheng Lin, Chih-Peng Lin et al., "Mirtazapine, in Orodispersible Form, for Patients with Preoperative Psychological Distress: A Pilot Study," *Acta Anaesthesiologica Taiwanica* 54 (2016): 16–23.

8 Christopher J. McDougle, Robyn P. Thom, Caitlin T. Ravichandran et al., "A Randomized Double-Blind, Placebo-Controlled Pilot Trial of Mirtazapine for Anxiety in Children and Adolescents with Autism Spectrum Disorder," *Neuropsychopharmacology* 47 (2022): 1263–70.

9 Arash Mowla and Haniyeh Baniasadipour, "Is Mirtazapine Augmentation Effective for Patients with Obsessive-Compulsive Disorder Who Failed to Respond to Sertraline Monotherapy? A Placebo-Controlled, Double-Blind, Clinical Trial," *International Clinical Psychopharmacology* 38 (2023): 4–8.

10 Anne Ostenfeld, Tonny Studsgaard Petersen, Lars Henning Pedersen et al., "Mirtazapine Exposure in Pregnancy and Fetal Safety: A Nationwide Cohort Study," *Acta Psychiatrica Scandinavica* 145, no. 6 (2022): 557–67.

Music Therapy

1 Jaclyn Bradley Palmer, Deforia Lane, Diane Mayo et al., "Effects of Music Therapy on Anesthesia Requirements and Anxiety in Women Undergoing Ambulatory Breast Surgery for Cancer Diagnosis and Treatment: A Randomized. Controlled Trial," *Journal of Clinical Oncology* 33, no. 28 (October 1, 2015): 3162–8.

2 Avinash Gogoularadja and Satvinder Singh Bakshi, "A Randomized Study on the Efficacy of Music Therapy on Pain and Anxiety in Nasal Septal Surgery," *International Archives of Otorhinolaryngology* 24, no. 2 (2020): e232–e236.

3 Keiichiro Wakana, Yukifumi Kimura, Yukie Nitta, and Toshiaki Fujisawa, "The Effect of Music on Preoperative Anxiety in an Operating Room: A Single-Blind Randomized Controlled Trial," *Anesthesia Progress* 69, no. 1 (2022): 24–30.

4 Ali Sait Kavakli, Nilgun Kavrut Oztruk, Hilal Yavuzel Adas et al., "The Effects of Music on Anxiety and Pain in Patients During Carotid Endarterectomy Under Regional Anesthesia: A Randomized Controlled Trial," *Complementary Therapies in Medicine* 44 (June 2019): 94–101.

5 Andrea Chirico, Patrizia Maiorano, Paola Indovina et al., "Virtual Reality and Music Therapy as Distraction Interventions to Alleviate Anxiety and Improve Mood States in Breast Cancer Patients During Chemotherapy," *Journal of Cellular Physiology* 235, no. 6 (June 2020): 5353–62.

6 Guangli Lu, Ruiying Jia, Dandan Liang et al., "Effects of Music Therapy on Anxiety: A Meta-Analysis of Randomized Controlled Trials," *Psychiatry Research* 304 (October 2021): 114137.

7 Michele Umbrello, Tiziana Sorrenti, Giovanni Mistraletti et al., "Music Therapy Reduces Stress and Anxiety in Critically Ill Patients: A Systematic Review of Randomized Clinical Trials," *Minerva Anestesiologica* 85, no. 8 (August 2019): 886–98.

8 Philip Hepp, Carsten Hagenbeck, Julius Gilles et al., "Effects of Music Intervention During Caesarean Delivery on Anxiety and Stress of the Mother a Controlled, Randomized Study," *BMC Pregnancy and Childbirth* 18 (2018): 435.

9 Dilruba Çelebi, Emel Yilmaz, Semra Tutcu Sahin, and Hakan Baydur, "The Effect of Music Therapy During Colonoscopy on Pain, Anxiety and Patient Comfort: A Randomized Controlled Trial," *Complementary Therapies in Clinical Practice* 38 (2020): 101084.

10 Mayara K. A. Ribeiro, Tereza R. M. Alcântara-Silva, Jordana C. M. Oliveira et al., "Music Therapy Intervention in Cardiac Autonomic Modulation, Anxiety, and Depression in Mothers of Preterms: Randomized Controlled Trial," *BMC Psychology* 6 (2018): 57.

11 Selina M. Kehl, Pearl La Marca-Ghaemmaghami, Marina Haller et al., "Creative Music Therapy with Premature Infants and Their Parents: A Mixed-Method Pilot Study on Parents' Anxiety, Stress and Depressive Symptoms and Parent-Infant Attachment," *International Journal of Environmental Research and Public Health* 18, no. 1 (2021): 265.

12 Orti de la Rubia, José Enrique, Maria Pilar Garcia-Pardo, Carmen Cabañés Iranzo et al., "Does Music Therapy Improve Anxiety and Depression in Alzheimer's Patients?" *The Journal of Alternative and Complementary Medicine* 42, no. 1 (2018): 33–6.

Probiotics

1 International Probiotics Association. https://internationalprobiotics.org.

2 International Probiotics Association. https://internationalprobiotics.org.

3 American Gastroenterology Association. https://gastro.org.

4 Lee-Ching Lew, Yan-Yan Hor, Nur Asmaa et al., "Probiotic *Lactobacillus plantarum* P8 Alleviated Stress and Anxiety While Enhancing Memory and Cognition in Stressed Adults: A Randomised, Double-Blind, Placebo-Controlled Study," *Clinical Nutrition* 38 (2019): 2053–64.

5 Beibei Yang, Jinbao Wei, Peijun Ju, and Jinghong Chen, "Effects of Regulating Intestinal Microbiota on Anxiety Symptoms: A Systematic Review," *General Psychiatry* 32 (2019): e100056.

6 R. F. Slykerman, F. Hood, K. Wickens et al., "Effects of *Lactobacillus rhamnosus* HN001 in Pregnancy on Postpartum Symptoms of Depression and Anxiety: A Randomised Double-Blind Placebo-Controlled Trial," *EBioMedicine* 24 (2017): 159–65.

7 Nhan Tran, Masha Zhebrak, Christine Yacoub et al., "The Gut-Brain Relatioship: Investigating the Effect of Multispecies Probiotics on Anxiety in a Randomized Placebo-Controlled Trial of Healthy Young Adults," *Journal of Affective Disorders* 252 (2019): 271–7.

8 Ebrahim Kouchaki, Omid Reza Tamtaji et al., "Clinical and Metabolic Response to Probiotic Supplementation in Patients with Multiple Sclerosis: A Randomized, Double-Blind, Placebo-Controlled Trial," *Clinical Nutrition* 36 (2017): 1245–9.

9 A. A. Mohammadi, S. Jazaueri, K. Khosravi-Darani et al., "The Effects of Probiotics on Mental Health and Hypothalamic-Pituitary-Adrenal Axis: A Randomized, Double-Blind, Placebo-Controlled Trial in Petrochemical Workers," *Nutritional Neuroscience* 19, no. 9 (November 2016): 387–95.

10 A. Venket Rao, Alison C. Bested, Tracey M. Beaulne et al., "A Randomized, Double-Blind, Placebo-Controlled Pilot Study of a Probiotic in Emotional Symptoms off Chronic Fatigue Syndrome," *Gut Pathogens* 1, no. 1 (2009): 6.

11 Richard Liu, Rachel F. L. Walsh, and Ana E. Sheehan, "Prebiotics and Probiotics for Depression and Anxiety: A Systematic Review and Meta-Analysis of Controlled Clinical Trials," *Neuroscience & Biobehavioral Reviews* 102 (July 2019): 13–23.

12 Charlotte Le Morvan de Sequeira, Marie Kaeber, Sila Elif Cekin et al., "The Effects of Probiotics on Quality of Life, Depression and Anxiety in Patients with Irritable Bowel Syndrome: A Systematic Review and Meta-Analysis," *Journal of Clinical Medicine* 10, no. 16 (August 8, 2021): 3497.

Psilocybin

1 Matthew W. Johnson and Roland R. Griffiths, "Potential Therapeutic Effects of Psilocybin," *Neurotherapeutics* 14 (2017): 734–40.

2 Charles S. Grob, Alicia L. Danforth, Gurpreet S. Chopra et al., "Pilot Study of Psilocybin Treatment for Anxiety in Patients with Advanced-Stage Cancer," *Archives of General Psychiatry* 68, no. 1 (January 2011): 71–8.

3 Stephen Ross, Anthony Bossis, Jeffrey Guss et al., "Rapid and Sustained Symptoms Reduction Following Psilocybin Treatment for Anxiety and Depression in Patients with Life-Threatening Cancer: A Randomized Controlled Trial," *Journal of Psychopharmacology* 30, no. 12 (2016): 1165–80.

4 G. I. Agin-Liebes, T. Malone, M. M. Yalch et al., "Long-Term Follow-up of Psilocybin-Assisted Psychotherapy for Psychiatric and Existential Distress in Patients with Life-Threatening Cancer," *Journal of Psychopharmacology* 34, no. 2 (February 2020): 155–66.

5 Roland R. Griffiths, Matthew W. Johnson, Michael A. Carducci et al., "Psilocybin Produces Substantial and Sustained Decreases in Depression and Anxiety in

Patients with Life-Threatening Cancer: A Randomized Double-Blind Trial," *Journal of Psychopharmacology* 30, no. 12 (2016): 1181–97.

6 Francisco A. Moreno, Christopher B. Wiegand, E. Keolani Taitano, and Pedro L. Delgado, "Safety, Tolerability, and Efficacy of Psilocybin in Nine Patients with Obsessive-Compulsive Disorder," *Journal of Clinical Psychiatry* 67 (2006): 1735–40.

7 Agustin Lugo-Radillo and Jorge Luis Cortes-Lopez, "Long-Term Amelioration of OCD Symptoms in a Patient with Chronic Consumption of Psilocybin-Containing Mushrooms," *Journal of Psychoactive Drugs* 53, no. 2 (2021): 146–8.

8 Joseph M. Rootman, Pamela Kryskow, Kalin Harvey et al., "Adults Who Microdose Psychedelics Report Health Related Motivations and Lower Levels of Anxiety and Depression Compared to Non-Microdosers," *Scientific Reports* 11 (2021): 22479.

9 E. I. Kopra, J.A. Ferris, A. R. Winstock et al., "Adverse Experiences Resulting in Emergency Medical Treatment Seeking Following the Use of Magic Mushrooms," *Journal of Psychopharmacology* 36, no. 8 (2022): 965–73.

10 Emma Honyiglo, Angélique Franchi, Nathalie Cartiser et al., "Unpredictable Behavior Under the Influence of 'Magic Mushrooms': A Case Report and Review of the Literature," *Journal of Forensic Sciences* 64, no. 4 (2018): 1266–70.

Reflexology

1 Take Charge of Your Well-Being. University of Minnesota. https://www.takingcharge.csh.umn.edu/reflexology.

2 Lisa Blackburn, Catherine Hill, Amy L. Lindsey et al., "Effect of Foot Reflexology and Aromatherapy on Anxiety and Pain During Brachytherapy for Cervical Cancer," *Oncology Nursing Forum* 48, no. 3 (May 2021): 265–76.

3 Zohre Rahmani Vasokolaei, Nahid Rajeh, Majideh Heravi-Karimooi et al., "Comparison of the Effects of Hand Reflexology versus Acupressure on Anxiety and Vital Signs in Female Patients with Coronary Artery Diseases," *Healthcare* 7, no. 1 (March 2019): 26.

4 S. Moghimi-Hanjani, Z. Mehdizadeh-Tourzani, and M. Shoghi, "The Effect of Foot Reflexology on Anxiety, Pain, and Outcomes of the Labor in Primigravida Women," *Acta Medica Iranica* 53, no. 8 (2015): 507–11.

5 I. Levy, S. Attias, T. S Lavee et al., "The Effectiveness of Foot Reflexology in Reducing Anxiety and Duration of Labor in Primiparas: An Open-Label Randomized Controlled Trial," *Complementary Therapies in Clinical Practice* 38 (February 2020): 101085.

6 Wei-Li Wang, Hao-Yuan Hung, Ying-Ren Chen et al., "Effect of Foot Reflexology Intervention on Depression, Anxiety, and Sleep Quality in Adults: A Meta-

Analysis and Metaregression of Randomized Controlled Trials," *Evidence-Based Complementary and Alternative Medicine* (2020): Article ID 2654353.

7 Reza Alinia-najjar, Masoumeh Bagheri-Nesami, Seyed Afshin Shorofi et al., "The Effect of Foot Reflexology Massage on Burn-Specific Pain Anxiety and Sleep Quality and Quantity of Patients Hospitalized in the Burn Intensive Care Unit (ICU)," *Burns* 46 (2020): 1942–51.

8 Tahereh Bahrami, Nahid Rejeh, Majideh Heravi-Karimooi et al., "The Effect of Foot Reflexology on Hospital Anxiety and Depression in Female Older Adults: A Randomized Controlled Trial," *International Journal of Therapeutic Massage and Bodywork* 12, no. 3 (September 2019): 16–21.

9 Rusen Öztürk, Ümran Sevil, Asuman Sargin, and M. Sait Yücebilgin, "The Effects of Reflexology on Anxiety and Pain in Patients After Abdominal Hysterectomy: A Randomized Controlled Trial," *Complementary Therapies in Medicine* 36 (2018): 107–12.

10 E. Ernst, P. Posadzki, and M. S. Lee, "Reflexology: An Update of a Systematic Review of Randomised Clinical Trials," *Maturitas* 68, no. 2 (February 2011): 116–20.

Selective Serotonin Reuptake Inhibitors (SSRIs)

1 Greta A. Bushnell, Moira A. Rynn, Stephen Crystal et al., "Simultaneous Benzodiazepine and SSRI Initiation in Young People with Anxiety Disorders," *Journal of Clinical Psychiatry* 82, no. 6 (November–December 2021): 20m13863.

2 Laiana Quagliato, Rafael C. Freire, and Antonio E. Nardi, "Risks and Benefits of Medications for Panic Disorder: A Comparison of SSRIs and Benzodiazepines," *Expert Opinion on Drug Safety* 17, no. 3 (March 2018): 315–24.

3 M. G. Koren Gilboa, R. Katz et al., "Anxiolytic Treatment But Not Anxiety Itself Causes Hyponatremia Among Anxious Patients," *Medicine* 98, no. 5 (February 2019): e14334.

4 Boris Birmaher, David A. Axelson, Kelly Monk et al., "Fluoxetine for the Treatment of Childhood Anxiety Disorders," *Journal of the American Academy of Child & Adolescent Psychiatry* 42, no. 4 (April 2003): 415–23.

5 Chuan Zou, Xiang Ding, Joseph H. Flaherty, and Birong Dong, "Clinical Efficacy and Safety of Fluoxetine in Generalized Anxiety Disorder in Chinese Patients," *Neuropsychiatric Disease and Treatment* 9 (2013): 1661–70.

6 Dinah S. Reddhough, Catherine Marraffa, Anissa Mouti et al., "Effect of Fluoxetine on Obsessive-Compulsive Behaviors in Children and Adolescents with Autism Spectrum Disorders," *JAMA* 322, no. 16 (October 22, 2019): 1561–9.

7   Beilin Zhang, Chao Wang, Lexiang Cui et al., "Short-Term Efficacy and Tolerability of Paroxetine Versus Placebo for Panic Disorder: A Meta-Analysis of Randomized Controlled Trials," *Frontiers in Pharmacology* 11 (March 2020): Article 275.

8   Michael A. Sugarman, Amy M. Loree, Boris B. Baltes et al., "The Effect of Paroxetine and Placebo on Treating Anxiety and Depression: A Meta-Analysis of Change on the Hamilton Rating Scales," *PLoS ONE* 9, no. 8 (August 27, 2014): e106337.

9   Xinyuan Li, Yanbo Hou, Yingying et al., "Efficacy and Tolerability of Paroxetine in Adults with Social Anxiety Disorder," *Medicine* 99, no. 14 (2020): e19573.

10 John T. Walkup, Anne Marie Albano, John Piacentini et al., "Cognitive Behavioral Therapy, Sertraline, or a Combination in Childhood Anxiety," *New England Journal of Medicine* 359, no. 26 (December 25, 2008): 2753–66.

11 Belinda Graham, Natalie M. Garcia, Hannah E. Bergman et al., "Prolonged Exposure and Sertraline Treatments for Posttraumatic Stress Disorder Also Improve Multiple Indicators of Social Functioning," *Journal of Traumatic Stress* 33, no. 4 (August 2020): 488–99.

12 Y. Panahi, B. Rezazadeh Moghaddam, A. Sahebkar et al., "A Randomized, Double-Blind, Placebo-Controlled Trial on the efficacy and Tolerability of Sertraline in Iranian Veterans with Post-Traumatic Stress Disorder," *Psychological Medicine* 41 (2011): 2159–66.

13 Sayed Hamzeh Hosseini, Fatemeh Espahbodi, and Sayed Mohammad Mehdi Mirzadeh Goudarzi, "Citalopram Verses Psychological Training for Depression and Anxiety Symptoms in Hemodialysis Patients," *Iranian Journal of Kidney Diseases* 6 (2012): 446–51.

14 Faruk Uguz, "Citalopram in Treatment of Pregnant Women with Panic Disorder: A Retrospective Study," *Journal of Clinical Psychopharmacology* 40, no. 6 (November/December 2020): 615–17.

15 Tal Carthy, Noa Benaroya-Milshtein, Avi Valevski, and Alan Apter, "Emotional Reactivity and Regulation Following Citalopram Therapy in Children and Adolescents with Anxiety Disorders," *Journal of Child and Adolescent Psychopharmacology* 27, no. 1 (2017): 43–51.

16 Sayed Alamy, Wei Zhang, Indu Varia et al., "'Escitalopram in Specific Phobia' Results in Placebo-Controlled Pilot Trial," *Journal of Psychopharmacology* 22, no. 2 (2008): 157–61.

17 Kensuke Miyazaki, "Perospirone Augmentation of Escitalopram in the Treatment of an Adolescent Sophophobia (Fear of Learning) Patient," *Neuropharmacology Reports*, First Published May 4, 2022.

18 Satoshi Asakura, Taiji Hayano, Atsushi Hagino, and Tsukasa Koyama, "A Randomized, Double-Blind, Placebo-Controlled Study of Escitalopram in Patients with Society Anxiety Disorder in Japan," *Current Medical Research and Opinion* 32, no. 4 (2016): 749–57.

19 Ryan Fung, Dean Elbe, and Evelyn Stewart, "Retrospective Review of Fluvoxamine-Clomipramine Combination Therapy in Obsessive-Compulsive Disorder in Children and Adolescents," *Journal of the Canadian Academy of Child and Adolescent Psychiatry* 30, no. 3 (August 2021): 150–5.

20 Satoshi Asakura, Osamu Tajima, and Tsukasa Koyama, "Fluvoxamine Treatment of Generalized Social Anxiety Disorder in Japan: A Randomized Double-Blind, Placebo-Controlled Study," *International Journal of Neuropsychopharmacology* 10, no. 2 (2007): 263–74.

21 Xue Liu, Xinyuan Li, Congxiao Zhang et al., "Efficacy and Tolerability of Fluvoxamine in Adults with Social Anxiety Disorder: A Meta-Analysis," *Medicine* 97, no. 28 (2018): e11547.

22 Suresh Durgam, Carol Gommoll, Giovanna Forero et al., "Efficacy and Safety of Vilazodone in Patients with Generalized Anxiety Disorder: A Randomized, Double-Blind, Placebo-Controlled, Flexible-Dose Trial," *Journal of Clinical Psychiatry* 77, no. 12 (2016): 1687–94.

23 Sriram Ramaswamy, David Driscoll, Christopher Reist et al., "A Double-Blind, Placebo-Controlled Randomized Trial of Vilazodone in the Treatment of Posttraumatic Stress Disorder and Comorbid Depression," *Primary Care Companion for CNS Disorders* 19, no. 4 (2017): 17m02138.

24 Franklin R. Schneier, Danielle M. Moskow, Tse-Hwei Choo et al., "A Randomized Controlled Pilot Trial of Vilazodone for Adult Separation Anxiety Disorder," *Depression and Anxiety* 34, no. 12 (December 2017): 1085–95.

25 Chi-Un Pae, Sheng-Min Wang, Changsu Han et al., "Vortioxetine, a Multimodel Antidepressant for Generalized Anxiety Disorder: A Systematic Review and Meta-Analysis," *Journal of Psychiatric Research* 64 (2015): 88–98.

26 M. C. Christensen, H. Loft, I. Florea, and R. S. McIntyre, "Efficacy of Vortioxetine in Working Patients with Generalized Anxiety Disorder," *CNS Spectrums* 24(2019): 249–57.

27 Takeshi Inoue, Shinji Fujimoto, Tatsuro Marumoto et al., "Therapeutic Potential of Vortioxetine for Anxious Depression: A Post Hoc Analysis of Data from a Clinical Trial Conducted in Japan," *Neuropsychiatric Disease and Treatment* 17 (2021): 3781–90.

Serotonin and Norepinephrine Reuptakedate Inhibitors (SNRIs)

1 Moira Rynn, James Russell, Janelle Erickson et al., "Efficacy and Safety of Duloxetine in the Treatment of Generalized Anxiety Disorder: A Flexible-Dose, Progressive-Titration, Placebo-Controlled Trial," *Depression and Anxiety* 25 (2008): 182–9.

2   Karla J. Alaka, William Noble, Angel Montejo et al., "Efficacy and Safety of Duloxetine in the Treatment of Older Adult Patients with Generalized Anxiety Disorder: A Randomized, Double-Blind, Placebo-Controlled Trial," *International Journal of Geriatric Society* 29 (201): 978–86.

3   Arash Mowla, Sanaz Boostani, and Seyed Ali Dastgheib, "Duloxetine Augmentation in Resistant Obsessive-Compulsive Disorder: A Double-Blind Controlled Clinical Trial," *Journal of Clinical Psychopharmacology* 36, no. 6 (December 2016): 720–3.

4   Damiaan Denys, Nic van der Wee, Harold J. G. M. van Megen, and Herman G. M. Westenberg, "A Double-Blind Comparison of Venlafaxine and Paroxetine in Obsessive-Compulsive Disorder," *Journal of Clinical Psychopharmacology* 23, no. 6 (December 2003): 568–75.

5   S. Kasserman Walderhaug, D. Aikins et al., "Effects of Duloxetine in Treatment-Refractory Men with Posttraumatic Stress Disorder," *Pharmacopsychiatry* 43, no. 2 (March 2010): 45–9.

6   A. J. Gelenberg, R. B. Lydiard, R. L. Rudolph et al., "Efficacy of Venlafaxine Extended-Release Capsules in Nondepressed Outpatients with Generalized Anxiety Disorder: A 6-Month Randomized Controlled Trial," *JAMA* 283, no. 23 (June 21, 2000): 3082–8.

7   Jingjing Zhang, Hongbing Xu, and Zhiqing Chen, "Pharmacoeconomic Evaluation of Venlafaxine Compared with Citalopram in Generalized Anxiety Disorder," *Experimental and Therapeutic Medicine* 5 (2013): 840–4.

8   Jacques Bradwejn, Antti Ahokas, Dan J. Stein et al., "Venlafaxine Extended-Release Capsules in Panic Disorder," *British Journal of Psychiatry* 187 (2005): 353–9.

9   Jonathan Davidson, David Baldwin, Dan J. Stein et al., "Treatment of Posttraumatic Stress Disorder with Venlafaxine Extended Release: A 6-Month Randomized Controlled Trial," *Archives of General Psychiatry* 63, no. 10 (2006): 1158–65.

10 H. NIcolini, D. Bakish, H. Duenas et al., "Improvement of Psychic and Somatic Symptoms in Adult Patients with Generalized Anxiety Disorder: Examination from a Duloxetine, Venlafaxine Extended-Release and Placebo-Controlled Trial," *Psychological Medicine* 39 (2008): 267–76.

11 Giovanni A. Fava, Giada Benasi, Marcella Lucente et al., "Withdrawal Symptoms After Serotonin-Noradrenaline Reuptake Inhibitor Discontinuation: Systematic Review," *Psychotherapy and Psychosomatics* 87 (2018): 195–203.

Tai Chi

1   https://www.statista.com/statistics/191622/participants-in-tai-chi-in-the-us-since-2008/.

2 Jen-Chen Tsai, Wei-Hsin Wang, Paul Chan et al., "The Beneficial Effects of *Tai Chi Chuan* on Blood Pressure and Lipid Profile and Anxiety Status in a Randomized Controlled Trial," *Journal of Alternative and Complementary Medicine* 9, no. 5 (2003): 747–54.

3 Manoj Sharma and Taj Haider, "Tai Chi as an Alternative and Complementary Therapy for Anxiety: A Systematic Review," *Journal of Evidence-Based Complementary & Alternative Medicine* 20, no. 2 (April 2015): 143–53.

4 Xuan Liu, Ru Li, Jiabao Cui et al., "The Effects of Tai Chi and Qigong Exercise on Psychological Status in Adolescents: A Systematic Review and Meta-Analysis," *Frontiers in Psychology* 12 (November 2021): Article 746975.

5 Julia Novelli, Karin Cinalioglu, Angela Potes et al., "Tai Chi/Qigong in Adults with Depression and Anxiety: A Pilot Retrospective Study," *Integrative Medicine Reports* 1, no. 1 (August 2022): 131–9.

6 Tiffany Field, Miguel Diego, and Maria Hernandez-Reif, "Tai Chi/Yoga Effects on Anxiety, Heartrate, EEG, and Math Computations," *Complementary Therapies in Clinical Practice* 16 (2010): 235–8.

7 Qian Cai, Shu-bin Cai, Jian-kun Chen et al., "Tai Chi for Anxiety and Depression Symptoms in Cancer, Stroke, Heart Failure, and Chronic Obstructive Pulmonary Disease: A Systematic Review and Meta-Analysis," *Complementary Therapies in Clinical Practice* 46 (2022): 101510.

8 D. E. Barrow, A. Bedford, G. Ives et al., "An Evaluation of the Effects of Tai Chi Chuan and Chi Kung Training in Patients with Symptomatic Heart Failure: A Randomised Controlled Pilot Study," *Postgraduate Medical Journal* 83 (2007): 717–21.

9 Putai Jin, "Efficacy of Tai Chi, Brisk Walking, Meditation, and Reading in Reducing Mental and Emotional Stress," *Journal of Psychosomatic Research* 36, no. 4 (1992): 361–70.

10 S. Y. Cetin, B. B. Calik, and A. Ayan, "Investigation of the Effectiveness of Tai Chi Exercise Program in Patients with Scleroderma: A Randomized Controlled Study," *Complementary Therapies in Clinical Practice* 40 (2020): 101181.

Vitamin D

1 M. Bičíková, M. Dušková, J. Vítku et al., "Vitamin D in Anxiety and Affective Disorders," *Physiological Research* 64, Supplement 2 (2015): S101–S103.

2 Cuizhen Zhu, Yu Zhang, Ting Wang et al., "Vitamin D Supplementation Improves Anxiety But Not Depression Symptoms in Patients with Vitamin D Deficiency," *Brain and Behavior* 10 (2020): e01760.

3 Alaa Eid, Sawsan Khoja, Shareefa AlGhamdi et al., "Vitamin D Supplementation Ameliorates Severity of Generalized Anxiety Disorder (GAD)," *Metabolic Brain Disease* 34 (2019): 1781–6.

4 F. Al Anouti, W. B. Grant, J. Thomas et al., "Associations Between Dietary Intake of Vitamin D, Sun Exposure, and Generalized Anxiety Among College Women," *Nutrients* 14 (2022): 5327.

5 Chen Liu, Weiqing Jiang, Mingzhu Deng et al., "Lower Vitamin D Levels in Panic Attacks in Shanghai: A Case-Control Study," *Asian Journal of Psychiatry* 51 (2020): 101948.

6 Donatella Marazziti, Filippo M. Barberi, Leonardo Fontenelle et al., "Decreased Vitamin D Levels in Obsessive-Compulsive Disorder Patients," *CNS Spectrums* 28, no. 5 (2023): 606–13.

7 Erman Esnafoglu and Elif Yaman, "Vitamin B12, Folic Acid, Homocysteine and Vitamin D Levels in Children and Adolescents with Obsessive Compulsive Disorder," *Psychiatry Research* 254 (2017): 232–7.

8 Dan Pu, Jing Luo, Yanhua Wang et al., "Prevalence of Depression and Anxiety in Rheumatoid Arthritis Patients and Their Associations with Serum Vitamin D Level," *Clinical Rheumatology* 37 (2018): 179–84.

9 Mana Miyamoto, Yuko Hanatani, and Kenichi Shibuya, "Increased Vitamin D Intake May Reduce Psychological Anxiety and the Incidence of Menstrual Irregularities in Female Athletes," *PeerJ* 10 (November 21, 2022): e14456.

10 Evangelia Zaromytidou, Theocharis Koufakis, Georgios Dimakopoulos et al., "Vitamin D Alleviates Anxiety and Depression in Elderly People with Prediabetes: A Randomized Controlled Study," *Metabolites* 12 (2022): 884.

11 Mohammed Al-Wardat, Nuha Alwardat, Gemma Lou De Santis et al., "The Association Between Serum Vitamin D and Mood Disorders in a Cohort of Lipedema Patients," *Hormone Molecular Biology and Clinical Investigation* 42, no. 4 (July 29, 2021): 351–5.

12 John P. Lee, Michael Tansey, Jennifer G. Jetton, and Matthew D. Krasowski, "Vitamin D Toxicity: A 16-Year Retrospective Study at an Academic Medical Center," *Laboratory Medicine* 49, no. 2 (May 2018): 123–9.

Index

acupressure   11
  and acute injured athletes   17
  administration   12
  and anxiety   13
  and anxiety associated with
      hemodialysis   16
  and anxiety in burn patients   17
  and anxiety in children   15
  and Cesarean Section anxiety   14
  and Chinese medicine   11
  costs   12
  during pregnancy   13
  prior to thoracoscopic surgery   15
  regulation   12
  risks   12
  side effects   12
  and students with mild anxiety   18
  types of acupressure   11
acupuncture   21
  administration   22
  for anxiety from Parkinson
      disease   23
  costs   22
  to help with *in vitro* fertilization
      anxiety   28
  regulation   22
  risks   22
  side effects   22
  and traditional Chinese medicine   21
  as treatment for anxiety   23
  as treatment for anxiety in
      children   24
  as treatment for preoperative
      anxiety   24
  as treatment for PTSD   25
  for treatment of anxiety in irritable
      bowel syndrome   26
acute coronary syndrome   235
adolescents   1, 7, 24, 38, 82, 87, 93, 129,
      130, 149, 150, 184, 189, 191, 193,
      241–5, 251, 254, 265, 278, 290

aerobic exercise   99
agoraphobia   1, 2, 51, 66, 95, 126, 189,
      271, 301
alcohol withdrawal   41
Alzheimer's disease   180
Amsterdam Pre-Operative Anxiety and
      Information Scale   25
anaerobic exercise   99
animal therapy   31
  administration   32
  for adolescents with anxiety   38
  for anxiety in nursing students   36
  for anxiety in students   33
  costs   32
  dog therapy   33
  equine therapy for youth   36
  farm animals as treatment   37
  for hospitalized adults   49
  for hospitalized children   34
  introduction   31
  for nurses at work   37
  regulation   32
  risks   33
  side effects   33
  therapy animals   32
  use of dogs   34
anxiety disorders   1
  diagnosis   4
  prevalence   1
anxiety risk factors   4
Apgar scores   44
aromatherapy   124–5, 128, 232
arrhythmias   14, 185
attention deficit hyperactivity
      disorder   31, 145
autism spectrum disorder   31, 73, 192

Bacillus   207
barbiturates   43, 44, 274
Beck Anxiety Inventory   23, 37, 129, 205
Beck Anxiety Scale   160

benzodiazepines   41
   administration   42
   alprazolam   43
   clonazepam   43
      compared to paroxetine for panic
         disorder   50
      for social anxiety disorder   51
   costs   42
   dependence on   42
   diazepam   43
      driving safely and diazepam   52
   efficacy compared to SSRIs and
      SNRIs   47
   efficacy of alprazolam compared to
      diazepam   50
   efficacy of alprazolam compared to
      lorazepam   49
   increased risk of fractures in
      children   46
   introduction   41
   long-term use in elderly   46
   lorazepam   43
   misuse   44
   overdose   44
   regulation   42
   risks   42
   safe driving with lorazepam   54
   side effects   44
   use during pregnancy   48
   use in the elderly   45
   use of alprazolam during
      pregnancy   48
   use of diazepam for anxiety   53
   use of lorazepam in children   53
   use of lorazepam in the elderly   55
beta-blockers   59
   administration   60
   alters response to anxiety   59
   anxiety helped by atenolol   61
   costs   60
   and dental anxiety   65
   and induced anxiety   65
   introduction   58
   propranolol
      anxiety and   66
      performance anxiety and   62
      PTSD and   63, 64
   regulation   60
   risks   60
   side-effects   60

Bifidobacterium   208
Black Box warning   42, 189, 242, 265
breast cancer   93–4, 110–11, 181–2, 199,
   220, 280
breast milk   61, 70, 110, 136
bromazepam   138
burn   17, 54, 64, 124–5, 235
buspirone   69
   administration   69
   costs   69
   introduction   69
   regulation   69
   risks   70
   side effects   70
   use in adolescents with OCD   75
   use in panic disorder   74
   use in Parkinson's Disease   73
   use in youth with autism   73
   usefulness for anxiety disorder   71

cannabinoids   79–82
cannabis and CBD   79
   administration   80
   costs   80
   forms of cannabis   81
   forms of CBD   81
   and improvements in anxiety   86
   increased use of marijuana in social
      anxiety disorder   86
   medical cannabis use for PTSD   85
   regulation   80
   relationship of cannabis use to
      anxiety   87
   risks   81
   side effects   81
   use of CBD in youth   83
   usefulness for acute stress   83
   usefulness for PTSD   84
   utility of CBD for anxiety   82
Cannabis sativa   79
carotid endarterectomy   201
cataract surgery   171–2
CBD   79–87, 102, 109, 172–4, 200,
   301–2, 311, 331
cesarean section   14
chamomile   119, 121–2, 124–5
Chi   21, 99, 275–82, 320
Chinese medicine   12, 118, 275
citalopram   239–41, 250–2, 267,
   271

The Clinical Global Impression (CGI)
    Scale 4
clomipramine 254
Cognitive Behavioral Therapy 89
    administration 89
    compared to mindfulness 94
    costs 89
    introduction 89
    and negative side effects 96
    regulation 89
    risks 90
    side effects 90
    and telemedicine 106
    use for anxiety 91
    use for anxiety in children and
        adolescents 93
    use for panic disorder 95
    use for social anxiety disorder
        96
Cohen's Perceived Stress Scale 210
college students 18, 112, 179–80, 206,
    211
colonoscopy 204
controlled substances 42
coronary artery disease 151, 185
Covid-19 139
Crohn's disease 156, 209, 285

DASS-21 5, 28, 210
dementia 44, 136, 145, 165, 236, 321
dental anxiety 65, 201
dental extraction 146–7
Depression and Anxiety Stress Scales 5,
    103
desvenlafaxine 263
diabetes 13, 16, 19, 31, 60, 156, 165, 185,
    210, 236, 275
discontinuation syndrome 189, 266
dog therapy 34–7
Drug Enforcement Administration
    (DEA) 218
duloxetine 257, 263, 265–8, 270, 272,
    275–6
dyslipidemia 185

Edinburgh Postnatal Depression
    Scale 161
endocannabinoid system (ECS) 79
Enterococcus 208
Epidiolex 80

Escherichia 208
escitalopram 183, 239, 241, 252–4
exercise 99
    administration 100
    for anxiety and fibromyalgia 104
    for breast cancer survivors 105
    costs 100
    for general anxiety disorder 101
    introduction 99
    for obsessive compulsive
        disorder 101
    for PTSD 103
    regulation 100
    risks 100
    side effects 100
    for state anxiety 102
    for those living with HIV 104
    for those with low back pain and
        anxiety 106
    use of walking for anxiety 102

the Faces Anxiety Scale 5
falling 2, 45, 70, 158, 165, 243
fat-soluble vitamin 285
fibromyalgia 92, 93, 95, 97, 103, 118,
    173, 275, 304
fluoxetine 115, 190, 223, 239, 240,
    245–6, 267
fluvoxamine 224, 239, 241, 254–6,
    267
FODMAP 210
Food and Drug Administration 48, 59,
    69, 80, 82, 97–8, 119, 135, 155,
    166, 187, 208, 263, 296

GABA 41, 100, 165
gabapentin 109
    administration 110
    and breast cancer anxiety 111
    costs 110
    introduction 109
    and performance anxiety 112
    regulation 110
    risks 110
    side effects 110
    and surgery related anxiety 112
    and use in OCD 116
    and use in panic disorder 115
    and use in PTSD 115
    and use in social phobia 113

generalized anxiety disorder   2
Generalized Anxiety Disorder-7 Scale
    6, 99
grapefruit   69–70

Hamilton Anxiety Rating Scale   4, 6, 45,
    49–50, 82, 99, 137, 152, 267,
    273, 288
hemodialysis   16, 184–5, 250
hemp   79–80
herbal medicine   119
    administration   120
    chamomile   122
    costs   120
    introduction   119
    kava kava   122
    lavender   122
    passionflower   121
    regulation   120
    risks   121
    saffron   121
    side effects   121
    St. John's Wort   123
    types   121
    use for patients with burns   124
    use of chamomile for generalized
        anxiety disorder   123
    use of kava kava for anxiety   126
    use of lavender for anxiety   127
    use of passionflower for anxiety   128
    use of saffron for anxiety   129
    use of St. John's Wort for anxiety and
        depression   131
    use of St. John's Wort for social
        phobia   130
hip arthroplasty   92
HIV   92, 95, 103, 122, 129, 304
Hospital Anxiety and Depression
    Scale   6, 86, 99, 130, 150, 157,
    159–61, 193, 280
hot flashes   83, 97, 116
hydroxyzine   135
    administration   135
    anxiety from pain   138
    costs   135
    introduction   135
    and neurodevelopment   142
    and panic disorder   141
    and pediatric dental patients   141

and preoperative anxiety   139
    reduces anxiety   136
    regulation   135
    risks   136
    side effects   136
    and surgery   138
hyperhidrosis   160–1
hypnosis   15–16, 45
    administration   145
    and burn patients   148
    and cancer patients   149
    and chronic disease   152
    and cognitive impairment   147
    during coronary angiography   151
    costs   145
    and dental extraction   146
    and hot flashes   150
    introduction   145
    for patients in intensive care   152
    and patients with COPD   150
    regulation   145
    risks   146
    side effects   146

in vitro fertilization   28
irritable bowel syndrome (IBS)   26, 145,
    214

Jon Kabat-Zinn   177

kava kava   119, 121, 125–7

Lactobacillus   208
lavender   103, 119, 122, 125, 128, 133–4,
    305–6
levomilnacipran   263
Liebowitz Social Anxiety Scale   86, 131,
    191, 253

Maastricht Acute Stress Test   84
magic mushrooms   217–18, 225–6
magnesium   155
    administration   155
    costs   155
    and dietary intake   159
    for generalized anxiety disorder   158
    and heart surgery patients   157
    and hyperhidrosis   160
    introduction   155

and obsessive-compulsive disorder
162
and postpartum anxiety 161
for premenstrual symptoms 158
regulation 155
and restless leg syndrome 162
risks 156
side effects 156
marijuana 65, 67–8, 72–3, 301
Marinol 80
medical students 27–8
melatonin 165
administration 166
and adverse events 165
and cataract surgery 171
and circadian rhythms 175
costs 166
before dental surgery 168
and extraction of wisdom teeth 170
introduction 165
and preoperative anxiety 167
and presurgical anxiety 171
regulation 166
risks 166
side effects 166
and supplement labels 172
and tourniquet pain 170
midazolam 128–9, 140, 167–9
milnacipran 263
mindfulness 94–5
mindfulness meditation 203
administration 204
and anxiety 205
and cancer related anxiety 208
for children and adolescents 210
compared to SSRI 209
costs 204
introduction 203
for patients undergoing
hemodialysis 210
regulation 204
risks 205
side effects 205
and social anxiety disorder 208
and stress 206
and women with breast cancer 207
mirtazapine 187
administration 187
and autism spectrum disorder 193

costs 187
introduction 187
and obsessive-compulsive
disorder 194
and panic disorder 189
and pregnancy 194
and preoperative anxiety 193
and PTSD 191
regulation 187
risks 188
side effects 188
and social anxiety disorder 190
monoamine oxidase inhibitor 70, 188
Multidimensional Anxiety Scale for
Children 93
music therapy 197
administration 197
and Alzheimer patients 205
and cesarean delivery 202
and colonscopy 203
costs 197
and critically ill patients 223
introduction 197
and mothers of preterm infants 203
Native Americans 144
and parents of preterm infants 204
regulation 197
and relief of anxiety 202
risks 199
side effects 199
and surgical anxiety 199
and treatment for breast cancer 201

neurotransmitters 41, 59, 69, 97, 155,
165, 187, 239, 263
nursing 15, 36–7, 61, 136, 181, 198, 236

ophophobia 253
oxazepam 50, 128

palliative sedation 41
panic attacks 7, 50–1, 74, 142, 189–90,
219, 225, 247, 272, 289
panic disorder 2–3, 6–7, 45–6, 50–1,
66, 74–5, 91–2, 95–6, 102–3,
116, 142, 187, 189–90, 239–41,
243–4, 247–9, 251, 271–2
Panic Disorder Severity Scale 7, 99
Parkinson's disease 73–4

paroxetine   50–1, 142, 239–40, 247–8, 268
passionflower   103, 120–1, 128, 132, 306
Penn State Worry Questionnaire   101
peripheral vascular disease   185
phobia   1, 3, 65–6, 92, 102–3, 112–13, 125, 130–1, 190, 245, 249, 252–3
Physician's Global Impression Scale   50
pineal gland   166
post-traumatic stress disorder (PTSD)   3
preoperative anxiety   24–5, 54, 117–18, 139, 147, 167, 169, 198, 200
probiotics   207
   administration   208
   and adolescents with anxiety   211
   and anxiety relief   210
   and chronic fatigue syndrome   213
   costs   208
   introduction   207
   and irritable bowel syndrome   214
   and multiple sclerosis   212
   and petrochemical workers   212
   and postpartum anxiety   211
   regulation   208
   risks   209
   side effects   209
psilocybin   217
   administration   218
   costs   218
   and dangerous behaviors   226
   and depression in cancer patients   221
   introduction   217
   and microdoses   224
   and obsessive-compulsive disorder   223
   regulation   218
   risks   219
   and safety   225
   side effects   219
   and use in cancer patients   220
PTSD Checklist   7–8, 99, 270
public speaking   111

Recommended Dietary Allowance   156
reflexology   229
   and acute coronary syndrome   235
   administration   230
   after hysterectomy   235
   and anxiety   232
   and burn issues   234
   and coronary artery disease   235
   costs   230
   introduction   229
   and labor   233
   regulation   230
   risks   231
   side effects   231
   and sleep   234
   theory   229
restless leg syndrome   97, 162
rheumatoid arthritis   118, 210, 290–1

Saccharomyces   207
saffron   119–21
salivary cortisol   206
scleroderma   282
seizures   9, 41, 44, 70, 97–8, 113, 136, 167, 219, 225, 242, 265
selective serotonin reuptake inhibitors (SSRIs)   239
   administration   240
   for child and adolescent anxiety   259
   citalopram   240
      for anxiety   250
      for panic disorder   251
   costs   249
   escitalopram   241
      for fear of learning   253
      for phobias   252
      for social anxiety disorder   280
   fluoxetine   240
      for obsessive-compulsive disorder   246
      efficacy for anxiety   245
   fluvoxamine   241
      for obsessive compulsive disorder   254
      for social anxiety disorder   255
   introduction   239
   and panic disorder   244
   paroxetine   240
      for anxiety disorders   247
      for panic disorder   247
   for PTSD   249
   regulation   240

risk for hyponatremia 244
risks 242
sertraline 241
side effects 242
for social anxiety disorder 248
vilazodone 241
for generalized anxiety
disorder 256
for separation anxiety
disorder 257
vortioxetine 242
for anxious depression 258
and generalized anxiety
disorder 257
separation anxiety disorder 1, 3, 92, 94,
245, 249, 257
serotonin 46, 69–70, 76, 97, 136, 165,
172, 187–8, 192, 194, 217, 239,
242–3, 255, 263, 265, 267
serotonin and norepinephrine reuptake
inhibitors (SNRIs) 263
administration 263
costs 263
duloxetine 263
for obsessive compulsive
disorder 267
for generalized anxiety
disorder 270
for PTSD 268
introduction 263
regulation 263
risks 265
side effects 265
venlafaxine 263
for obsessive compulsive
disorder 268
for generalized anxiety
disorder 271
for panic disorder 271
for PTSD 272
XR for anxiety 270
serotonin syndrome 70, 188, 243, 255,
265
sertraline 71, 191–2, 194, 239, 241,
249–50, 267
social anxiety disorder 3
Spielberger's State-Trait Anxiety
Inventory 2, 8, 14, 27, 99,
127

St. John's wort 119–20, 122, 126–7,
130–1, 242
Streptococcus 208
suicidal ideation 179, 189, 267
suicidal thoughts 98, 265
Symptom Check List 52
Syndros 80

Tai Chi 275
administration 276
and anxiety and depression 279
and anxiety relief 278
costs 278
with heart failure 280
and hypertension 277
introduction 275
and medical issues 280
regulation 276
risks 277
side effects 277
theory 275
used in schleroderma patients 282
used with yoga 279
THC 81
therapy animals 32
therapy dog 31–2, 34, 37–9
triclofos 140

undergraduates 27, 86

venlafaxine ER 271–3
vilazodone 239, 241, 256–7
visual analog scale (VAS) 18, 139, 167,
201, 204, 223
vitamin B6 159
vitamin D 285
administration 286
costs 286
and generalized anxiety disorder
288
introduction 285
and obsessive compulsive
disorder 289
and panic attacks 289
regulation 286
and rheumatoid arthritis 290
risk 286
side effects 286
and toxicity 292

as treatment for anxiety 287,
288
and use in athletes 291
and use in patients with
prediabetes 291
vortioxetine 239, 242, 257–9

water soluble vitamins 285

xerostmia 188

Yale-Brown Obsessive Compulsive
Scale 8–9, 93, 99, 115, 162,
194, 223, 267–8, 290, 295
yoga 94, 279–80

zone therapy 229

About the Authors

Myrna Chandler Goldstein, MA, has been a freelance writer and independent scholar for more than thirty years. She is the author of Greenwood's *Pain Management: Fact versus Fiction*, *Dietary Supplements: Fact versus Fiction*, and other Greenwood books.

Mark A. Goldstein, MD, is the founding chief emeritus of the Division of Adolescent and Young Adult Medicine at Massachusetts General Hospital and Associate Professor of Pediatrics at Harvard Medical School. He is working on a book on how physicians face challenges, and he is also the editor in chief of *Current Pediatrics Reports*.